Lecture Notes on Clinical Pharmacology

Lecture Notes on Clinical Pharmacology

JOHN L. REID DM FRCP
Regius Professor of Medicine and Therapeutics
University of Glasgow

PETER C. RUBIN DM FRCP
Professor of Therapeutics
University of Nottingham

BRIAN WHITING MD FRCP FFPM
Professor of Medicine and Therapeutics
Dean, Faculty of Medicine
University of Glasgow

FOURTH EDITION

OXFORD
BLACKWELL SCIENTIFIC PUBLICATIONS
LONDON EDINBURGH BOSTON
MELBOURNE PARIS BERLIN VIENNA

© 1982, 1985, 1989, 1992 by
Blackwell Scientific Publications
Editorial Offices:
Osney Mead, Oxford OX2 0EL
25 John Street, London WC1N 2BL
23 Ainslie Place, Edinburgh EH3 6AJ
238 Main Street, Cambridge
Massachusetts 02142, USA
54 University Street, Carlton
Victoria 3053, Australia

Other Editorial Offices:
Librairie Arnette SA
1, rue de Lille
75007 Paris
France

Blackwell Wissenschafts-Verlag GmbH
Kurfürstendamm 57
10707 Berlin
Germany

Blackwell MZV
Feldgasse 13
1238 Wien
Austria

All rights reserved. No part of this publication may be reproduced, stored in a retrieval system, or transmitted, in any form or by any means, electronic, mechanical, photocopying, recording or otherwise, except as permitted by the UK Copyright, Designs and Patents Act 1988, without the prior permission of the copyright owner.

First published, 1982
Second edition 1985
Reprinted 1987, 1988
Third edition 1989
Reprinted 1990, 1991
Fourth edition 1992
Reprinted 1993, 1994 (twice)
Four Dragons edition 1992
Reprinted 1993, 1994 (twice)

Set by Semantic Graphics, Singapore
Printed and bound in Great Britain
by Hartnolls Ltd, Bodmin, Cornwall

DISTRIBUTORS

Marston Book Services Ltd
PO Box 87
Oxford OX2 0DT
(*Orders:* Tel: 0865 791155
Fax: 0865 791927
Telex: 837515)

USA
Blackwell Scientific Publications, Inc.
238 Main Street,
Cambridge, MA 02142
(*Orders:* Tel: 800 759-6102
617 876-7000)

Canada
Times Mirror Professional Publishing, Ltd
130 Flaska Drive
Markham, Ontario L6G 1B8
(*Orders:* Tel: 800 268-4178
416 470-6739)

Australia
Blackwell Scientific Publications Pty Ltd
54 University Street
Carlton, Victoria 3053
(*Orders:* Tel: 03 347-5552)

A catalogue record for this book is available from the British Library

ISBN 0–632–03404–1
ISBN 0–632–03407–6 (Four Dragons)

Contents

Contributors

The following contributed substantially to the revision and rewriting of chapters in this edition:

Cytotoxic Drugs and Immunopharmacology
   Mr J.A. Bradley, *Department of Surgery, Western Infirmary, Glasgow.*
Cardiac Arrhythmias
   Professor S. Cobbe, *Department of Medical Cardiology, Royal Infirmary, Glasgow.*
Drugs and Endocrine Disease
   Dr J.M.C. Connell, *MRC Blood Pressure Unit, Western Infirmary, Glasgow.*
Heart Failure and Angina Pectoris
   Dr H.J. Dargie, *Department of Cardiology, Western Infirmary, Glasgow.*
Drugs and Gastrointestinal Disease
   Professor C.W. Howden, *Division of Digestive Diseases, University of South Carolina School of Medicine, Columbia, South Carolina.*
Cytotoxic Drugs and Immunopharmacology
   Professor S. Kaye, *Department of Clinical Oncology, The University of Glasgow, Glasgow.*
Adverse Drug Reactions
   Professor D.H. Lawson, *Department of Medicine, Royal Infirmary, Glasgow.*
Drugs at the Extremes of Age
   Dr P.J.W. Scott, *Department of Geriatric Medicine, Stobhill Hospital, Glasgow.*

Colleagues from the Department of Medicine and Therapeutics at the University of Glasgow contributed to the following chapters:

Drugs and Respiratory Disease
   Dr G.J. Addis
Drugs and Neurological Disease
   Dr M.J. Brodie
Corticosteroids
   Dr H.L. Elliott
Thrombosis and Coagulation
   Dr W.S. Hillis

Preface

Clinical pharmacology is a specialty which has grown in importance with the increase in both the number and the complexity of drugs. Bridging the gap between laboratory science and the practice of medicine at the bedside, clinical pharmacology has as its primary aim the promotion of safe and effective drug use: to optimize benefits and minimize risks.

Developments in medicine, pharmacology and physiology have led to a better understanding of disease processes and a more rational use of drugs. Recent years have seen the development of drugs designed to interact with specific receptors or enzyme systems. In addition the application of biochemical and immunological techniques has led to a clearer appreciation of the mechanisms involved in adverse drug reactions and interactions. With this understanding has come the potential to reduce greatly the number of unwanted drug effects. The intensity of drug action is often related to plasma concentration, and recent advances in analytical techniques have enabled rapid and accurate determination of the plasma concentrations of many drugs. This provides an added dimension to the optimization of drug use.

For many years we have taught clinical pharmacology to medical practitioners and undergraduate students. We were persuaded by our students that there was a need for a brief, clearly written and up to date review of clinical pharmacology. *Lecture Notes on Clinical Pharmacology* was prepared to meet this need in 1981 and now enters its fourth edition. The book has been extensively revised and updated: several chapters have been re-written. A new section on immunopharmacology has been added and a chapter on Drugs and Endocrine Disease has been restored following many protests. We have not attempted to be comprehensive, but have tried to emphasize the principles of clinical pharmacology, areas which are developing rapidly and topics which are of particular clinical importance. The book is based on the course of lectures and seminars in clinical pharmacology and therapeutics for medical students at the University of Glasgow. In addition, we have drawn on our experience of organizing courses for postgraduate students, general practitioners and medical specialists. Thus, while intended primarily for medical students, we believe this book will also be of use to those preparing for higher examinations and doctors in established practice who wish to remain well informed of current concepts in clinical pharmacology.

For all who use it, we hope this book will provide a clear understanding not only of *how* but also *when* to use drugs.

April 1992

John Reid
Peter Rubin
Brian Whiting

Acknowledgements

We are very grateful to colleagues who have given their time to provide valuable assistance in reviewing and updating chapters relating to their special interest: Dr John Asbury, Dr Ian Bone, Dr David Davies, Dr Lishel Horn, Dr Kennedy Lees, Ms Janet McCabe, Dr Angus Mackay, Mr Paul O'Donnell, Professor Douglas Sleigh, Professor Roger Sturrock, Dr Alison Thomson, Dr Neil Thomson and Professor Martin Whittle.

We owe a great debt of gratitude to Mrs Mary Wood and Miss Nan Scott for their considerable efforts in typing and collating the original text and revisions. Mrs Randa Reid prepared the index. Mr Peter Saugman and Mr Robert Campbell of Blackwell Scientific Publications have advised, guided and encouraged us throughout and to them we also offer our thanks.

We ourselves accept full responsibility for the contents of the volume and for any mistakes or misunderstandings.

John Reid
Peter Rubin
Brian Whiting

Section 1

Chapter 1
Principles of Clinical Pharmacology

Until the twentieth century, medical practice depended largely on the administration of mixtures of natural plant or animal substances. These preparations contained a number of pharmacologically active agents in variable amounts. Their actions and indications were empirical and based on historical or traditional experience. Their use was rarely based on an understanding of the mechanism of disease or careful critical measurement of effect.

During the last 80 years, an increased understanding of biochemical and pathophysiological factors in disease has developed. The chemical synthesis of agents with well characterized, specific actions on cellular mechanisms has led to the introduction of many powerful and effective drugs.

1.1 PRINCIPLES OF DRUG ACTION

Pharmacological agents are used in therapeutics to:

1 Cure disease:
 (a) Chemotherapy in cancer or leukaemia.
 (b) Antibiotics in specific bacterial infections.

2 Alleviate symptoms:
 (a) Antacids in dyspepsia.
 (b) Non-steroidal anti-inflammatory drugs in rheumatoid arthritis.

3 Replace deficiencies: restoration of normal function by the replacement of a deficiency in an endogenous hormone, enzyme or transmitter.

A *drug* is a single chemical entity that may be one of the constituents of a medicine.

A *medicine* may contain one or more active constituents (drugs) together with additives to facilitate administration.

Mechanism of drug action

Action on a receptor

A receptor is a specific macromolecule, usually a protein, to which a specific group of drugs or naturally occurring substances such as neurotransmitters or hormones can bind.

An agonist is a substance which stimulates or activates the receptor to produce an effect.

Table 1.1. Some receptors involved in the action of commonly used drugs

Receptor	Subtype	Main actions of natural agonist	Drug agonist	Drug antagonist
Adrenoceptor	α_1	Vasoconstriction		Prazosin
	α_2	Hypotension, sedation	Clonidine	
	β_1	Heart rate	Dopamine, Dobutamine	Atenolol Metoprolol
	β_2	Bronchodilation Vasodilation Uterine relaxation	Salbutamol Terbutaline Ritodrine	
Cholinergic	Muscarinic	Heart rate Secretion Gut motility Bronchoconstriction		Atropine Benztropine Orphenadrine Ipratropium
	Nicotinic	Contraction of striated muscle		Suxamethonium Tubocurarine
Histamine	H_1	Bronchoconstriction, capillary dilation		Chlorpheniramine, terfenadine
	H_2	↑ Gastric acid		Cimetidine Ranitidine
Dopamine		CNS neurotransmitter	Bromocriptine	Chlorpromazine Haloperidol Thioridazine
Opioid		CNS neurotransmitter	Morphine, pethidine, etc.	Naloxone

An antagonist prevents the action of an agonist but does not have any effect itself unless it also possesses partial agonist activity.

The biochemical events which result from an agonist–receptor interaction and which produce an effect are still to be determined.

There are many types of receptors and in several cases subtypes have been identified which are also of therapeutic importance (Table 1.1).

Action on an enzyme

Enzymes, like receptors, are protein macromolecules with which substrates interact to produce activation or inhibition. Drugs in common clinical use which exert their effect through enzyme action generally do so by inhibition.

Digoxin inhibits the membrane bound Na^+/K^+ ATPase.

Aspirin inhibits platelet cyclo-oxygenase.

Captopril inhibits angiotensin converting enzyme.

Phenelzine inhibits monoamine oxidase.

Carbidopa inhibits decarboxylase.

Allopurinol inhibits xanthine oxidase.

Drug receptor antagonists and enzyme inhibitors can act as competitive reversible antagonists or as non-competitive irreversible antagonists. The duration of the effect of drugs of the latter type is much longer than that of the former. Effects of competitive antagonists can be overcome by increasing the dose of endogenous or exogenous agonist while effects of irreversible antagonists cannot usually be overcome.

Propranolol is a competitive β-adrenoceptor antagonist used in hypertension and angina. Its effects last for hours and can be overcome by administering an appropriate dose of a β-receptor agonist like isoprenaline.

Phenelzine is an irreversible non-competitive monoamine oxidase inhibitor used in depression. Its action and adverse effects may persist for 2–3 weeks.

Action on membrane ionic channels

The conduction of impulses in nerve tissues and electromechanical coupling in muscle depends on the movement of ions, particularly sodium, calcium and potassium, through membrane channels. Several groups of drugs interfere with these processes:

Antiarrhythmic drugs (Chapter 6).
Calcium slow channel antagonists (Chapter 8).
General and local anaesthetics (Chapter 18).
Anticonvulsants (Chapter 20).

Cytotoxic actions

Drugs used in cancer or in the treatment of infections may kill malignant cells or microorganisms. Often the mechanisms have been defined in terms of effects on specific receptors or enzymes. In other cases, chemical action (alkylation) damages DNA or other macromolecules and results in cell death or failure of cell division.

Dose–response relationship

Dose–response relationships in clinical practice rarely follow the classical sigmoid pattern of experimental studies. It is uncommon for the upper plateau or maximum effect to be reached in man or to be relevant therapeutically. Dose–response relationships may be steep or flat. The former implies a marked increase in response with modest increases in dose, while the latter implies little increase in response over a wide dose range (Fig. 1.1).

The potency of a drug is relatively unimportant; what matters is its efficacy or the maximum effect that can be obtained.

In clinical practice the maximum therapeutic effect may often be unobtainable because of the appearance of adverse or unwanted effects: few, if any, drugs cause a single pharmacological response. The dose–adverse response relationship is often different in shape and position to that of the dose–therapeutic response relationship. The difference between the dose which will produce the desired effect and that which will cause adverse effects is called the therapeutic index and is a measure of the selectivity of a drug (Fig. 1.2).

The shape and position of dose–response curves in a group of patients is variable because of genetic, environmental and disease factors, but this variability is not solely an expression of differences in response to drugs. It has two important components, the dose–plasma concentration relationship and the plasma concentration–effect relationship

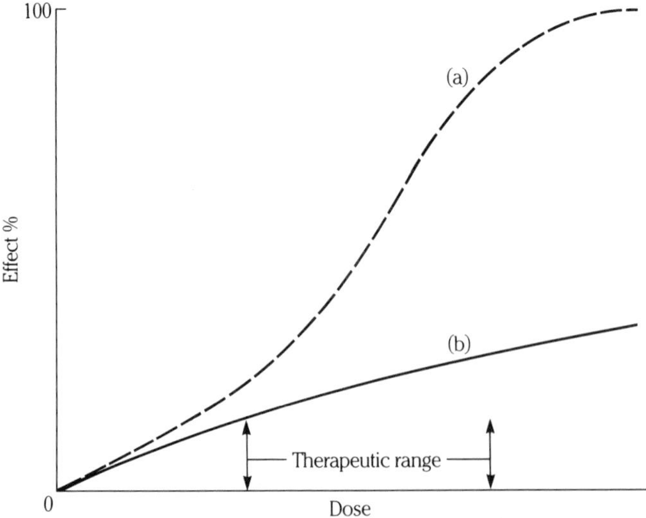

Fig. 1.1. Schematic examples of a drug (a) with a steep dose–response relationship in the therapeutic range, e.g. warfarin as an oral anticoagulant, and (b) a flat dose–response relationship within the therapeutic range, e.g. thiazide diuretics in hypertension.

Dose → Concentration → Effect

With the development of specific and sensitive chemical assays for drugs in body fluids, it has been possible to characterize the dose–plasma concentration relationships in individual patients so that this component of the variability in response can be largely accounted for. This is pharmacokinetics (Chapter 1, Section 1.2), and its application in clinical practice is clinical pharmacokinetics

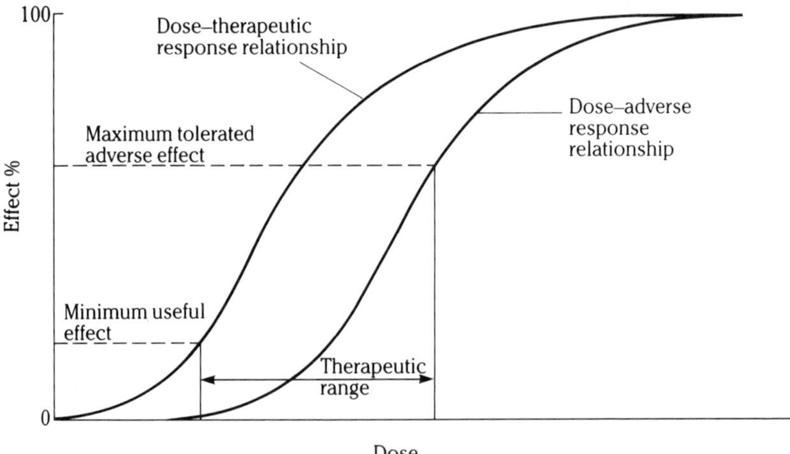

Fig. 1.2. Schematic diagram of the dose–response relationship for the desired effect (dose–therapeutic response) and for an undesired adverse effect. The therapeutic index is the extent of displacement of the two curves within the therapeutic dose range.

(Chapter 2). The residual variability in the dose–response relationship characterized by the concentration–effect component is a true expression of drug response or, in quantitative terms, a good measure of the sensitivity of a patient to a drug. This is the province of pharmacodynamics and the exploration of the factors which underlie the variability in both pharmacokinetics and pharmacodynamics is the basis of clinical pharmacology.

1.2 PRINCIPLES OF PHARMACOKINETICS

Clearance

When a drug is given continuously by intravenous infusion or repetitively by mouth, a balance is eventually achieved between input (dose rate) and output (the amount eliminated over a given period of time). This balance gives rise to a constant amount of drug in the body, reflected in the plasma as a steady state concentration (C_{pss}). During a constant rate infusion the C_{pss} will remain constant; with repetitive oral dosing, it will fluctuate between peaks and troughs.

The relationship between C_{pss}, drug input and output can be written

$$C_{pss} = \frac{\text{Input}}{\text{Output}} = \frac{\text{Dose rate}}{\text{Clearance}} \qquad \text{(Eqn. 1.1)}$$

where 'clearance' is the net result of all eliminating processes, principally determined by the liver and/or kidneys. Since the dose rate has units of amount/time(e.g. mg/h) and C_{pss} has units of amount/volume (e.g. mg/l), clearance has units of volume/time, thus

$$\text{Clearance} = \frac{\text{Dose rate}}{C_{pss}} \qquad \text{(Eqn. 1.2)}$$

and represents the theoretical volume of fluid from which a drug is completely removed in a given period of time.

Clearance depends critically on the efficiency with which the liver and/or kidneys can eliminate a drug; it will vary in disease states which affect these organs *per se* or which affect the blood flow to these organs. Equation 1.1 shows that the C_{pss} will vary inversely with clearance if the dose rate is not altered to compensate for a change in clearance. In stable clinical conditions, however, clearance remains constant and Eqn. 1.1 shows that the C_{pss} is directly proportional to dose rate. The important clinical implication is that if the dose rate is doubled, the C_{pss} doubles: if the dose rate is halved, the C_{pss} is halved. This is illustrated in Fig. 1.3. If each C_{pss} is plotted against its corresponding dose rate, the direct proportionality becomes obvious (Fig. 1.4) and the slope of the line (a constant) is the reciprocal of clearance (C_{pss}/Dose rate). In pharmacokinetic terms, this is referred to as a first-order or linear process, and results from the fact that the rate of elimination is proportional to the amount of drug present in the body.

A constant rate intravenous infusion will clearly yield a constant C_{pss}, often referred to as the average steady state concentration. If a drug is administered orally at regular intervals, the average C_{pss} may be approximated by the concentration

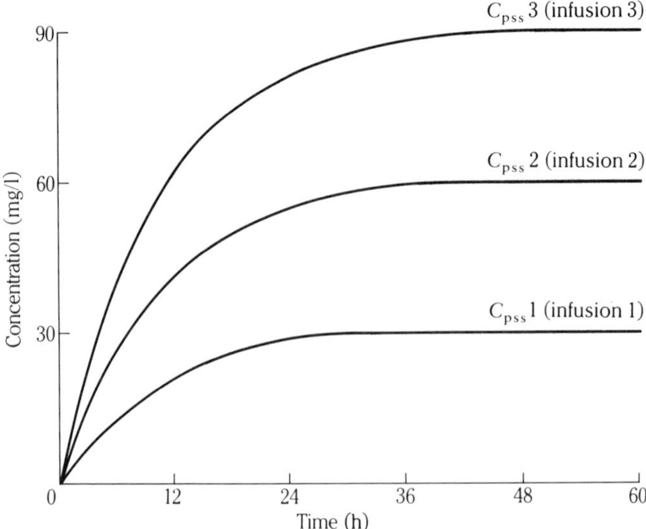

Fig. 1.3. Plots of concentration vs. time for three infusions allowed to reach steady state. Infusion 2 is at a rate twice that of infusion 1. Infusion 3 is at a rate three times that of infusion 1. The three steady state concentrations (C_{pss} 1, 2 and 3) are directly proportional to the corresponding infusion rates.

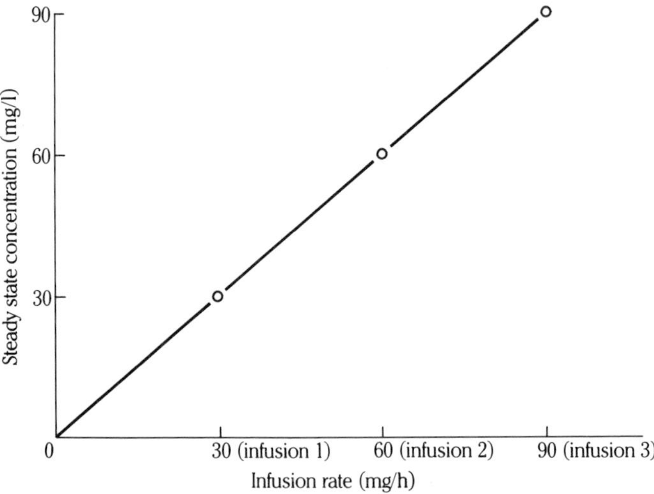

Fig. 1.4. Three steady state concentrations plotted against corresponding infusion rates. The equation of the line is $C_{pss} = 1/Cl \cdot$ infusion rate, so that the slope of the line is the reciprocal of clearance.

which is one-third of the way between a trough and a peak in any dosage interval.

Equation 1.1 also highlights the important fact that if an estimate of clearance is available, it can be used to determine the maintenance dose rate for any desired C_{pss}, thus

$$\text{Maintenance dose rate} = \text{Clearance} \times \text{Desired } C_{pss} \qquad \text{(Eqn. 1.3)}$$

Volume of distribution

Once a drug has gained access to the bloodstream it is distributed to a greater or lesser extent to other tissues and the processes of metabolism and elimination begin. In the blood, a proportion of the drug is bound to plasma proteins—notably albumin. Only the unbound, or free, fraction distributes because the protein bound complex is too large to pass through all the membranes. Movement of the drug between the blood and other tissues proceeds until an equilibrium is established between the unbound drug in plasma and the drug in tissues. The volume of distribution, V, is conceived of as the volume of fluid into which a drug apparently distributes based on the amount of drug in the body and the measured concentration in the plasma. If a drug was wholly confined to the plasma, then V would assume a value equal to that of the volume of the plasma—approximately 3 litre in an adult. If, on the other hand, it was distributed throughout all body water, then V would have a value of approximately 42 litre. In reality, drugs are rarely distributed into volumes which have these precise physiological values. Indeed, some drugs have apparent volumes of distribution far in excess of total body water and this emphasizes that distribution is not only a matter of dilution throughout fluid but also of sequestration or binding by various body tissues, e.g. muscle and fat. The pK_a of a drug, its partition coefficient in fatty tissue and regional blood flow also play a part. The volume of distribution can vary, therefore, from relatively small values, e.g. an average of 0.14 l/kg body weight for aspirin, to large values, e.g. an average of 7.0 l/kg body weight for digoxin (Table 1.2).

In general, a small V occurs when:

1. Lipid solubility is low.
2. There is a high degree of plasma protein binding.
3. There is a low level of tissue binding.

Table 1.2. Average volumes of distribution of some commonly used drugs

Drug	Volume of distribution (l/kg)
Nortriptyline	20
Digoxin	7
Propranolol	4
Lignocaine	1.5
Phenytoin	0.65
Theophylline	0.5
Gentamicin	0.23
Aspirin	0.14
Warfarin	0.1

A high V occurs when:

1 Lipid solubility is high.
2 There is a low degree of plasma protein binding.
3 There is a high level of tissue binding.

Knowledge of volumes of distribution is important for a number of reasons:

Calculation of the size of a loading dose

This may sometimes be appropriate if an immediate response to treatment is required. Therapeutic success depends on a close relationship between plasma concentration and response together with the absence of adverse effects if a relatively large dose is suddenly administered. A loading dose can be calculated as follows

$$\text{Loading dose} = V \times \text{Desired concentration} \qquad \text{(Eqn. 1.4)}$$

and this is sometimes employed when drug response would take many hours or days to develop if the regular maintenance dose was given from the outset, e.g. digoxin.

Estimation of peak and trough levels

It may be important to estimate the concentration–time profile during repetitive drug administration, principally in terms of the peak (maximum) and trough (minimum) levels achieved. These are determined by the size of the dose, its rate of absorption, the volume of distribution and clearance. For many drugs, dosage regimens should be designed to maintain concentrations within a therapeutic range by avoiding excessively high (potentially toxic) peaks or low ineffective troughs.

Single intravenous bolus dose

A number of other important pharmacokinetic principles can be appreciated by considering the plasma concentrations which result from a single i.v. bolus dose. If we assume that the drug distributes instantaneously into its volume of distribution, V, then its concentration will decline exponentially as shown in Fig. 1.5(a). This is based on the concept that the body can be depicted as a single homogeneous compartment of volume, V, as shown in Fig. 1.6. The initial concentration, C_o, depends only on the dose (D) and V, thus

$$C_o = \frac{D}{V} \qquad \text{(Eqn. 1.5)}$$

while the subsequent decline in concentrations can be described by the exponential expression

$$C(t) = \frac{D}{V} e^{-kt} \qquad \text{(Eqn. 1.6)}$$

where k is the elimination rate constant of the drug, t is any time after drug administration and e^{-kt} is the fraction of drug remaining at time t. If the

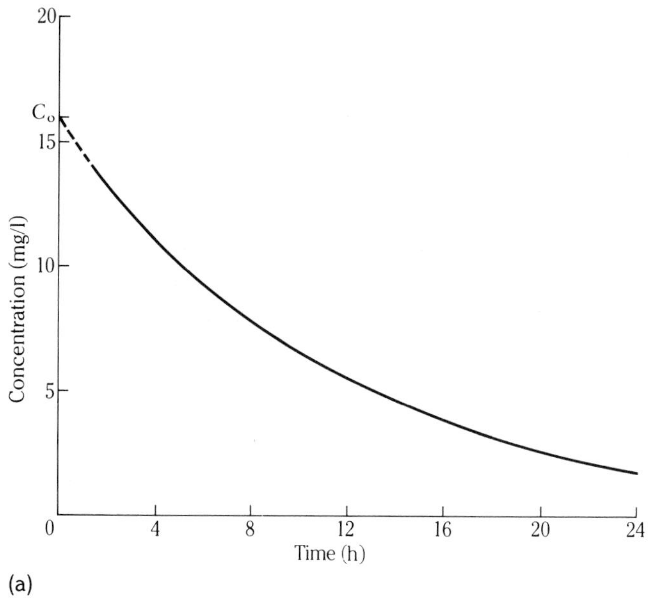

(a)

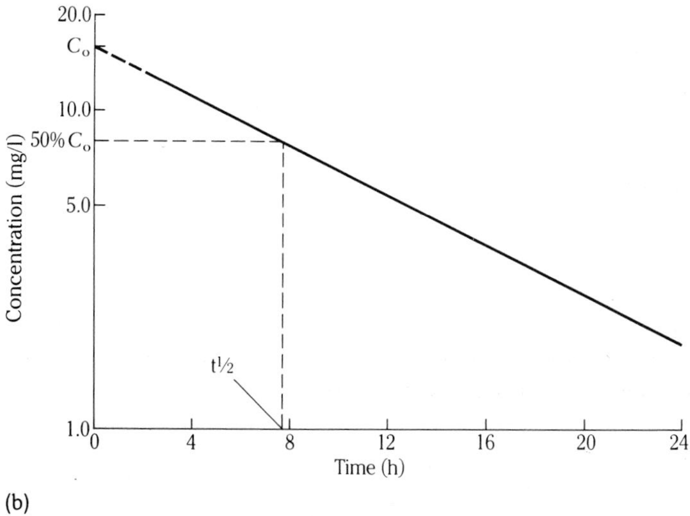

(b)

Fig. 1.5. (a) Plot of concentration vs. time after a bolus intravenous injection. The interception on the *y* (concentration) axis, C_o, is the concentration resulting from the instantaneous injection of the bolus dose. (b) Semi-logarithmic plot of concentration vs. time after a bolus intravenous injection. The slope of this line is *k*; the elimination rate constant (Eqns 1.6 and 1.7) and the elimination half-life of the drug can be determined easily from such a plot by noting the time at which the concentration has fallen to half its original value.

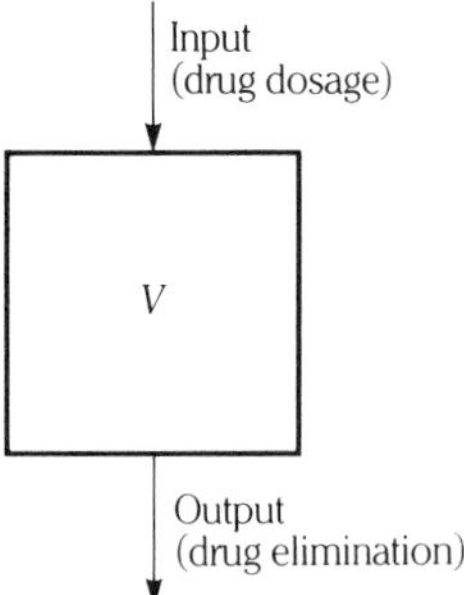

Fig. 1.6. The body depicted as a simple compartment of volume V.

concentrations are plotted on a logarithmic scale, a linear decline will be obtained [Fig. 1.5(b)], according to the following equation

$$\ln C(t) = \ln \frac{D}{V} - kt \qquad \text{(Eqn. 1.7)}$$

where the slope of this line is k. This represents the constant fraction of the volume of distribution from which drug is eliminated in a given period of time and is therefore determined by clearance and volume of distribution, thus

$$k = \frac{\text{Clearance}}{\text{Volume of distribution}} \qquad \text{(Eqn. 1.8)}$$

k can also be expressed in terms of the half-life of a drug. The half-life $t_{1/2}$ is the time required for the plasma concentration to fall to one-half of its original value and can be derived either graphically [Fig. 1.5(b)] or from the expression

$$t_{1/2} = \frac{\ln 2}{k} \qquad \text{(Eqn. 1.9)}$$

where ln 2 is the natural logarithm of 2, or 0.693. It can be used to predict the time at which steady state will be achieved after starting a regular treatment schedule or after any change in dose. As a rule, in the absence of a loading dose, steady state is attained after four to five half-lives. Further, when toxic drug levels have been inadvertently produced, it is very useful to estimate how long it takes for such levels to reach the therapeutic range, or how long it takes for all the drug to be eliminated once the drug has been stopped. Usually, elimination is effectively complete after four to five half-lives.

Bioavailability

After oral administration, all parent drug may not reach the systemic circulation. Equations 1.1–1.3 should be modified to reflect this by introducing a reduction factor that accounts for the proportion of drug which does reach the systemic circulation, i.e. its bioavailability, designated F, with a value ranging from 0 to 1 (0–100%). Equations 1.1–1.3 then become

$$C_{pss} = \frac{F \times \text{Dose rate}}{\text{Clearance}} \qquad \text{(Eqn. 1.10)}$$

$$\frac{\text{Clearance}}{F} = \frac{\text{Dose rate}}{C_{pss}} \qquad \text{(Eqn. 1.11)}$$

$$\text{Dose rate} = \frac{\text{Clearance} \times C_{pss}}{F} \qquad \text{(Eqn. 1.12)}$$

This implies that if F is not known with certainty (and it rarely is) then clearance estimates based on oral dosing can at best be only estimates of clearance/F. Similarly, any maintenance dose rate calculations based on Eqns 1.1–1.3 must take the uncertainty in F into account.

After oral administration, numerous factors can prevent complete absorption—tablet factors such as formulation design and solubility, the presence of food and other drugs in the gut and first-pass metabolism.

First-pass metabolism

First-pass or presystemic metabolism refers to metabolism of a drug that occurs *en route* from the gut lumen to the systemic circulation. For the majority of drugs given orally, absorption occurs across that portion of gastrointestinal epithelium that is drained by veins forming part of the hepatoportal system. Before reaching the systemic circulation such drugs must pass through the liver and are, therefore, exposed to enzymes in that organ which metabolize drugs. For drugs that are susceptible to extensive hepatic metabolism, a substantial proportion of an orally administered dose can be metabolized before it ever reaches its site of pharmacological action.

Drugs with a high first-pass metabolism are listed in Table 1.3.

Table 1.3. Some drugs which undergo extensive first-pass metabolism

Analgesics	*Drugs acting on CNS*
Aspirin	Chlormethiazole
Morphine	Chlorpromazine
Paracetamol	Imipramine
Pentazocine	Levodopa
Pethidine	Nortriptyline
Cardiovascular drugs	*Respiratory drugs*
Glyceryl trinitrate	Salbutamol
Isoprenaline	Terbutaline
Isosorbide dinitrate	
Labetalol	*Oral contraceptives*
Lignocaine	
Metoprolol	
Nifedipine	
Prazosin	
Propranolol	
Verapamil	

The importance of first-pass metabolism is twofold:

1 It is one of the reasons for apparent differences in drug absorption between individuals. Even healthy people show considerable variation in liver metabolizing capacity.

2 In patients with severe liver disease, first-pass metabolism may be dramatically reduced, leading to the absorption of greater amounts of parent drug.

Linear vs. non-linear kinetics

In the discussion on clearance, it was pointed out that the hallmark of linear kinetics is the proportionality between dose rate and steady state concentration. This arises because the rate of elimination is proportional to the amount of drug in the body, while the clearance remains constant. This is not, however, always the case, as is exemplified by the drug phenytoin. When the enzymes responsible for

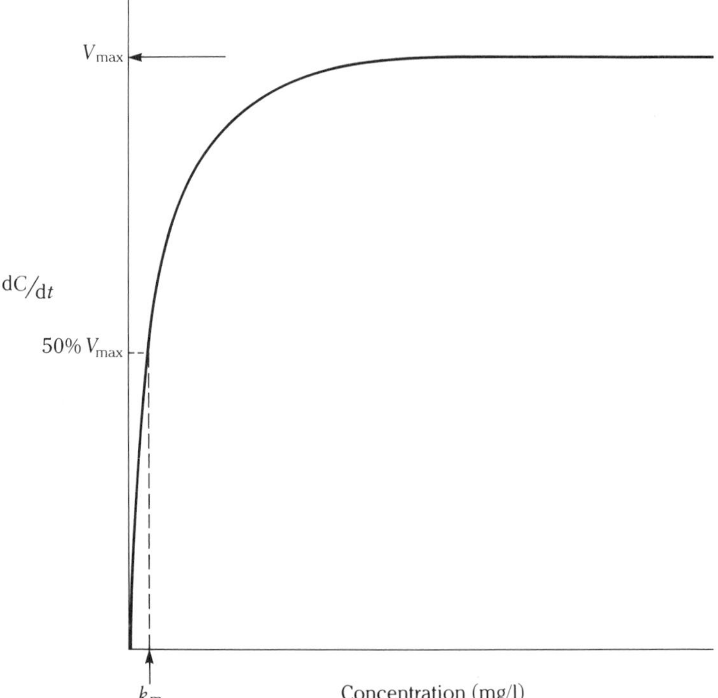

Fig. 1.7. Diagrammatic representation of the general relationship between drug concentration, C, and the rate of change of drug concentration, dC/dt. V_{max} is the maximum velocity at which the drug metabolizing enzyme can function and is a constant (with units of mass/time). k_m is the concentration at which V_{max} is 50%. The k_m is usually much higher than therapeutic concentrations and dC/dt vs. C is essentially linear (Eqn. 1.15). With a few drugs, notably phenytoin, therapeutic plasma concentrations are in the region of $k_m = 50$ so that the dC/dt vs. C relationship is non-linear, governed by the relationship shown in Eqn. 1.13.

metabolism reach a point of saturation, the rate of elimination—in terms of amount of drug eliminated in a given period of time—becomes constant and does not increase further in response to an increase in plasma concentration (or an increase in the amount of drug in the body due to an increase in dose). This gives rise to non-linear or zero-order kinetics.

The general relationship between drug concentration (C) and rate of change of concentration (dC/dt) is shown in Fig. 1.7. The maximum rate at which the enzymes can function, V_{max}, corresponds to the plateau attained by the curve. For phenytoin, V_{max} has a typical value of 7 mg/kg/day. k_m is the steady state concentration at which 50% V_{max} is attained, and has a typical value of 4 mg/l.

The equation relating dC/dt to C is the Michaelis–Menten equation

$$\frac{dC}{dt} = \frac{-V_{max} \times C}{k_m + C} \qquad \text{(Eqn. 1.13)}$$

and the fundamental difference between linear and non-linear kinetics can be appreciated by considering two extreme cases.

1 The plasma concentration is considerably less than k_m. In this case, the Michaelis–Menten equation can be approximated to

$$\frac{dC}{dt} = \frac{-V_{max} \times C}{k_m} \qquad \text{(Eqn. 1.14)}$$

or

$$\frac{dC}{dt} = \frac{-V_{max}}{k_m} \cdot C \qquad \text{(Eqn. 1.15)}$$

where V_{max}/k_m is a constant. This means that the rate of change of concentration is then proportional to the concentration (linear kinetics). In other words, the concentrations achieved by most drugs in clinical practice are far less than the k_m values, and the kinetics are linear.

2 The plasma concentration is considerably greater than k_m. In this case, the Michaelis–Menten equation can be approximated to

$$\frac{dC}{dt} = V_{max} \qquad \text{(Eqn. 1.16)}$$

which indicates that the rate of elimination is constant and will not change in response to a change in concentration. The consequence of this is that if the dose rate approaches, or exceeds, V_{max}, a change in dose will be associated with a disproportionate change in concentration. This can be seen in Fig. 1.8. If, as in the case of phenytoin, the working range of concentrations encompasses and exceeds k_m, the relationship between the steady state concentration and dose rate will alter as the concentration changes. At low concentrations, the increase in concentration will be proportional to the dose rate (linear pharmacokinetics). At higher concentrations, the increase will not be proportional, but will be much greater than would have been anticipated (non-linear pharmacokinetics).

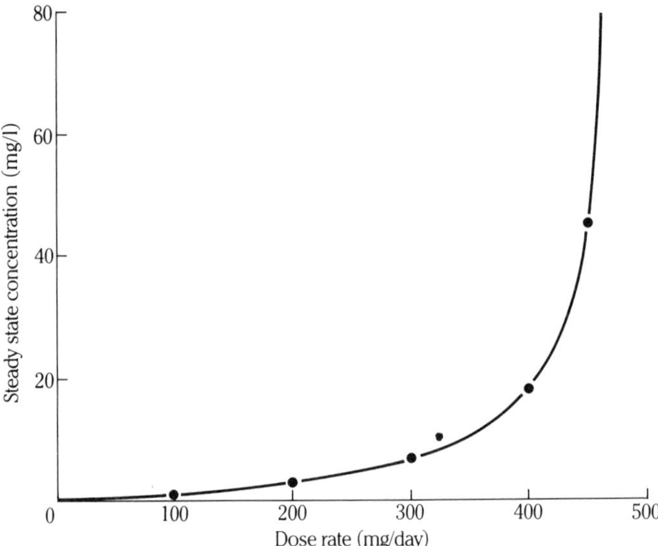

Fig. 1.8. The C_{pss}/dose rate relationship governed by Michaelis–Menten kinetics (Eqn. 1.13).

Comment

The practical importance of non-linear kinetics is that a small increase in dose can lead to a large increase in concentration. This is particularly important when toxic side effects are closely related to concentration, as with phenytoin.

1.3 PRINCIPLES OF DRUG ELIMINATION

Drug metabolism

Drugs are eliminated from the body by two principal mechanisms: liver metabolism and renal excretion. Drugs that are already water-soluble are generally excreted unchanged by the kidney. Lipid-soluble drugs are not easily excreted by the kidney because, following glomerular filtration, they are largely reabsorbed from the proximal tubule. The first step in the elimination of such lipid-soluble drugs is metabolism to more polar (water-soluble) compounds. This is achieved mainly in the liver, and generally occurs in two phases:

1 Mainly oxidation (sometimes reduction or hydrolysis) to a more polar compound.

2 Conjugation, usually with glucuronic acid or sulphate.

Phase 1 metabolism

Oxidation can occur in various ways: hydroxylation, oxygenation at carbon, nitrogen or sulphur atoms, *N*- and *O*-dealkylation or deamination. These reactions are catalysed by the mixed function oxidases of the endoplasmic reticulum, which comprise at least four types of enzymes: cytochrome P-450 and b5 with their corresponding reductases. The biochemistry of the mixed function oxidase system has not been fully elucidated. It is known, however, that there are multiple forms of cytochrome P-450, which can act on numerous substrates.

Phase 1 metabolites usually have only minor structural differences from the parent drug but may exhibit totally different pharmacological actions. For example, the aromatic hydroxylation of phenobarbitone abolishes its hypnotic activity, while metabolism of azathioprine produces the powerful antimetabolite 6-mercaptopurine.

Phase 2 reactions

These involve the addition of small endogenous molecules to the phase 1 metabolite, and almost always lead to abolition of pharmacological activity. Like phase 1 reactions, the liver is the major site but conjugation can occur in the gut wall where it can contribute to first-pass metabolism.

Metabolic drug interactions

The wide range of drugs metabolized by the mixed function oxidase system provides the opportunity for interactions of two types:

1 Induction (Table 1.4). Enzyme activity increases by stimulation of synthesis of new enzyme protein as the concentration of substrate increases. A drug may induce its own metabolism or, if two drugs which are metabolized by the same enzyme are given together, each can influence the metabolism of the other. For example, the anticonvulsants phenytoin, carbamazepine and phenobarbitone are all metabolized by the same enzymes that metabolize the constituents of oral contraceptives. If a woman receiving an oral contraceptive starts taking one of these anticonvulsants, the metabolism of the oestrogen and progestogen in the oral contraceptive increases with the risk of contraceptive failure. This phenomenon is not limited to drug administration. Cigarette smoking, for example, results in enzyme induction with increased metabolism of theophylline.

Table 1.4. Some drugs which induce metabolizing enzymes in the liver

Carbamazepine
Griseofulvin
Phenobarbitone
Phenytoin
Rifampicin

2 Inhibition (Table 1.5). Concurrently administered drugs can also lead to an inhibition of enzyme activity. Cimetidine, for example, decreases the metabolism of theophylline, leading to potentially dangerous adverse effects, e.g. arrhythmias and fits.

Comment

Enzyme induction produces clinical effects over days or weeks: the consequences of enzyme inhibition are usually immediate.

Table 1.5. Some drugs which inhibit metabolizing enzymes in the liver

Allopurinol
Azapropazone
Chloramphenicol
Cimetidine
Ciproflaxacin
Disulfiram
Erythromycin
Isoniazid

Genetic factors in metabolism

The rate at which healthy people metabolize drugs is variable. Studies with monozygotic and dizygotic twins have shown this variability to have a strong genetic basis, although environmental factors also make a contribution. There are a number of specific examples which are clinically important:

1 Acetylation in the liver is under genetic polymorphic control, the activity of *N*-acetyltransferase being determined by a recessive gene. Approximately 50% of Caucasians are slow acetylators and several drugs are known to be cleared from the body more slowly in such people (Table 1.6). Slow acetylators are more likely to develop concentration related adverse effects, e.g. the lupus erythematosus syndrome with hydralazine or procainamide. These patients should receive lower doses of drug than fast acetylators or, if possible, avoid these drugs.

2 Oxidation at a carbon atom also shows genetic polymorphism, but here the number of poor metabolizers is small: about 9% of the Caucasian population. The best documented clinical example consists of patients who are unable to metabolize debrisoquine (an adrenergic neurone blocker) and show an excessive fall in blood pressure following this drug. Other drugs showing impaired metabolism in this group of patients include nortriptyline and metoprolol. The clinical importance of oxidative polymorphism has yet to be established.

Table 1.6. Some drugs which are metabolized by acetylation

Dapsone
Hydralazine
Isoniazid
Phenelzine
Procainamide
Nitrazepam
Sulphasalazine
Other sulphonamides

Renal excretion

Three processes are implicated in renal excretion of drugs.

1 Glomerular filtration. This is the most common route of renal elimination. The free drug is cleared by filtration, and the protein bound drug remains in the circulation where some dissociates to restore equilibrium.

2 Active secretion in the proximal tubule. Both weak acids and weak bases have specific secretory sites in proximal tubular cells. Penicillins are eliminated by this route, as is about 60% of procainamide.
3 Passive reabsorption in the distal tubule. This occurs only with unionized, i.e. lipid-soluble, drugs. Whether or not weak acids and bases are reabsorbed depends on the urine pH, which determines the degree of ionization.

If renal function is impaired, e.g. by disease or old age, then the clearance of drugs which normally undergo renal excretion is decreased (Chapter 3).

Chapter 2
Clinical Pharmacokinetics: Therapeutic Drug Monitoring

2.1 JUSTIFICATION FOR THERAPEUTIC DRUG MONITORING

Drug concentrations in blood following a particular dose can vary widely between patients for several reasons:

1 Individual differences in absorption, first-pass metabolism, volume of distribution and clearance.

2 Altered pharmacokinetics because of gastrointestinal, hepatic, renal or cardiac disease.

3 Drug interactions.

4 Poor compliance with drug therapy.

In many cases, it is relatively easy to evaluate the pharmacological effects of a drug by clinical observation, and dosage regimens can be changed to increase therapeutic effect or to eliminate unwanted effects. Measurement of drug concentrations in blood is performed when the desired therapeutic actions or possible toxicity cannot be evaluated readily or safely from direct clinical observation (Table 2.1).

Table 2.1. Drugs for which plasma level measurements may be a useful guide to dosage

Antiarrhythmics (Chapter 6)	*Anticonvulsants* (Chapter 20)
Digoxin	Phenytoin
Disopyramide	Carbamazepine
Lignocaine	Phenobarbitone
Mexiletine	
Quinidine	*Miscellaneous*
	Theophylline (Chapter 11)
Antibiotics (Chapter 10)	Methotrexate (Chapter 13)
Gentamicin	Lithium (Chapter 19)
Tobramycin	Tricyclic antidepressants (Chapter 19)
Netilmicin	Cyclosporin (Chapter 13)
Vancomycin	

From drug concentration measurements, the following questions can be addressed:

1 Does the concentration reflect the present dose? (e.g. is it truly representative of steady state?).

Table 2.2. Examples of therapeutic ranges

Drug	Accepted therapeutic range (mg/l)	(μmol/l)
Digoxin	0.8–2	1–2.6
Disopyramide	2–5	6–15
Lignocaine	1.5–5	6–21
Carbamazepine	4–12	20–50
Phenobarbitone	10–30	50–150
Phenytoin	10–20	40–80
Gentamicin	Trough < 2; peak 5–12	Molecular units not applicable
Theophylline	8–20	44–111

2 Is the concentration within the 'therapeutic' or 'target' range, i.e. the range of concentrations below which the drug is usually ineffective and above which it is usually toxic (Table 2.2)?

3 If the concentration is not satisfactory or the patient is not responding, or has toxicity, what steps should be taken to arrive at a more appropriate dose?

Low concentrations for which there is no other explanation usually indicate poor compliance with therapy.

2.2 USE OF CLEARANCE ESTIMATES

The concept of clearance was introduced in Chapter 1 and it is important to recognize the significance of clearance in determining an individual patient's maintenance dose requirements. It is also important to note that clearance varies not only between individuals but also within an individual in response to his or her changes in clinical condition.

The physiological and pathological factors which affect clearance depend to a large extent on which organ is primarily responsible for elimination. For example, clearance of the bronchodilator theophylline, a drug which is eliminated by hepatic metabolism, is influenced by age, weight, alcohol consumption, cigarette smoking, other drugs, congestive cardiac failure, hepatic cirrhosis, acute pulmonary oedema and severe chronic obstructive airways disease.

Clearance in any individual therefore results from the interaction of a number of factors and is best determined directly from concentration measurements. Good estimates, however, can be made if relationships have previously been established between drug clearance and the sort of patient factors listed above. Again considering theophylline, the average population value for clearance is 0.04 l/h/kg, based on lean or ideal body weight. The way in which other factors alter this value is shown in Table 2.3. The final value for clearance is determined by multiplying 0.04 l/h/kg by the product of all factors present. This means that, on average, smokers require 1.6 times the theophylline dose of non-smokers and patients with cirrhosis require half the dose of patients without cirrhosis.

Table 2.3. Factors influencing theophylline clearance

Factor	Adjustments required
Smoking	× 1.6
Congestive cardiac failure	× 0.4
Hepatic cirrhosis	× 0.5
Acute pulmonary oedema	× 0.5
Severe chronic obstructive airways disease	× 0.8

For drugs primarily excreted by the kidney, e.g. digoxin, creatinine clearance closely reflects drug clearance, but congestive cardiac failure may also have to be taken into account as it influences cardiac output and therefore renal function. Thus digoxin clearance in a 70 kg patient without cardiac failure can be estimated from the equation

$$\text{Digoxin clearance (ml/min)} = 1.02 \times \text{Creatinine clearance} + 57\ \text{ml/min} \qquad \text{(Eqn. 2.1)}$$

whereas if the patient has cardiac failure, the equation is

$$\text{Digoxin clearance (ml/min)} = 0.88 \times \text{Creatinine clearance} + 23\ \text{ml/min} \qquad \text{(Eqn. 2.2)}$$

The 57 and 23 ml/min in these equations represent the net clearance of digoxin by routes other than the kidney, such as metabolism and clearance by the hepatobiliary system.

2.3 INTERPRETATION OF PLASMA LEVELS

Whenever a plasma concentration is measured it is essential to determine whether or not it is representative of a true steady state. This requires that at least four to five half-lives have elapsed since treatment started or since any change in dose and that no doses have been omitted. If these conditions can be satisfied and the kinetics can be assumed to be linear, Eqn. 1.11 can be used to determine clearance and this can be used to manipulate dosage. Alternatively, the concentration can be used to adjust the dose by simple proportionality.

Concentrations not at steady state cannot be used in this way and if a sensible interpretation is to be made it may be necessary to use more sophisticated mathematical techniques. It is also essential to remember that drugs with non-linear kinetics (such as phenytoin) require special consideration and different techniques are applied to the interpretation of their concentrations. An example is given on p. 26.

Successful interpretation of a concentration measurement depends on accurate information. The minimum usually required consists of the following:

1 Time of sample collection with respect to the previous dose.

2 An accurate and detailed dosage history—drug dose, frequency and route of administration.

3 Total duration of therapy to assess whether or not steady state has been achieved.

4 Relevant patient details such as age, sex, weight, serum creatinine or creatinine clearance and assessments of cardiac and hepatic function.

In addition, the reason for requesting a drug analysis should be considered carefully. 'Routine' requests made simply because analyses are available are of little value and are a waste of valuable resources.

2.4 EXAMPLES OF THERAPEUTIC DRUG MONITORING

Digoxin

A 68 year old man weighing 72 kg is taking 0.25 mg digoxin daily to control atrial fibrillation and congestive cardiac failure. Anorexia and nausea have developed and digoxin toxicity is suspected. A concentration of 2.6 μg/l is measured just before his daily dose (i.e. a trough concentration) and this indicates that the dose is inappropriately high. His creatinine clearance is 28 ml/min. The questions therefore are—what should the dose be and how long will it take for concentrations to decline to 'therapeutic' levels? To answer these questions, clearance, volume of distribution and half-life have to be determined.

Clearance

As the drug is being taken orally, absorption is incomplete and the dose should be multiplied by the appropriate bioavailability factor, in this case 0.6 (i.e. dose = 0.6×0.25 mg). The clearance equation (Eqn. 1.11) requires that the average steady state concentration (C_{pss}) is used in the denominator. This is not the measured trough (2.6 μg/l in this case) but a value a little higher—approximately one-third of the distance between the steady state trough and peak concentrations. In the case of digoxin, this is approximately 0.5 μg/l and the average C_{pss} is therefore 2.8 μg/l. If the dosage interval is 24 h

$$\text{Clearance} = \frac{0.6 \times 0.25 \times 1000}{2.8 \times 24}$$
$$= 2.2 \text{ l/h (or 37 ml/min)}$$

Volume of distribution

Although there is a simple proportional relationship between the volume of distribution of digoxin (V_{dig}) and body weight ($V_{dig} = 7$ l/kg, Chapter 1, Table 1.2), V_{dig} also depends to some extent on renal function, as is shown by the following equation

$$V_{dig}(\text{l/kg}) = 3.12 \times \text{Creatinine clearance (ml/min/kg)} + 3.84 \qquad \text{(Eqn. 2.3)}$$

which implies that as creatinine clearance falls V_{dig} also falls. In this patient, V_{dig} is therefore more appropriately calculated from this equation because of the low value of creatinine clearance:

$$V_{dig} = 3.12 \times \frac{28}{72} + 384$$
$$= 5.05 \text{ l/kg}$$
$$= 364 \text{ litre}$$

Half-life is calculated from the relationship

$$t_{1/2} = \frac{0.639}{\text{Clearance}} \times V$$
$$= \frac{0.693 \times 364}{2.2}$$
$$= 115 \text{ h (4.8 days)} \qquad \text{(Eqn. 2.4)}$$

As a trough level of 1.3 μg/l would represent a satisfactory concentration (i.e. 50% of the previously observed trough of 2.6 μg/l), it is clear that this will be achieved if the drug is withheld for one half-life, or about 5 days.

The new maintenance dose required to achieve a C_{pss} of 1.5 μg/l is calculated by substituting the estimated clearance (2.2 l/h) and the bioavailability (0.6) into Eqn. 1.12, thus

$$\text{Dose} = \frac{2.2 \times 1.5 \times 24}{0.6}$$
$$= 132\ \mu\text{g/day}$$
$$= 0.132 \text{ mg/day}$$

Because of the dosage limitations imposed by commercially available tablets, the options are 0.125 mg daily to produce an average C_{pss} of 1.4 μg/l or 0.1875 mg daily to produce a level of 2.1 μg/l. The decision as to which dose to use depends on the patient's response to the drug.

This example illustrates how an estimate of clearance can be obtained from routine measurements at steady state. It is subject to various errors, mainly in the form of uncertainty about the extent of bioavailability, the actual dosage history (raising the question of compliance) and the time of sampling. It is always interesting, however, to compare this estimate with one obtained indirectly from an equation predicting clearance from other clinical data, such as creatinine clearance and cardiac status (Eqns 2.1 and 2.2). In this case, the concentration measurement gives a clearance estimate of 37 ml/min whereas Eqn. 2.2 gives an estimate of 48 ml/min. This serves to illustrate the approximate nature of these calculations, the importance of recognizing sources of error and the limitations of using equations without taking biological variability into account. The change in dose could, of course, have been quickly determined by multiplying the incorrect dose by the ratio of the desired C_{pss} to that observed. Thus

$$\text{Dose} = 0.25 \times \frac{1.5}{2.8} \text{ mg/day}$$

which would lead to the same choice as above, i.e. 0.125 mg daily.

Phenytoin

A 30 year old man, weighing 70 kg, with epilepsy (grand mal) had been given phenytoin, but a dose of 350 mg daily had failed to control his fits adequately. Confident that he had taken the dose regularly for a number of weeks and that steady state had been achieved, his phenytoin plasma concentration was found to be 9 mg/l. What dose should now be recommended?

To answer this, two things should be borne in mind. Firstly, it appears that a steady state concentration of 9 mg/l is too low and a target concentration within the range 10–20 mg/l would be more appropriate. To make the correct adjustment, a specific target should be chosen—say 15 mg/l (a 67% increase in concentration). Secondly, it would be wrong to increase the dose by an equivalent amount because at this level the relationship between dose rate and steady state concentration is not linear.

The problem is solved by returning to the Michaelis–Menten equation (Eqn. 1.13) and rewriting it in terms of steady state concentrations

$$\text{Dose rate} = \frac{V_{max} \times C_{pss}}{k_m + C_{pss}} \qquad \text{(Eqn. 2.5)}$$

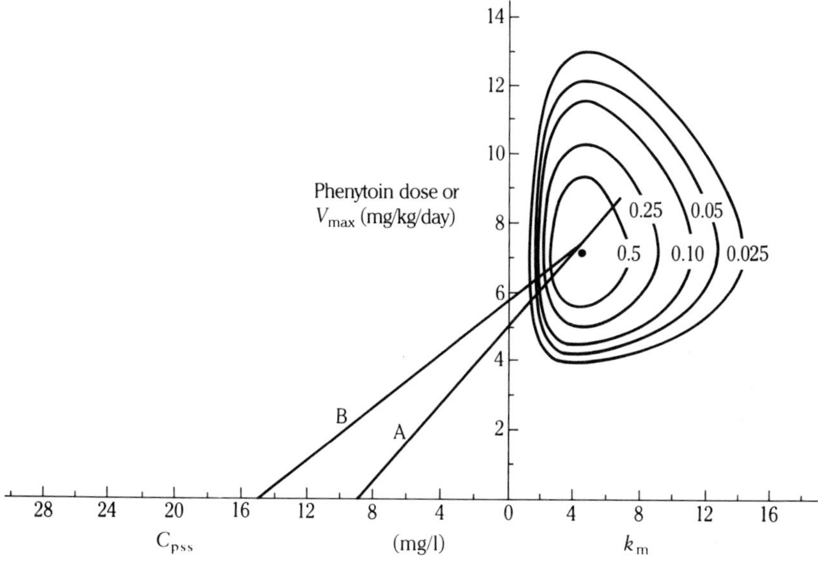

Fig. 2.1. Nomogram used to estimate the most probable values of V_{max} and k_m in a patient from a steady state concentration measurement and known dosage history. The 'orbits' represent the proportion of patients whose V_{max} and k_m values lie within that orbit.

Line A is drawn connecting the daily dose of phenytoin (mg/kg/day) to the corresponding steady state concentration and extrapolated so that it crosses the orbits. The coordinate of the midpoint of the line crossing the innermost orbit gives the most likely values for V_{max} and k_m in that patient.

A new maintenance dose is determined by drawing line B from this point to the desired steady state concentration and reading off the point of intersection on the *y* (mg/kg/day) axis. In this figure, line A represents a dose of 350 mg daily and a C_{pss} of 9 mg/l (μg/ml). The V_{max} is 7.5 mg/kg/day; k_m is 4.2 mg/l. Line B is drawn from this point to a C_{pss} of 15 mg/l, indicating a new maintenance dose of 5.7 mg/kg/day, or 400 mg/day.

From Vozeh, S. *et al.* (1981). Predicting individual phenytoin dosage. *Journal of Pharmacokinetics and Biopharmaceutics* **9**, 131.

If k_m is assumed to be 4 mg/l then V_{max} can be calculated by rearranging Eqn. 2.5 thus

$$V_{max} = \frac{\text{Dose rate } (4 + C_{pss})}{C_{pss}}$$

i.e. for a dose rate of 350 mg/day and C_{pss} of 9 mg/l, V_{max} is 506 mg/day (assuming complete bioavailability).

To calculate the new dose, the desired C_{pss}, V_{max} and k_m can be substituted into Eqn. 2.5 thus

$$\text{Dose rate} = \frac{506 \times 15}{4 + 15} = 400 \text{ mg/day}$$

Note that a 14% increase in dose produces a 67% increase in C_{pss}. The same result can be arrived at using a convenient nomogram (Fig. 2.1).

Comment

These examples illustrate steady state situations, one linear and one non-linear. The mathematical approaches used are straightforward. When interpretation of non-steady state concentrations is required, more sophisticated techniques are employed to estimate values such as clearance and volume of distribution because simple proportionality, based on concentration measurements, cannot be used to change dose. If the kinetics are linear, however, the clearance estimate immediately facilitates choice of dose if a target concentration can be specified (Eqn. 1.12).

Chapter 3
Influence of Disease on Pharmacokinetics and Pharmacodynamics

Drugs are usually considered in terms of their effect on disease processes. However, several diseases can influence the pharmacokinetics of a drug or its pharmacodynamic effect on target organs. This is of considerable clinical importance when diseases of the liver or kidney modify drug elimination, or when drug distribution and elimination are altered in congestive cardiac failure.

3.1 INFLUENCE OF GASTROINTESTINAL DISEASE

Achlorhydria

Achlorhydria occurs in the elderly population: gastric pH increases and gastric acid secretion is thought to decrease to 25–35% of that in a 20 year old. Achlorhydria, however, has no effect on cephalexin, penicillin V, tetracycline or paracetamol, whereas aspirin absorption is increased because the higher pH increases its rate of dissolution, an effect secondary to an increase in the amount of aspirin in ionized form.

Coeliac disease

There are several pathophysiological factors that can influence drug absorption. In addition to the considerable loss of absorptive surface, the rate of gastric emptying is increased, intraluminal pH is increased, the enterohepatic circulation is decreased, permeability of the gut wall is increased, intestinal drug metabolism is decreased and activity of various enzymes such as esterases is decreased. The outcome is complex: some drugs show decreased absorption, e.g. amoxycillin and pivampicillin; others show increased absorption, e.g. cephalexin; decreased absorption of dietary folate may increase the risk of bone marrow toxicity from co-trimoxazole; some show no change, e.g. ampicillin.

Crohn's disease

Again there are several changes that can influence drug absorption. The absorptive surface area is decreased, the gut wall is thickened and bacterial flora is altered. The absorption of the two components of co-trimoxazole is affected in opposite ways: that of trimethoprim is decreased, while sulphamethoxazole absorption is increased.

Comment

Many factors can influence drug absorption when the gastrointestinal tract is abnormal. The presence of a malabsorption syndrome does not imply that drugs are necessarily malabsorbed: the absorption of some can actually increase. There is currently insufficient information to comment on the clinical importance of these changes, but theoretically treatment failure may occur because of malabsorption, and drug toxicity may result from increased absorption.

3.2 INFLUENCE OF IMPAIRED RENAL FUNCTION

Impaired renal function can influence drug therapy for the following reasons:

1 Pharmacokinetics may be altered.

(a) Decreased elimination of drugs that are normally excreted entirely or mainly by the kidneys.

(b) Decreased protein binding.

2 Drug effect may be altered.

3 Existing clinical condition may be worsened.

4 Adverse effects may be enhanced.

Each of these factors is now considered in more detail.

Altered pharmacokinetics

Elimination

Since the kidney represents one of the major routes of drug elimination, a decrease in normal function can influence the clearance of many drugs. If a drug normally cleared by the kidney is given to someone with decreased renal function without altering the dose, the steady state blood concentrations of that drug increase. This is of considerable importance in the case of drugs showing concentration related adverse effects, particularly those in which toxic effects occur just above the therapeutic range.

When such drugs are given to patients with renal dysfunction, therefore, the aim is to achieve the same concentrations as seen in patients with normal kidneys. This is achieved by:

1 Determining renal function, either by measuring creatinine clearance (based on a 24 h urine collection) or by estimating creatinine clearance from the serum creatinine concentration, body weight, age and sex.

2 Modifying the dose, either by increasing the dosage interval or by giving less drug at the usual frequency. In severe renal failure these two approaches are often combined: less drug is given less often than usual. The necessary extent and precision of dose modification depends very much on the toxicity of the drug concerned. In the case of aminoglycosides, even minor impairment of renal function requires some modification of dose while the dose of penicillins need only be reduced in severe renal failure (creatinine clearance, 10 ml/min). Guidance on dosage reduction is readily available for most commonly used drugs.

3 Giving a loading dose. This may be necessary if therapeutic concentrations have to be established rapidly, since about five half-lives are required to achieve steady state drug concentrations: the prolonged half-life resulting from renal impairment delays the attainment of steady state.

4 Monitoring drug concentrations. This is mandatory for drugs with serious concentration related adverse effects, e.g. aminoglycosides and digoxin. Nomograms are useful guides to the doses likely to be appropriate, but every patient is different. Measured concentrations of drugs in the blood must be used to assess the altered kinetics and to determine the most appropriate dose. This is discussed further in Chapter 2, Section 2.1.

Decreased protein binding

The following changes occur in patients with impaired renal function:

1 Acidic drugs are less bound but the binding of basic drugs undergoes little or no change.

2 The decrease in binding is correlated with the severity of renal impairment.

3 Haemodialysis does not return binding to normal but renal transplantation does.

4 The structure of albumin is changed in renal failure and this probably largely explains the changes in binding.

The clinical relevance of decreased protein binding is demonstrated by the interpretation of serum phenytoin concentrations in renal failure. The usually quoted therapeutic range of phenytoin is 10–20 mg/l, which represents total (bound and unbound) drug. In renal failure the proportion of bound drug falls and the free phenytoin fraction increases. An equilibrium is therefore established in renal failure where bound phenytoin is reduced but free phenytoin concentration is unchanged. Since it is the free phenytoin which is pharmacologically active, the concentration of phenytoin necessary to produce a therapeutic effect is reached at a lower total phenytoin concentration. Putting this in numerical terms, the therapeutic range for phenytoin in severe renal failure is 5–10 mg/l.

Altered drug effect

Independent of changes in pharmacokinetics there are several examples of increased sensitivity to drug effects in renal failure. Opiates, barbiturates, phenothiazines and benzodiazepines all show greater central nervous system effects in patients with renal failure compared to those with normal renal function. The reason is not known, but meningeal permeability is increased in renal failure and this could be one explanation.

Various antihypertensive drugs have a greater postural effect in renal failure. Again the reasons are not clear but changes in sodium balance and autonomic dysfunction may be partly responsible.

Worsening of the existing clinical condition

Drug therapy can result in deterioration of the clinical condition in the following ways:

1 By further impairing renal function. In patients with renal failure it is clearly desirable to avoid drugs that are known to be nephrotoxic and for which alternatives are available. Examples include cephaloridine, cephalothin, penicillamine and gold.

2 By causing fluid retention. Fluid balance is a major problem in the more severe forms of renal failure. Drugs that cause fluid retention should therefore be avoided, e.g. carbenoxolone and anti-inflammatory drugs such as indomethacin.

3 By increasing the degree of uraemia. Tetracyclines, except doxycycline, have an antianabolic effect and should be avoided.

Enhancement of drug adverse effects

1 Digoxin. In addition to the decreased elimination referred to earlier, digoxin is more likely to cause adverse effects in patients with severe renal failure if there are substantial electrolyte abnormalities, particularly hypercalcaemia and/or hypokalaemia.

2 Potassium sparing diuretics. Since potassium elimination is impaired in renal failure, diuretics which also conserve potassium (amiloride, spironolactone) are more likely to cause hyperkalaemia.

3.3 INFLUENCE OF LIVER DISEASE

Impaired liver function can influence the response to treatment in several ways:

1 Altered pharmacokinetics:
   (a) Increased bioavailability resulting from reduced first-pass metabolism.
   (b) Decreased protein binding.
   (c) Decreased elimination.

2 Altered drug effect.

3 Worsening of metabolic state.

Altered pharmacokinetics

The liver is the largest organ in the body, has a substantial blood supply (around 1.5 l/min) and is interposed between the gastrointestinal tract and the systemic circulation. For these reasons it is uniquely suited for the purpose of influencing drug metabolism.

Decreased first-pass metabolism

A decrease in hepatocellular function decreases the capacity of the liver to perform metabolic processes, while portosystemic shunting directs drugs away from sites of metabolism. Both factors are usually present in patients with severe cirrhosis.

Knowledge of the drugs that undergo first-pass metabolism is important in situations where it is decreased as the result of disease. Considerably more active drug then reaches the site of action and any given dose of drug has unexpectedly intense effects.

Examples for patients with severe cirrhosis are:

Chlormethiazole (bioavailability, tenfold increase).

Labetalol (twofold increase).

Paracetamol (50% increase).

Pentazocine (fourfold increase).

Pethidine (twofold increase).
Propranolol (twofold increase).

Decreased protein binding and decreased elimination by liver metabolism

These aspects are interdependent and should therefore be considered together.

In this context, drugs can be classified according to the ability of the liver to metabolize them.

High extraction drugs

These are drugs that the liver metabolizes at a very high rate. Their clearance is dependent only on the rate at which drug is delivered to the enzyme systems and is proportional to liver blood flow. The clearance of these drugs is sensitive to factors which can influence hepatic blood flow, such as congestive cardiac failure.

Examples include: lignocaine, propranolol, pethidine, pentazocine, nortriptyline and morphine.

Low extraction drugs

The rate of metabolism of drugs in this case is sufficiently low that hepatic clearance is not limited by the amount of drug delivered to the liver but is dependent on the capacity of the liver enzymes to metabolize the drugs concerned. The rate of metabolism of these drugs is dependent on the concentration of drug at the enzyme receptor site which is, in turn, proportional to the free concentration of drug in plasma.

Examples include: diazepam, warfarin, chlorpromazine, theophylline and paracetamol.

The influence of liver disease on drug elimination is complex: the type of liver disease is critical. In acute viral hepatitis the major change is in hepatocellular function, but drug metabolizing ability usually remains intact and hepatic blood flow can actually increase. Mild to moderate cirrhosis tends to result in decreased hepatic blood flow and portosystemic shunting, while severe cirrhosis usually shows reductions both in cellular function and blood flow.

Comment

Unlike the measurement of creatinine clearance in renal disease, there is no simple test that can predict the extent to which drug metabolism is decreased in liver disease. At best, a low serum albumin, raised bilirubin and prolonged prothrombin time give a rough guide.

The fact that a drug is metabolized by the liver does not necessarily mean that its kinetics are altered by liver disease. It is not possible, therefore, to extrapolate the findings from one drug to another. This is presumably because superficially similar metabolic pathways are mediated by different forms of cytochrome P-450.

The documentation of modestly altered kinetics does not necessarily imply clinical importance. Even normal subjects show quite wide variations in kinetic indices and, in addition, kinetics should not be viewed in isolation from alterations in drug effect, which are usually much more difficult to assess. However, if a drug is known to be subject to substantial kinetic changes, the clinical significance is much more likely.

If it is clinically desirable to give a drug that is eliminated by liver metabolism to a patient with cirrhosis, it should be started at a low dose and drug levels or effect should be monitored very closely.

Altered drug effect

Deranged brain function

The more severe forms of liver disease are accompanied by poorly understood derangements of brain function which ultimately result in the syndrome of hepatic encephalopathy. However, even before encephalopathy develops, the brain is extremely sensitive to the effects of centrally acting drugs.

This is independent of changes in drug kinetics. A state of coma can result from administering 'normal' doses of opiates or barbiturates to such patients.

Decreased clotting factors

Patients with liver disease also show increased sensitivity to oral anticoagulants. These drugs exert their effect by decreasing the vitamin K dependent synthesis of clotting factors II, VII, IX and X. When the production of these factors is already reduced by liver disease, a given dose of oral anticoagulant has a greater effect than in subjects with normal liver function.

Worsening of metabolic state

Drug induced alkalosis

Excessive use of diuretics can precipitate encephalopathy. The mechanism involves hypokalaemic alkalosis, which results in conversion of NH_4^+ to NH_3, the unionized ammonia crossing easily into the CNS to worsen or precipitate encephalopathy.

Fluid overload

Patients with advanced liver disease often have oedema and ascites secondary to hypoalbuminaemia and portal hypertension. This problem can be worsened by drugs that cause fluid retention, e.g. carbenoxolone, antacids that contain large amounts of sodium and non-steroidal anti-inflammatory agents. This last group of drugs should be avoided anyway because of the increased risk of gastrointestinal bleeding.

Hepatotoxic drugs (Table 3.1)

Where an acceptable alternative exists, it is wise to avoid drugs that can cause liver damage, e.g. oral contraceptives, rifampicin and repeated exposure to halothane anaesthesia.

3.4 INFLUENCE OF CONGESTIVE HEART FAILURE

Congestive heart failure can influence drug kinetics in the following ways:

1 Decreased rate or extent of gastrointestinal absorption, e.g., hydrochlorthiazide and metolazone.

Table 3.1. Drugs that can cause liver damage

Hepatitis
Halothane (repeated exposure)
Isoniazid
Methyldopa
Phenelzine
Cholestasis with a mild hepatic component
Phenothiazines
Tricyclic antidepressants
Non-steroidal anti-inflammatory drugs (especially phenylbutazone)
Rifampicin, ethambutol, pyrazinamide
Sulphonylureas
Sulphonamides, ampicillin, nitrofurantoin; erythromycin estolate
Oral contraceptives (stasis without hepatitis)
Cirrhosis
Methotrexate

2 Decreased volume of distribution, e.g. lignocaine and procainamide.
3 Decreased elimination, e.g. lignocaine and theophylline.

Altered pharmacokinetics

Decreased gastrointestinal absorption

The main factors involved are:
1 Mucosal oedema.
2 Reduced epithelial blood supply.
3 Splanchnic vasoconstriction.

Decreased volume of distribution

This is thought to result from decreased tissue perfusion. It is clearly documented for lignocaine (reduced by about 50% in severe failure). Therefore, for any given dose, correspondingly higher blood concentrations are achieved. The corollary and practical importance of this is that initial loading doses should be reduced correspondingly.

Decreased elimination

The main factors involved are, for the liver:
1 Decreased perfusion.
2 Decreased oxidizing capacity because of hypoxia.
3 Decreased metabolizing capacity because of congestion.
For the kidney they are:
1 Decreased glomerular filtration rate.
2 Increased tubular reabsorption.

The clearance of lignocaine is dependent on liver blood flow and in heart failure can be reduced by up to 50%. For theophylline the metabolic capacity of the liver is important and again clearance is reduced in heart failure (Chapter 2, Table 2.3) as these drugs have concentration related toxicity:

1 The rate of administration must be reduced in heart failure.

2 Therapeutic drug monitoring may be used to adjust therapy.

3.5 INFLUENCE OF THYROID DISEASE

Thyroid disease alters a patient's response to digoxin. Hyperthyroid patients are relatively resistant to the drug while hypothyroid patients are extremely sensitive to it. The reasons are in part kinetic and in part dynamic. The clearance of digoxin is roughly proportional to thyroid function so, for any given dose, lower concentrations are achieved in hyperthyroid patients and higher concentrations are achieved in hypothyroid patients compared to normals. These effects are influenced by the volume of distribution decreasing in hypothyroidism and increasing in hyperthyroidism (Chapter 6). In addition, hypothyroidism increases the sensitivity of cardiac tissue to digoxin but the mechanism is not understood.

Lithium can cause hypothyroidism apparently by inhibiting the release of thyroid hormone from the gland. It is important to recognize this complication in order to avoid mistaking hypothyroidism for a relapse in the depressive illness. Thyroxine can be prescribed concurrently with lithium.

Chapter 4
Drugs at the Extremes of Age

Most information in clinical pharmacology has been derived from experiments and observations in young or middle-aged patients or healthy volunteers. However, most drug use is concentrated in children and those over the age of 65 years. In Scotland, for example, approximately 20% of prescriptions are issued for those aged less than 16 years and 40% for those over 65 years. Relatively little information is available about drug absorption, effect and elimination at these extremes of age.

4.1 USE OF DRUGS IN NEONATES

Drug distribution

Compared to the adult a much higher percentage of neonatal body mass is water: 75% is water in the full-term neonate, while 85% is the figure in premature babies. In a premature infant only 1% of body weight is accounted for by fat, while in the full-term neonate the figure is 15%.

Membrane permeability is generally greater in the neonate compared to the adult, and this is particularly true of the blood–brain barrier.

Protein binding is considerably less in the neonate compared to the adult. Possible reasons for this include the presence of competing endogenous substances (bilirubin, free fatty acids, steroids), differences in pH and differences in the molecular species of binding proteins. A decrease in protein binding and increased volume of distribution have been demonstrated in the neonate for salicylates, benzylpenicillin, ampicillin and digoxin.

Drug metabolism

Liver drug metabolizing activity is reduced in the neonate, but it is difficult to generalize as different pathways develop at different rates. Hydroxylation and glucuronidation are very slow to develop while sulphate conjugation is much faster. Many commonly used drugs have been shown to have substantially prolonged half-lives in the neonate: diazepam, phenobarbitone, nortriptyline, tolbutamide, theophylline and chloramphenicol. The decreased metabolism of chloramphenicol can cause an adverse reaction characterized by cardiovascular collapse, coma and cyanosis if serum concentration exceeds 25 mg/l.

Drug excretion

Glomerular filtration at birth is approximately 30–40% that of the adult when corrected for body surface area, while at the fifth day of life glomerular filtration rate has increased to about 50% of adult values. This decreased renal function has the predictable effect of decreasing the clearance of drugs that undergo renal elimination. Benzylpenicillin is cleared from premature infants at about 30% of the rate seen in adults when adjusted for body weight. The same observations have been made with other penicillins and the aminoglycosides.

Drug effect

One method of assessing drug effect is to compare the LD_{50} in neonatal and mature animals. Using this technique various central nervous system depressants such as barbiturates, chlorpromazine and the opiates have been shown to have a substantially greater effect on a mg/kg dose basis in neonatal compared to mature animals. On the other hand, some clinically important drugs are less potent in the neonate, e.g. digoxin and phenytoin. The increased volume of distribution of digoxin cannot by itself explain the greater dose per kilogram needed in the neonate since studies on isolated cardiac tissue have shown that there is an intrinsic decrease in sensitivity to digoxin in the neonatal period. Therefore, these drugs are given on a greater mg/kg dose regimen than in the adult.

Comment

These differences in distribution, elimination and effect between neonates and adults, between premature and full-term neonates and between drugs in babies of the same maturity mean that no hard and fast rules can be applied to drug dosing. In general, effective and safe doses have been arrived at by experience, and guidance is found in standard textbooks of paediatrics. Therapeutic drug monitoring may provide useful information (aminoglycosides, digoxin and theophylline).

4.2 USE OF DRUGS IN CHILDREN

Drug metabolism

Several drugs that are cleared by liver metabolism undergo more rapid elimination in late infancy and early childhood compared to the adult.

Examples include: phenytoin, theophylline, carbamazepine and phenobarbitone.

Drug excretion

Glomerular filtration reaches adult rates by about 5 months of age while tubular secretion and reabsorption achieve adult levels by about 7 months. Digoxin appears to have a greater clearance in children than adults: the effective daily dose in childhood is around 10–15 μg/kg compared with approximately 3.5 μg/kg in adults.

Therapeutic drug concentration monitoring

The indication for drug concentration monitoring should be the same as in adults.

However, the results must be interpreted in the light of considerable ignorance about concentration–effect relationships in children.

Drug doses

There is no entirely satisfactory method of calculating drug dose in children because of differences in elimination and possibly also drug effect compared to adults. It is certainly not satisfactory simply to scale down adult doses, since children generally need more on a mg/kg basis. Working from a knowledge of surface area tends to be more reliable, but this requires estimation from nomograms after obtaining height and weight

$$\text{Dose} = \frac{\text{Surface area (m}^2)}{1.8} \times \text{Adult dose}$$

However, this should still be regarded as an approximation.

Comment

For most commonly used drugs detailed guidelines are available in textbooks and practical guides to paediatrics. *If you are prescribing for a child, check the dose schedule first.*

4.3 DRUGS AND THE ELDERLY

The elderly (age 65 years and over) constitute approximately 14% of the population yet they consume 40% of drug prescriptions in the UK. This high consumption of drugs is related to an increasing prevalence of acute and chronic disease. Multiple drug prescribing leads to problems with drug compliance and, perhaps more importantly, is directly related to the incidence of side effects. The overall incidence of drug side effects in the elderly is up to three times that seen in the young. Adverse drug reactions in the elderly tend to be dose related rather than idiosyncratic. This suggests that side effects may be related to changes in pharmacokinetics and (or) pharmacodynamics with increasing age.

Drug absorption, distribution, metabolism, excretion and activity can all change as a result of ageing. However, the common presence of multiple pathology in the old frequently has a greater effect than ageing alone.

Drug absorption

Ageing is associated with increased gastric pH, delayed gastric emptying, decreased intestinal motility and reduced splanchnic blood flow. Despite these changes there is little evidence to suggest that intestinal drug absorption changes with age. The rate of absorption of digoxin is slower in the elderly but the overall bioavailability remains the same.

Drug distribution

Age related changes in body composition, in protein binding and in organ blood flow all can affect drug disposition.

Ageing is associated with a relative increase in body fat and corresponding reduction in body water. The volume of distribution of water-soluble drugs is smaller and this tends to cause an increase in initial drug concentration (e.g. digoxin and cimetidine). Lipid-soluble drugs tend to have an increased volume of distribution (e.g. nitrazepam and diazepam) which prolongs the elimination half-life and may prolong effect.

The extent of plasma protein–drug binding changes little with age but the plasma albumin concentration may fall considerably with the onset of disease.

Acidic drugs tend to bind to albumin. A fall in plasma albumin concentration can lead to increased levels of free active drug. This often results in drug toxicity (usually due to increased therapeutic response) even though the overall plasma drug concentration remains within a defined 'therapeutic range' (e.g. phenytoin). In theory, a reduction in protein binding could also increase the risk of adverse drug interactions, e.g. increased displacement of warfarin from plasma protein binding sites by some non-steroidal anti-inflammatory drugs. There is no strong evidence that this type of interaction is a more significant problem in the elderly than in the young.

Many basic drugs bind to plasma α_1-acid glycoprotein. The concentration of this glycoprotein tends to rise with disease. The resultant increase in protein binding of drugs (e.g. lignocaine and disopyramide) does not appear to have any clinical significance.

Drug metabolism and age

There is evidence for age related changes in the rates of metabolism of some drugs. In general, drugs which undergo microsomal oxidation (e.g. chlordiazepoxide) are likely to be metabolized more slowly in the elderly. Despite this, there is no evidence that the concentration or activity of hepatic microsomal oxidizing enzymes is reduced in the elderly. The age related reduction in oxidizing capacity may be related to the reduction in hepatic volume and blood flow that occurs in the elderly. Conjugation pathways do not appear to be affected by age.

First-pass metabolism may be reduced considerably in the elderly. This is probably the consequence of the age associated reduction in liver mass and blood flow. As a result, drugs which undergo extensive first-pass metabolism (e.g. labetalol and propranolol) may show considerably increased bioavailability in the elderly.

This effect is amplified by the presence of chronic liver disease.

Renal excretion

In old age there is a fall in both renal blood flow and renal function. Glomerular filtration falls by approximately 30% by the age of 65, compared with young adults. Digoxin and the aminoglycoside antibiotics are excreted mainly by glomerular filtration and these will tend to accumulate in the elderly if the dose is not reduced. Renal tubular function also declines and drugs such as penicillin and procainamide, which undergo active tubular secretion, have a marked reduction in clearance. In addition, the elderly are more likely to suffer a further reduction in renal function as a result of renal tract disease such as infection. Illness in the elderly is frequently accompanied by dehydration and this reduces renal function even further. The overall effect of physiological ageing and disease considerably diminishes the elderly kidney's capacity to excrete drugs.

Receptor sensitivity

In practice it is very difficult to assess accurately drug receptor numbers or sensitivity. In most cases information is derived from drug effect related to drug plasma concentration. Using this approach it can be shown that the elderly are more sensitive to the effects of benzodiazepine drugs such as nitrazepam, temazepam and diazepam. Warfarin is more potent in the elderly because of a greater effect on coagulation factor synthesis.

Perhaps most is known about the effects of ageing on autonomic receptors. There is a decline in the tachycardia produced by stimulation of β_1-adrenergic receptors. On the other hand, there appears to be no age-related change in β_2-adrenoceptor mediated vascular or bronchial relaxation. The effect of the vasoconstrictor α_1-adrenoceptor is also unchanged with age.

Impairment of homeostasis

The effect of drugs in the elderly may be affected by a loss of homeostatic control that is often seen in the elderly patient.

Cardiovascular postural reflexes are commonly less effective in the aged. Elderly patients tend to fall more easily than the young and this is made worse by the use of drugs that cause postural hypotension. There are many such drugs including diuretics, antihypertensive agents and sedatives.

The elderly have impaired thermoregulation. Many of the major tranquillizers may precipitate hypothermia. This is partly due to a direct hypothermic effect but also due to a reduction in physical activity.

Compliance

There is no evidence that an elderly patient whose mental function is normal is more likely to make mistakes with their medication than a younger patient. However, one of the main contributory factors to poor drug compliance at all ages is polypharmacy—the rate of errors when three drugs are prescribed is approximately 20% but it is close to 100% when 10 drugs are prescribed—and the high consumption of drugs in the elderly results in a greater opportunity to make errors. This is often made worse by the prevalence of mental impairment, which is as high as 25% in those over the age of 85 years. Physical handicap can also contribute to poor compliance. Arthritic hands have great difficulty in opening 'child-proof' containers or 'bubble-packed' drugs.

Rules for prescribing drugs for the elderly

1 Make an accurate diagnosis. The presentation of disease in the elderly is often non-specific (e.g. confusion, dizziness and incontinence). It is important to make an accurate diagnosis to allow appropriate therapy.

2 Treat only important disorders. Elderly patients frequently have multiple pathology. This can lead to polypharmacy with resultant increase in side effects and poor compliance.

3 Avoid ineffective drugs. Prescriptions for marginally effective or ineffective drugs can only lead to side effects and poor compliance. It should be remembered that there is no drug treatment for dementia and those advertised for the treatment of atherosclerosis or urinary incontinence have little, if any, measurable effect.
4 Review drugs regularly. It is important to review the need for each prescription. If a drug is considered necessary, make sure the minimum dose required is used.
5 Understand the changes in pharmacology with age for each drug used. All new drugs released for use in the UK must specify any special precautions or dosage changes that are necessary for the elderly patient. If no such information is available then it is better to keep the dose as low as possible, remembering that relative renal insufficiency is very common in the elderly.

Chapter 5
Drugs in Pregnant and Breast Feeding Women

Nearly 40% of women in the UK take at least one drug during pregnancy, excluding iron, vitamins and drugs used during delivery. Once in the maternal circulation, drugs are separated from the fetus by a lipid placental membrane which any given drug crosses to a greater or lesser extent depending on the physicochemical properties of the molecule.

Drugs in pregnancy can be viewed from two standpoints:

1 Effect of drugs on the fetus.

2 Effect of pregnancy on the drug.

5.1 EFFECT OF DRUGS ON THE FETUS

Drugs can influence fetal development at three separate stages:

1 Fertilization and implantation period: conception to about 17 days gestation.

2 Organogenesis: 18–55 days.

3 Growth and development: 56 days onward.

The possible consequences of drug exposure are quite different at each stage. In addition, drugs given at the end of pregnancy can influence structure or function in the neonate.

Fertilization and implantation period

Interference by a drug with either of these processes clearly leads to failure of the pregnancy at a very early and probably subclinical stage. Therefore, very little is known about drugs that influence this process in the human.

Organogenesis

It is during this period that the developing embryo shows great sensitivity to the teratogenic effects of drugs. A teratogen is any substance (virus, environmental toxin or drug) that produces deformity. Before discussing the teratogenic properties of certain drugs, the following points must be appreciated:

1 Teratogenesis in the human is very difficult to predict from animal studies because of considerable species variation. Thalidomide, the most notorious drug teratogen of recent times, showed no teratogenicity in mice and rats.

2 Serious congenital deformities are present in 1–2% of all babies, therefore, a drug is only readily identified as teratogenic if its effects are frequent, unusual

Table 5.1. Drugs which are known to be teratogenic

Drug	Deformity
Danazol	Virilization of female fetus
Lithium	Cardiac (Ebstein's complex)
Phenytoin	Craniofacial; limb
Carbamazepine	Craniofacial; limb
Primidone	Facial clefting; cardiac
Retinoic acid	CNS
Sodium valproate	Neural tube
Stilboestrol	Adenocarcinoma of vagina in teenage years
Warfarin	Multiple defects; chondrodysplasia punctata

and/or serious. A low-grade teratogen that infrequently causes minor deformities is likely to pass unnoticed.

Table 5.1 lists some drugs which are known to be teratogenic. It is important to realize that, even for known teratogens, first trimester use often results in a normal baby: e.g. lithium is teratogenic in about 10% of exposures and warfarin in about 5%. Also, there will be occasions, such as the use of warfarin in women with prosthetic heart valves, where the risks to the mother of not using the drug outweigh the risks of exposure in the fetus.

Comment

The greatest risk of teratogenesis occurs at a time when a woman might not even be aware that she is pregnant. Only a few drugs are known definitely to be teratogenic, but many more could be under certain circumstances. When prescribing for a woman of childbearing age, remember that she might be pregnant and ask yourself if the benefits of drug use outweigh the risks, however small, of teratogenesis.

Growth and development

During this stage major body structures have been formed, and it is their subsequent development and function that can be affected:

1 Antithyroid drugs cross the placenta and can cause fetal and neonatal hypothyroidism.

2 Tetracyclines inhibit bone growth and discolour teeth.

3 Drugs with dependence potential, e.g. benzodiazepines, opiates and dextropropoxyphene, which are taken regularly during pregnancy can result in withdrawal symptoms in the neonate.

Drugs given at the end of pregnancy

1 Aspirin in analgesic doses can cause haemorrhage in the neonate.

2 Indomethacin (and possibly high doses of aspirin) cause premature closure of the ductus arteriosus with resulting pulmonary hypertension.

3 CNS depressant drugs (e.g. opiates, benzodiazepines) can cause hypotension, respiratory depression and hypothermia in the neonate.

5.2 EFFECT OF PREGNANCY ON DRUG ABSORPTION, DISTRIBUTION AND ELIMINATION

The substantial physiological changes that occur in pregnancy can influence drug disposition while pathological conditions in pregnancy can accentuate these changes.

Absorption

There is a decrease in gastrointestinal motility during the later part of pregnancy, and this can either increase the absorption of poorly soluble drugs such as digoxin or decrease the absorption of drugs that undergo metabolism in the gut wall, such as chlorpromazine.

Drug distribution

Maternal plasma volume and extracellular fluid volume increase by about 50% by the last trimester, and this should decrease the steady state concentration of drugs with a small volume of distribution. Considerable changes in protein concentration occur during the last trimester, with serum albumin falling by about 20% while α_1-acid glycoprotein increases in concentration by about 40% in normal pregnancies. These changes are accentuated in pre-eclampsia with albumin concentration falling by about 34% and glycoprotein rising by as much as 100%. This means that the free fraction of acidic drugs can substantially increase while that of basic drugs can be greatly decreased in the last trimester. Diazepam, phenytoin and sodium valproate have been shown to have significantly elevated free fractions in the last trimester.

Drug elimination

Effective renal plasma flow doubles by the end of pregnancy but this has only been shown to be important in a few cases; for example, the clearance of ampicillin doubles and the dose must also be doubled for systemic (but of course not for renal tract) infections. The hepatic microsomal mixed function oxidase system undergoes induction in pregnancy, probably as the result of high circulating levels of progesterone. This leads to an increased clearance of drugs that undergo metabolism by this pathway, and there is evidence that the steady state concentrations of the anticonvulsants sodium valproate, phenytoin, carbamazepine and phenobarbitone are decreased to a clinically significant extent during the second and third trimesters. Therefore, higher doses are required as the pregnancy progresses, with careful monitoring of drug concentrations.

5.3 DRUG TREATMENT OF COMMON MEDICAL PROBLEMS DURING PREGNANCY

Infection

Urinary tract infections are common during pregnancy. Penicillins are the preferred treatment (subject to appropriate sensitivity testing), since these drugs have never been implicated in teratogenesis and are generally well tolerated. Nitrofurantoin is not harmful to the fetus but frequently causes nausea. Tetracyclines are contraindicated (Table 5.1). Co-trimoxazole should be avoided. In early pregnancy the trimethoprim component can possibly cause limb reduction and cleft palate, while at the end of pregnancy the sulphonamide component can cross the placenta and displace bilirubin from protein binding sites in the neonate.

Fortunately, severe infections in pregnancy are rare. Aminoglycosides cause fetal eighth nerve damage, and the benefits of their use must be seen in this context. At present there is no evidence to suggest fetal damage from cephalosporins, metronidazole or chloramphenicol. However, chloramphenicol can cause cardiovascular collapse in neonates and should not be used at the end of pregnancy unless absolutely necessary.

In the case of tuberculosis, both isoniazid and ethambutol have been used extensively during pregnancy, including the first trimester, with no fetal defects. The incidence of fetal deformity following rifampicin is three times greater than with isoniazid or ethambutol, and this drug should be avoided in the first trimester if possible. Streptomycin definitely causes auditory deficit and should not be used.

Diabetes mellitus

Diabetic pregnancies are associated with a twofold increase in perinatal mortality. Liveborn neonates are prone to respiratory distress syndrome, hypoglycaemia, hypocalcaemia and jaundice.

The aim of therapy is obsessionally to maintain pre-prandial blood glucose concentrations between 3 and 6 mmol/l (55–110 mg/100 ml). The adequacy of therapy in the short term is monitored by daily preprandial glucose estimation.

Gestational diabetes, i.e. the development of mild glucose intolerance during pregnancy, can sometimes be managed adequately by carbohydrate restriction. If this fails, insulin is used.

Insulin is usually given as twice daily injections of a highly purified preparation containing a mixture of short and intermediate acting types. Insulin-dependent diabetics who are on different regimens should be changed when they become pregnant or, preferably, before conception. Insulin requirements often increase from around the fifteenth to the thirtieth week of pregnancy, remain constant until delivery and then fall rapidly to prepregnancy levels. Therefore, daily monitoring of blood glucose is mandatory to maintain normoglycaemia.

Asthma

Poorly controlled asthma is associated with increased perinatal mortality. Maternal hypoxia and respiratory alkalosis are the major determinants of fetal distress in asthmatic pregnancies.

Theophylline, salbutamol by metered aerosol and steroids have good safety records at all stages of pregnancy. There has been little experience with newer bronchodilators.

Pregnancy should not alter the general approach to asthma as described in Chapter 11. It is important to control bronchospasm and avoid prolonged abnormalities of blood gases or acid–base balance.

Epilepsy

The main issues are possible teratogenicity associated with anticonvulsants and the need for therapeutic drug level monitoring to control fits.

The incidence of congenital malformations in children of epileptic mothers is about 6%, which is three times higher than the general population. In part, this could reflect a genetic predisposition, but anticonvulsants seem largely to be responsible. Cleft palate and congenital heart disease are the most common findings. Troxidone, phenytoin and phenobarbitone are almost certainly teratogenic. Sodium valproate probably increases the likelihood of neural tube defects. There are insufficient data on carbamazepine to be certain about its effects. Co-administration of anticonvulsants produces a greater risk than when either drug is used alone.

At the present time the following guidelines seem appropriate to the management of pregnant epileptics:

1 Management should begin before conception:

(a) If a woman has been seizure-free for 2–3 years, consider slowly stopping treatment.

(b) There is no justification for changing from, for example, phenobarbitone or phenytoin to a drug about which even less is known. However, control should be optimized on monotherapy if possible.

2 Discuss the possibility of a birth defect in the context of around a 95% likelihood of a normal child compared to 98% in the general population.

3 There is no point in changing treatment if a woman presents after the first 8–9 weeks of pregnancy as any damage will already have occurred.

4 A real time scan around 18 weeks is likely to detect major structural defects.

The pharmacokinetic changes associated with pregnancy are clinically important in the treatment of epilepsy. Anticonvulsant concentrations tend to fall during pregnancy (see above) and, although partially offset by a decrease in protein binding, this change in drug level can be accompanied by increased seizure frequency. Therefore, concentration monitoring is required at monthly intervals during pregnancy. The aim should be to maintain concentrations at the lower end of the therapeutic range, with doses being increased as necessary to achieve this. At postpartum there is a return to normal kinetics over 5–10 days and monitoring is again required to aid dosage adjustment.

A further issue concerns drug induced suppression of vitamin K dependent clotting factors. Mothers receiving anticonvulsants should be given 20 mg/day vitamim K for the last 2 weeks of pregnancy and vitamin K should also be given to the newborn baby.

Hypertension

Maternal high blood pressure is a leading cause of fetal loss, particularly when it is severe or accompanied by proteinuria. In addition, hypertension is a leading (though rare) cause of maternal death in the UK.

Bed rest and sedation have traditionally been used but neither is of proven value.

Among antihypertensive drugs, methyldopa has been most widely used. It significantly lowers blood pressure and reduces midtrimester abortions in patients with essential hypertension, but has not been shown to influence fetal outcome in hypertension developing later in pregnancy. Methyldopa is not teratogenic.

Beta-blockers successfully lower blood pressure in pregnancy, but have not been shown conclusively to improve fetal outcome. They are not teratogenic.

Hydralazine is often used to complement one of the above drugs and similarly causes no damage to the fetus but is of uncertain value in improving fetal outcome.

Diuretics are usually avoided in the management of hypertension during pregnancy because such patients are already volume depleted and diuresis could further impair perfusion of the fetoplacental unit.

Hyperthyroidism

Carbimazole crosses the placenta and appears in breast milk. The concentrations achieved in the fetus or neonate are sufficient to suppress thyroid function. Various approaches have been advocated:

1 The use of the lowest dose of carbimazole that controls the hyperthyroidism and reducing this towards term.

2 The administration of a beta-blocker alone to provide symptomatic relief until other treatment can be instituted after delivery.

3 Partial thyroidectomy if the condition is diagnosed in the first trimester.

5.4 BREAST FEEDING

Breast feeding has become popular again in Western countries. The factors that determine the transfer of drugs into breast milk are the same as those influencing drug distribution in general (Chapter 1, Section 1.2).

Most drugs enter breast milk to a greater or lesser extent but, because the concentration has been greatly reduced by distribution throughout the mother's body, the amount of drug actually received by the breast fed baby is usually clinically insignificant.

Drugs that can safely be given to breast feeding mothers include:

Penicillins, cephalosporins.
Theophylline, salbutamol by inhaler, prednisolone.
Valproate, carbamazepine, phenytoin.
Beta-blockers, methyldopa, hydralazine.
Warfarin, heparin.
Haloperidol, chlorpromazine.
Tricyclic antidepressants.

Low oestrogen dose oral contraceptives have no effect on established milk production or on breast fed babies.

Certain drugs achieve sufficient concentration in breast milk, and they are sufficiently potent that their use in breast feeding mothers should be avoided. These include:

Sulphonamides, chloramphenicol, isoniazid, tetracyclines.
Narcotic analgesics.
Benzodiazepines.

Lithium.
Antithyroid drugs, radioactive iodine.
Phenindione.
Antineoplastic drugs.

Comment
Most commonly used drugs can be safely used in women who are breast feeding. If in doubt, seek further information.

Section 2

Chapter 6
Cardiac Arrhythmias

The use of ambulatory electrocardiographic monitoring has emphasized the high prevalence of cardiac arrhythmias not only in patients with heart disease but also in normal subjects. However, not all electrocardiographically documented arrhythmias require treatment. In all instances, the physician must consider the balance between the symptomatic or prognostic significance of the arrhythmias and the potential side effects of therapy. In certain circumstances, the indications for drug treatment are clear:

1 Therapy and prophylaxis of recurrent life-threatening arrhythmias, e.g. ventricular tachycardia and fibrillation.

2 Arrhythmias producing major haemodynamic sequelae, e.g. hypotension and cardiac failure.

3 Troublesome symptomatic arrhythmias, e.g. recurrent supraventricular tachycardia.

The role of antiarrhythmic drugs in the treatment of 'warning arrhythmias' (ventricular premature beats or short runs of asymptomatic non-sustained tachycardia) remains controversial. Despite the theoretical attractions of this approach, it has not been shown to reduce mortality from subsequent ventricular fibrillation in either the short or long term following myocardial infarction.

The choice of the most appropriate antiarrhythmic drug depends on several factors:

1 Patient related:
(a) Electrocardiographic diagnosis.
(b) Possible mechanism of the arrhythmia.
(c) Nature of underlying cardiac disease (if any), especially left ventricular function.
(d) Requirement for acute or long-term therapy.

2 Drug related:
(a) Mechanism of drug action—primary and secondary.
(b) Pharmacokinetics.
(c) Haemodynamic effects of the drug.
(d) Non-cardiac effects of the drug.

Under different circumstances, the aims of the therapy may be termination of a tachycardia with restoration of sinus rhythm (e.g. supraventricular tachycardia), control of ventricular rate without restoration of sinus rhythm (e.g. atrial fibrillation) and prevention of recurrent episodes of tachycardia.

6.1 RELEVANT PATHOPHYSIOLOGY

Normal electrophysiology

Cardiac muscle may be divided into three electrophysiologically distinct types:

1 Tissue with spontaneous pacemaker activity, i.e. the sinoatrial (SA) and atrioventricular (AV) nodes.

2 Specialized high velocity conducting tissue—the His–Purkinje system.

3 'Working' atrial and ventricular myocardium.

The action potentials of SA and AV nodal cells show diastolic depolarization, which results in the generation of spontaneous action potentials. The upstroke of the cardiac action potential is dependent on the 'slow' inward calcium current. Conduction velocity in nodal tissue, e.g. AV node, is slow, accounting for the delay between atrial and ventricular contraction, and limiting the rate at which atrial impulses are transmitted to the ventricles.

Depolarization in His–Purkinje tissue and atrial and ventricular myocardium depends on the rapid inward sodium current. The action potential upstroke and therefore conduction velocity is much faster than that in nodal tissue, allowing electrical activation of the atria or ventricles in a short period of time and permitting coordinated contraction. Under normal circumstances, atrial and ventricular myocardium has no intrinsic automaticity, while that of the His–Purkinje network is slow (30 beats/min).

Mechanisms of arrhythmias

Arrhythmias may arise either from abnormal automaticity or from disorders of impulse conduction. The majority of clinically important arrhythmias depend on the latter mechanism and are examples of the 're-entry' phenomenon. Re-entry occurs when an advancing wave of depolarization finds one pathway temporarily inexcitable (refractory) as a result of acute ischaemia, prior ischaemic damage or prematurity. Depolarization may proceed by another route and reach the distal part of the area which was refractory after a long enough period to allow retrograde conduction, albeit slowly. If the time taken for the impulse to pass around such a circuit exceeds the refractory period of the normal tissue at the proximal site, this tissue will be re-excited and the potential for a continuous 'circus' movement will exist. It is now felt that atrial flutter and fibrillation, supraventricular tachycardias, recurrent ventricular tachycardia secondary to previous myocardial infarction and ventricular fibrillation are all examples of re-entry.

Abnormal automaticity is the likely basis for the arrhythmias of digitalis toxicity.

Classification of antiarrhythmic drugs

No completely satisfactory classification of antiarrhythmic drugs exists. They may be categorized according to their predominant site of action. Thus, some agents act predominantly on arrhythmias arising in the ventricles (e.g. lignocaine), some on those arising in the AV node (e.g. verapamil) and others have effects on both atrial and ventricular muscle (e.g. disopyramide). The most commonly used classification was proposed by Singh and Vaughan Williams, following observations on the electrophysiological effects of drugs on isolated tissues. Four principal modes of action have been identified (Table 6.1). It should be remembered, however, that individual drugs may have actions in more than one category. The antiarrhythmic actions of digitalis and adenine nucleotides are not included in this classification; they are considered separately in Sections 6.6 and 6.7.

Table 6.1. Classification of antiarrhythmic drug actions

Class	Drug
I: Fast sodium channel inhibitors	Ia: Quinidine, procainamide, disopyramide
	Ib: Lignocaine, phenytoin, mexiletine, tocainide
	Ic: Flecainide
II: Antisympathetic agents	Beta-blockers
III: Prolongation of action potential duration	Amiodarone, bretylium, sotalol
IV: Slow calcium channel antagonists	Verapamil, diltiazem
Not classified	Digoxin, adenine nucleotides

Class I action

These drugs interfere with the rapid sodium current, resulting in slowing of conduction, an increase in refractory period or both. This action is sometimes termed 'local anaesthetic' or 'membrane stabilizing'. Class I drugs have been subdivided according to their subsidiary properties. Class Ia agents lengthen action potential duration moderately and cause minor slowing of intracardiac conduction and widening of the QRS complex in therapeutic concentrations. Class Ib drugs shorten action potential duration and have no effect on intracardiac conduction or the QRS complex in sinus rhythm. Class Ic drugs have no net effect on action potential duration but exert their most powerful effect in two ways: by slowing intracardiac conduction and widening the QRS complex.

Class II action

Drugs with Class II action decrease the arrhythmogenic effects of catecholamines. This may occur by competitive antagonism at β-adrenoceptors (beta-blockers), by non-competitive adrenoceptor antagonism (amiodarone) or by inhibition of noradrenaline release at sympathetic nerve terminals (bretylium).

Class III action

Class III activity involves lengthening of action potential duration and effective refractory period without interference with the inward sodium current. Clinically available drugs in this category possess additional Class II (bretylium, sotalol) or both Class I and II (amiodarone) activity.

Class IV action

Inhibition of the slow inward Ca^{2+} current by this class of drugs results in slowed conduction and prolonged refractoriness in the atrioventricular node. This action is of particular value in blocking supraventricular tachycardia involving the AV node as one limb of a re-entry circuit.

6.2 CLASS I AGENTS

General

Since all Class I agents interfere with sodium channel activity and reduce Na^+ influx, they may reduce intracellular Na^+ concentrations which, by Na^+/Ca^{2+} exchange, results in a reduced intracellular Ca^{2+} concentration. Thus, all Class I agents have a potentially negative inotropic effect and need to be used with great caution in patients with overt or incipient heart failure. In some instances (e.g. quinidine) the negative inotropic effect may be balanced by peripheral vasodilation. Of the subgroups, Group Ib agents have the least negative inotropic action and Group Ia the most. Since Class I agents share a common mode of action, they should not be used in combination except in expert hands. The risks of producing conduction block or exacerbating arrhythmias are considerable.

Class Ia agents

Quinidine

Mechanism

Quinidine reduces the maximal rate of depolarization, depresses spontaneous phase 4 diastolic depolarization in automatic cells, slows conduction and also prolongs the effective refractory period of atrial, ventricular and Purkinje fibres.

Pharmacokinetics

Seventy per cent of the drug is absorbed from the gut. With conventional preparations, measurable levels are obtained within 15 min and the peak effect occurs between 1 and 3 h. However, because the average half-life is of the order of 6 h, slow-release preparations are more commonly used. It is 80–90% bound to plasma proteins and is metabolized by hydroxylation; the inactive metabolites are excreted in the urine. Antiarrhythmic effects are seen with drug levels of 2.3–5 mg/l. In cirrhosis, the clearance of quinidine is reduced. There is also less binding to plasma proteins and hence lower plasma levels are effective.

Adverse effects

Higher concentrations are associated with: decreased myocardial contractility; peripheral vasodilation and hypotension; electrophysiological effects with possible sinus arrest or sinoatrial block, progressive QRS and QT prolongation, which may lead to paroxysmal ventricular tachycardia with torsades de pointes. Toxic concentrations may also lead to AV dissociation. Other adverse effects include: gastrointestinal symptoms with nausea, vomiting and diarrhoea; cinchonism; hypersensitivity reactions with fever, purpura, thrombocytopaenia and hepatic dysfunction. Quinidine has a vagolytic action which increases AV conduction. This may lead to rapid conduction from atria to ventricles. In the treatment of atria tachycardia or atrial flutter, digitalis should be given before quinidine administration.

Drug interactions

Quinidine interacts with digoxin and may precipitate digoxin toxicity. Digoxin plasma levels are increased and the dose of digoxin must be reduced to compensate for this.

Clinical use and dose

Quinidine now has limited use, e.g. prophylaxis following cardioversion. The dose is 200–600 mg orally 6 hourly after an initial test dose.

Procainamide

Mechanism

Procainamide has similar electrophysiological properties to quinidine, with typical class I activity. It has also been shown experimentally to increase the ventricular fibrillation threshold.

Pharmacokinetics

Procainamide can be administered orally, being 75% bioavailable. Again, because it has a relatively short half-life of the order of 3.5 h, it is usually given as a slow-release preparation. The compound is metabolized to *N*-acetyl procainamide (NAPA), which has Class III antiarrhythmic activity in its own right. Antiarrhythmic activity of procainamide occurs at blood levels of 4–10 mg/l and toxic effects are likely with blood levels of 16 mg/l. Relatively high plasma levels of both parent drug and NAPA occur in renal impairment and cardiac failure.

The drug is metabolized by acetylation in the liver. The enzyme, which is bimodally distributed in the population, also metabolizes isoniazid and hydralazine; slow acetylators theoretically require smaller doses for antiarrhythmic activity than fast acetylators.

Adverse effects

These may follow rapid intravenous administration and include hypotension with vasodilatation and reduced cardiac output. Electrocardiogram (ECG) changes include QRS and QT prolongation. In higher doses PR prolongation may occur with delayed AV conduction, leading to heart block. On chronic oral therapy at high dosage many patients develop a drug induced lupus erythematosus syndrome with a positive antinuclear factor. However, there is usually an absence of renal effects. This is particularly common in slow acetylators.

Drug interactions

Procainamide reduces the antimicrobial effect of sulphonamides. The mechanism appears to be formation of *p*-aminobenzoic acid from procaine.

Clinical use and dose

It is useful in the full spectrum of arrhythmias arising from atrial, junctional and ventricular tissue, including lignocaine-resistant ventricular rhythms. It is administered intravenously, 50–100 mg every 5 min to a total dose of 1000 mg or until hypotension or QRS widening occurs. Oral dosage is 250–500 mg 3 hourly orally or by slow-release preparation.

Disopyramide

Mechanism

Disopyramide has electrophysiological properties similar to quinidine.

Pharmacokinetics

Disopyramide is 70–80% bioavailable. The half-life in normal subjects is 6–8 h. Fifty per cent is excreted unchanged in the urine; a further 25% is excreted in the form of the main metabolite—the *N*-dealkylated form of disopyramide. The dose should be reduced in severe renal failure when creatinine clearance levels are less than 25 ml/min. The therapeutic range is 2–5 mg/l.

Adverse effects

Disopyramide has marked negative inotropic actions and should be avoided in patients with incipient or overt cardiac failure. Other adverse effects are related primarily to anticholinergic activity with urinary retention, glaucoma and blurred vision. QT prolongation occurs with increasing plasma concentrations, and this may also predispose to re-entry arrhythmias. Relative contraindications to therapy include sick sinus syndrome and prostate hypertrophy.

Clinical use and dose

Disopyramide is used for atrial and ventricular arrhythmias, including those resistant to lignocaine. The dose is 100–200 mg 6 hourly orally or by slow-release preparation. It is also available for slow intravenous injection 2 mg/kg over 20 min.

Class Ib agents

Lignocaine

Mechanism

Lignocaine causes only marginal slowing of conduction velocity in Purkinje fibres and in ventricular muscle, but is selectively active in suppressing ventricular premature beats and ventricular tachycardia. It is the standard agent in ventricular arrhythmias following myocardial infarction and surgery. Like other Class Ib agents, it has no useful action against supraventricular tachycardias.

Pharmacokinetics

Lignocaine is not given orally because it is hydrolysed in the gastrointestinal tract and is submitted to extensive first-pass metabolism in the liver so that adequate blood levels are not achieved. Following intravenous administration, the elimination half-life is about 100 min. The clearance of lignocaine is reduced in cardiac failure and lower rates of infusion are required (Chapter 3, Section 3.4).

Adverse effects

Although therapeutic concentrations have little haemodynamic effect, high levels of lignocaine cause bradycardia, hypotension and even asystole. Gastrointestinal symptoms with nausea and vomiting may also occur. At levels higher than 5 mg/l, CNS adverse effects may occur with parasthesiae, twitching and even grand mal seizures.

Clinical use and dose

Lignocaine has no action on atrial arrhythmias but it is used in the termination of haemodynamically stable ventricular tachycardia and the prevention of recurrent ventricular tachycardia or fibrillation after myocardial infarction. Although the intramuscular route has been advocated in domiciliary practice, absorption tends to be erratic and blood levels achieved vary widely according to the haemodynamic status of the patient. Therefore, lignocaine is routinely given by the intravenous route: 1–2 mg/kg body weight is given by rapid injection followed by an infusion of 2 mg/min to maintain arrhythmia suppression. This dosage regimen, however, requires adjustment in the presence of cardiac failure or liver disease. Therapeutic blood levels are 1.5–5 mg/l.

Tocainide

Tocainide is a lignocaine analogue that is active after both intravenous and oral administration. Its haemodynamic and electrophysiological actions are similar to lignocaine and its potential use is as an alternative to this standard agent, with the advantage of long-term administration. However, it should be emphasized that ventricular arrhythmias occurring in the acute phase of myocardial infarction or after cardiac surgery do not normally require long-term prophylaxis.

Dose

The dose is 500–750 mg i.v. over 300 min followed by 600–800 mg orally. The maintenance dose is 1200–2400 mg daily in divided doses.

Adverse effects

Neurological side effects may limit usage. A significant risk of bone marrow depression has been reported and for this reason tocainide is no longer licensed in the UK except for life-threatening arrhythmias.

Mexiletine

Mechanism

This primary amine has similar electrophysiological action to lignocaine.

Pharmocokinetics

Mexiletine is active after both oral and intravenous administration. It is extensively metabolized to *p*-hydroxy- and hydroxymethylmexiletine and to their corresponding deaminated alcohols by hepatic metabolism. The half-life in normal subjects is 9–12 h. However, this may be increased, particularly following acute myocardial infarction. Oral absorption is reduced when given with morphine or diamorphine.

Adverse effects

Toxic effects include nausea, dizziness, drowsiness, tremor and hypotension, common at plasma levels above 2.0 mg/l.

Clinical use and dose

Mexiletine is used in the treatment of ventricular arrhythmias and is particularly useful as an alternative to lignocaine. Mexiletine is given initially as a 1–3 mg/kg i.v. bolus injection, then 20–45 μg/kg/min by intravenous infusion, followed by 0.6–1.2 g orally in 24 h. Effective plasma levels are 0.75–2.0 mg/l; the therapeutic range is narrow.

Phenytoin

Phenytoin has Class I activity but in addition in hypokalaemia it reduces the duration of the action potential in Purkinje and ventricular fibres. Haemodynamic adverse effects include dose related impairment of myocardial contractility following intravenous use. Adverse effects are reviewed on pp. 235–6. It finds occasional use as an alternative to lignocaine or in digoxin induced arrhythmias, given in 50–100 mg rapid intravenous doses over 5 min up to 1000 mg.

Class Ic agents

Flecainide

Mechanism

Flecainide slows conduction in the atria, His–Purkinje system, accessory pathways and ventricles. In therapeutic concentration it causes lengthening of the PR and QRS intervals. Flecainide is a powerful broad spectrum antiarrhythmic effective against atrial arrhythmias, tachycardias involving accessory pathways (Wolff–Parkinson–White syndrome) and ventricular arrhythmias.

Pharmacokinetics

Flecainide is well absorbed orally, and about 27% is excreted unchanged in the urine. The remainder undergoes biotransformation to active metabolites, but the plasma concentrations of the unconjugated pharmacologically active forms are considerably less than that of the parent drug itself. Flecainide is not extensively protein bound. The average elimination half-life in normal subjects is 14 h, permitting twice daily administration, but the half-life is increased in cardiac and renal failure.

Adverse effects

Flecainide may exacerbate pre-existing conduction disorders and should be used with great care in patients with sinoatrial disease, AV nodal disease or bundle branch block. It may cause an acute increase in the stimulation threshold in patients with implanted pacemakers, with the consequent risk of asystole. Paradoxical arrhythmogenic effects associated with exacerbation of ventricular arrhythmias may occur. These are not normally of the torsades de pointes type, but rather a sustained (often incessant) monomorphic ventricular tachycardia with gross widening of the QRS complex and a relatively slow rate (120–140/min).

Clinical use and dose

Flecainide is particularly useful in the maintenance treatment of recurrent atrial and ventricular arrhythmias and in the Wolff–Parkinson–White syndrome. Sustained oral doses range from 100 to 200 mg twice daily with target therapeutic plasma concentrations of 0.2–1.0 mg/l. Intravenous flecainide (up to 2 mg/kg) may be given by slow intravenous infusion over 30 min.

Other Class Ic agents

Flecainide should not be used for the suppression of asymptomatic unsustained ventricular arrhythmias. Its use in patients with prior myocardial infarction is potentially hazardous and should be restricted to specialized arrhythmia centres.

Several newer Class Ic agents are available in other countries and will be introduced into the UK in the near future.

Encainide

This agent has a similar antiarrhythmic spectrum to flecainide and is well tolerated orally. It appears to have a less negative inotropic action than flecainide. The pharmacokinetics are complex, with the majority of subjects metabolizing encainide rapidly to *O*-demethylencainide (ODE) and 3-methoxy-*O*-demethylencainide (MODE). Fortunately, both ODE and MODE have equal antiarrhythmic potency to the parent compound, and the plasma half-life of ODE and MODE in rapid metabolizers is similar to that of encainide in slow metabolizers. Thus, in practice, the half-life is the same irrespective of the metabolizer status.

Propafenone

This Class Ic agent has additional minor beta-blocking and calcium antagonist properties. It is effective against supraventricular and ventricular arrhythmias.

6.3 CLASS II AGENTS

β-Adrenoceptor antagonists

The pharmacokinetics, adverse effects and mechanisms of action are discussed in Chapter 8.

Clinical use

These compounds are particularly useful for the control of inappropriate sinus tachycardia or supraventricular arrhythmias provoked by conditions of high catecholamine excretion, including emotion, exercise or anaesthesia. For intravenous use, metoprolol, propranolol and acebutolol have all been used. Beta-blockers are also useful in the control of ventricular arrhythmias associated with a fast sinus rate in the absence of cardiac failure. Their prophylactic use in the reduction of sudden death after myocardial infarction has been suggested, and recent studies with timolol, propranolol, metoprolol and atenolol have been encouraging. Other clinical situations in which the beta-blockers are useful include mitral valve prolapse, hypertrophic obstructive cardiomyopathy and hereditary prolonged QT syndrome.

Bretylium

This agent has adrenergic neurone blocking activity and suppresses noradrenaline release. It is eliminated by the kidney with a half-life of 7–12 h. Bretylium also has Class III action on Purkinje fibres and is effective in ventricular arrhythmias, particularly ventricular fibrillation refractory to lignocaine or procainamide and repeated electrical defibrillation.

Adverse effects include hypotension.

It is administered by the intravenous route, 5–10 mg/kg, or by the intramuscular route, 5 mg/kg.

6.4 CLASS III AGENTS

Amiodarone

Mechanism

Amiodarone prolongs the action potential duration and effective refractory period in all cardiac tissues. It is also a non-competitive α- and β-adrenoceptor antagonist, and has Class I and Class II activity.

Pharmacokinetics

After oral administration, considerable accumulation occurs in muscle and fat, and the therapeutic action may take several weeks to develop fully. Amiodarone is metabolized in the liver to desethylamiodarone, which is also electrophysiologically active. The steady state therapeutic plasma concentrations of amiodarone and desethylamiodarone are 1–2 mg/l. Elimination of amiodarone is complex, with an initial relatively rapid half-life (1–2 days) and an extremely slow terminal half-life (more than 30 days).

Adverse effects

Amiodarone has little negative inotropic effect and is the best tolerated of all the antiarrhythmic agents in heart failure. Sinus node automaticity and intracardiac conduction are depressed, therefore it should be used with caution in the presence of SA or AV nodal disease. As with all drugs which prolong ventricular repolarization, arrhythmogenic effects with torsades de pointes ventricular tachycardia may occur. The use of amiodarone is principally limited by its non-cardiac side effects, of which the most important are pulmonary (alveolitis), hepatic (hepatitis), neurological (tremor, ataxia), thyroid (hyper- or hypothyroidism) and cutaneous (photosensitivity). The last effect occurs in a high percentage of patients, of whom a small minority develop a slate-grey discoloration of light-exposed areas, especially the nose and cheeks. Corneal microdeposits occur in almost all patients, but do not interfere with vision.

Clinical use and dose

Amiodarone is effective in a wide variety of supraventricular and ventricular arrhythmias, including those associated with the Wolff–Parkinson–White syndrome. An oral loading dose of 600–1200 mg daily is given for 2 weeks, which is then reduced to 100–400 mg daily. In view of its adverse effects, chronic amiodarone therapy should be used only in life-threatening or severely disabling arrhythmias, and should not be used unless conventional drugs have been shown to be ineffective. In contrast, intravenous amiodarone may be very effective in the acute conversion or control of troublesome supraventricular and ventricular arrhythmias. It often achieves chemical cardioversion in recent-onset atrial flutter and fibrillation. The initial dose is 300 mg i.v. given over 30 min to avoid hypotension, followed by up to 1200 mg/24 h. The intravenous preparation is irritant and should be given via a central vein.

Drug interactions

Amiodarone potentiates the effect of warfarin and increases plasma digoxin levels. Dose reduction is required in both cases.

Sotalol

Mechanism

Sotalol is a non-selective beta-blocker which also possesses Class III activity and thus prolongs atrial and ventricular action potential duration and refractory period. It has no Class I activity at therapeutic concentrations.

Clinical use

Sotalol appears to be more effective than other beta-blockers, particularly in supraventricular tachycardias involving accessory pathways and in ventricular arrhythmias. It may be used in the prophylaxis of recurrent ventricular tachycardia. The side effects are those of other beta-blockers (see Chapter 8) with the additional predisposition to torsades de pointes, principally when there is overdosage, coexisting potassium depletion or coadministration of other drugs which lengthen the QT interval. The dosage of sotalol in antiarrhythmic therapy ranges from 80 to 320 mg twice daily.

6.5 CLASS IV AGENTS

Verapamil

Mechanism

Electrophysiologically, the slow inward Ca^{2+} mediated current is inhibited, decreasing AV conduction and blocking intranodal re-entry circuits.

Pharmacokinetics

Bioavailability is 10–20%. It is eliminated by the kidneys.

Adverse effects

In view of its depressant effects on the SA and AV nodes, verapamil is contraindicated in heart block or sinoatrial disease. Verapamil has significant negative inotropic action and is contraindicated in heart failure. Additional effects include nausea, dizziness, facial flushing and constipation.

Drug interactions

Verapamil potentiates the negative effects of digoxin and beta-blockers on AV nodal conduction. Verapamil and beta-blockers in combination may cause high-grade AV block or asystole, particularly if either is administered intravenously. Beta-blockers also enhance the negative inotropic action of verapamil.

Clinical use and dose

Verapamil is particularly useful in re-entry supraventricular arrythmias by inhibiting one limb of the re-entry circuit. Increased AV block also allows control of the ventricular rate in atrial flutter and atrial fibrillation. It is mainly useful in supraventricular arrhythmias; there is little action on ventricular arrhythmias. Verapamil should not be used in the termination of undiagnosed wide-complex tachycardias where ventricular tachycardia cannot be excluded. Verapamil can be used by both oral and intravenous routes. Intravenous verapamil is administered by infusion or rapid injections of 5–10 mg, with infusion rates of 0.005 mg/kg/min. Oral dosage is 80–120 mg three times daily.

Diltiazem

This calcium channel blocker has similar antiarrhythmic properties to verapamil. Dosage is 60–120 mg thrice daily.

Comment

Calcium channel blockers of the dihydropyridine class (e.g. nifedipine) do not interfere with AV nodal conduction and have no antiarrhythmic action.

6.6 DIGITALIS GLYCOSIDES

The term digitalis or digitalis glycoside refers to any of the cardioactive steroids which share an aglycone ring structure and have positive inotropic and electrophysiological effects. In the UK, the vast majority of clinicians use the cardiac glycoside, digoxin.

Mechanism

A major effect is to decrease sodium transport out of the cardiac cell by inhibiting Na^+/K^+ ATPase (the sodium pump). The resulting accumulation of sodium results in an increase of intracellular calcium ions by Na^+/Ca^{2+} exchange, which is responsible for the positive inotropic effects of digitalis glycosides. In addition, the actions of these drugs at the membrane result in electrophysiological changes which decrease cardiac conduction at the AV node and sensitize the sinoatrial node to vagal impulses. At high concentrations, digitalis glycosides increase myocardial automaticity as a result of intracellular calcium overload.

The three major effects of digitalis glycosides on the heart are:

1 Positive inotropic effect.

2 Decreased ventricular rate in atrial fibrillation or flutter, by decreasing AV conduction.

3 Increased myocardial automaticity in high (toxic) concentrations, or at 'therapeutic' concentrations if other factors such as hypokalaemia are present.

Digoxin

Pharmacokinetics

Digoxin can be given orally or intravenously. The average volume of distribution is approximately 7.3 l/kg; this is decreased in patients with renal disease, hypothyroidism and in patients taking quinidine. It is increased in thyrotoxicosis. Clearance varies from individual to individual and is the result of both renal and metabolic elimination mechanisms. In healthy adults, the metabolic component is of the order of 40–60 ml/min/70 kg, and the renal component approximates creatinine clearance. Metabolic clearance is reduced in congestive cardiac failure. Clearance in any individual can be calculated by the equations discussed in Chapters 1 and 2.

In patients with normal renal function, the elimination half-life is approximately 2 days. In patients with severe renal disease, the half-life increases to approximately 4–6 days.

Adverse effects

Adverse effects are determined in part by plasma concentration (> 2.5 μg/l for digoxin) and in part by electrolyte balance. Digoxin and potassium compete for cardiac receptor sites and hypokalaemia can precipitate digitalis adverse effects. Hypercalcaemia also potentiates toxicity.

The common extracardiac adverse effects are:

1 Anorexia, nausea and vomiting.

2 Fatigue.

3 Weakness.

4 Diarrhoea.

5 Less commonly, neurological symptoms including difficulty in reading, confusion or even psychosis can occur. Abdominal pain is another less common manifestation.

The cardiac adverse effects are:

1 Sinus bradycardia or sinus arrest.

2 Various degrees of AV block, including complete heart block.

3 Junctional rhythm.

4 Atrial or ventricular tachycardia.

5 Premature ventricular ectopic beats or ventricular fibrillation.

Cardiac signs precede extracardiac signs in about 50% of cases. A common effect of digitalis glycosides on the ECG, i.e. prolonged PR interval and ST segment depression, does not indicate toxicity.

Drug interactions

Digoxin absorption is decreased by drugs that increase intestinal motility, e.g. metoclopramide, and increased by drugs such as propantheline that decrease motility. Many antacids, particularly magnesium trisilicate, reduce digoxin absorption. Digoxin levels increase if quinidine or amiodarone is coadministered, and toxicity can occur. The potential for toxicity is enhanced for all cardiac glycosides when diuretics are coadministered because of hypokalaemia.

Digitoxin and ouabain

Digitoxin is more lipid soluble than digoxin and is practically 100% absorbed from the gastrointestinal tract. It is given orally and intravenously. It is extensively metabolized by the liver, and the elimination half-life is 5–7 days. Renal impairment does not appreciably alter digitoxin kinetics but binding to plasma proteins, normally of the order of 90–97%, may be slightly decreased in uraemia.

It seems likely that digitoxin is excreted in the bile and is then reabsorbed to some extent, i.e. it has an enterohepatic circulation. Cholestyramine, which can bind cardiac glycosides in the gut, can interrupt the enterohepatic circulation; whether it can shorten the duration of digitoxin toxicity is still a matter for speculation.

Ouabain is poorly absorbed from the gut and is administered exclusively by the intravenous route. Its onset of action is rapid and it has a shorter half-life than digoxin, approximately 1 day. Elimination is mainly renal.

Clinical use and doses

The principal use of cardiac glycosides is in the control of ventricular rate in atrial fibrillation, particularly when a return to sinus rhythm is not expected (e.g. chronic mitral valve disease). The onset of action, even after intravenous administration, is delayed for several hours. Thus, if clinical circumstances require urgent control of ventricular rate, other approaches such as cardioversion or intravenous amiodarone may be more appropriate. Acute digitalization has been superseded by the use of intravenous verapamil in the termination of supraventricular tachycardias.

Cardiac glycosides are effective in the control of ventricular rate in chronic atrial fibrillation. Combination therapy with verapamil or beta-blockers provides better control of exercise heart rate with a lower risk of toxicity than high-dose glycosides but does not appear to produce superior exercise capacity compared with glycosides alone.

Although glycosides are a logical therapy in congestive heart failure associated with atrial fibrillation, their value in patients with heart failure in sinus rhythm is only modest. Given the availability of potent diuretics, cardiac glycosides are best regarded as second-line therapy, and indeed many would introduce angiotensin converting enzyme inhibitors before cardiac glycosides in view of the narrow therapeutic ratio of the latter.

The dosing schedules used with the cardiac glycosides depend not only on the pharmacokinetic properties of the drug but also on factors that determine individual susceptibility. The general approach is usually to introduce a loading dose of the glycoside and then to follow this by a maintenance dose. The loading dose is determined by the volume of distribution and the desired plasma concentration; the maintenance dose is determined by clearance (Chapters 1 and 2). If a maintenance dose is employed without a loading dose, drug accumulation and activity develop slowly because steady state is not reached for four to five half-lives. With digoxin, the major determinant of clearance is renal function and the maintenance dose for this glycoside must be reduced if renal function is subnormal and excretion is impaired. Nomograms and simple equations can be used to estimate the most appropriate loading and maintenance doses. However, these must remain approximations and the patient's clinical response must influence long-term management. The average loading dose of digoxin is 1.0–1.5 mg p.o., or 0.3–1.0 mg i.v. The usual oral maintenance dose in the presence of normal renal function is 0.125–0.25 mg daily.

The use of drug monitoring of the glycoside plasma levels has been useful, particularly in renal impairment and toxicity. The normal therapeutic range of digoxin is 1–2 μg/l. Venous sampling should be performed 3–4 h after an intravenous dose or 6–8 h after an oral dose. If blood levels are low then compliance should be checked, possible causes of malabsorption considered and, in the case of digitoxin, causes of interruption of the enterohepatic circulation or increased hepatic metabolism should be considered.

Treatment of digitalis induced toxicity

Treatment of digitalis induced arrhythmias is often difficult. The glycoside should be withdrawn and, if hypokalaemia is present, potassium chloride should be administered by infusion at a rate of 20 mmol/h (not exceeding 100 mmol total) with electrocardiographic and biochemical monitoring.

Ventricular arrhythmias may require lignocaine or phenytoin administration. Supraventricular arrhythmias may respond to beta-blockade or phenytoin. Care must be observed when using verapamil and procainamide, as increased degrees of heart block may occur. Temporary pacing may be required for heart block with haemodynamic effects or in the rare instance of SA node arrest. Intravenous amiodarone infusion has shown promise in digitoxic arrhythmias. Life-threatening digitalis intoxication may be treated with specific Fab antidigoxin antibodies, which bind and inactivate digoxin.

6.7 ADENINE NUCLEOTIDES

Mechanism

The adenine nucleotides adenosine and adenosine triphosphate (ATP) act via purinergic receptors situated in the SA and AV nodes. Stimulation of these receptors causes hyperpolarization of the cells, resulting in suppression of automaticity and conduction. This results in transient sinus bradycardia and AV block. Adenine nucleotides may interrupt the re-entrant circuit in AV nodal tachycardia or in atrioventricular tachycardia involving an accessory pathway, while increasing the degree of AV block in atrial flutter or fibrillation. ATP has been in clinical use in many European countries for several years. Adenosine has been licenced recently in the USA and the UK.

Pharmacokinetics

ATP is rapidly metabolized to adenosine in the plasma and probably exerts its antiarrhythmic effects as adenosine. Both nucleotides are inactive orally. The plasma half-life of adenosine is approximately 10 s, and both agents are given by intravenous bolus injection. Adenosine is metabolized to the inactive inosine.

Adverse effects

Adenine nucleotides are vasodilators, and produce a marked flushing. Bolus injection causes a transient increase followed by a small fall in blood pressure, but the duration of action of a bolus dose is normally insufficient to cause clinically significant hypotension. A feeling of chest tightness or sometimes chest pain is experienced, which may be very unpleasant but is transient. Adenine nucleotides may precipitate bronchoconstriction in asthmatics. Transient complete heart block lasting a few seconds may occur. This usually responds to coughing.

Clinical use and dose

Adenine nucleotides are given as bolus doses for the termination of regular supraventricular tachycardias as an alternative to intravenous verapamil. Tachycardias involving the AV node as an integral part of the re-entry circuit will be terminated, while atrial tachycardias will demonstrate transient slowing of the ventricular rate which may allow identification of the rhythm, e.g. atrial flutter. Dosing of adenosine is by rapid intravenous injection, starting with a bolus of 2.5 mg. The antiarrhythmic effect occurs shortly after the onset of flushing, usually 20–30 s after injection. If the initial dose is ineffective, repeat boluses of 5, 7.5, 10, 15 or 20 mg may be given at 2–3 min intervals until success is achieved or the dose is limited by patient tolerance.

Drug interactions

The effects of adenine nucleotides are inhibited by purinoceptor antagonists (methylxanthines) and accentuated by dipyridamole. Adenine nucleotides may be given safely to patients already receiving β-adrenoceptor antagonists or calcium channel blockers.

Chapter 7
Heart Failure and Angina Pectoris

7.1 HEART FAILURE

Aims

1 To improve cardiac performance.

2 To reduce symptoms caused by pulmonary venous congestion and peripheral oedema.

3 To improve survival.

Relevant pathophysiology

Cardiac performance is determined by:

1 Preload: ventricular end-diastolic pressure and volume. In normal hearts an increased preload leads to increased end-diastolic fibre length which in turn causes increased force of contraction. In heart failure this response is reduced or even reversed.

2 Force of cardiac contraction: determined largely by the intrinsic strength and integrity of the muscle cells. Force of contraction is decreased by:

(a) Ischaemic heart disease.

(b) Specific disorders affecting heart muscle, such as hypertension and myocarditis.

(c) Disorders of heart muscle of unknown cause, e.g. dilated cardiomyopathy.

3 Myocardial compliance: an important determinant of ventricular filling and therefore of cardiac output. Compliance is decreased by:

(a) Fibrosis.

(b) Hypertrophy.

(c) Ischaemia.

4 Afterload: the ventricular wall tension developed during ejection. Afterload is increased by:

(a) Increased arterial pressure.

(b) Obstruction to outflow, e.g. aortic stenosis.

Heart failure exists when cardiac output is insufficient to meet the requirements of tissue perfusion. In Western countries heart failure is usually caused by one of the following:

Ischaemic heart disease.

Hypertension (Chapter 8).

Heart muscle disorders.

Valvular heart disease.

In response to heart failure, compensatory mechanisms are activated:

1 Sodium and water retention; this has beneficial and adverse consequences.

(a) Beneficial: improves perfusion by increasing intravascular volume.

(b) Adverse: increases preload. In the failing heart the beneficial limits of increasing myocardial fibre length are eventually exceeded. Pulmonary congestion and peripheral oedema develop.

2 Increased activity of sympathetic nervous system and also renin–angiotensin–aldosterone system; this also has beneficial and adverse aspects.

(a) Beneficial: increased myocardial contractility; maintains cardiac output and blood pressure.

(b) Adverse: increased afterload and, therefore, myocardial oxygen demand; increased peripheral vascular resistance may reduce tissue perfusion; tachyarrhythmias.

Drugs used in heart failure

1 Diuretics: thiazides, loop diuretics.

(a) Decrease peripheral and pulmonary oedema.

(b) Decrease preload by reduction in circulatory volume.

2 Drugs with a positive inotropic effect: cardiac glycosides (mainly chronic heart failure); β-adrenoceptor agonists (acute heart failure only).

3 Drugs that offload the ventricles:

(a) Mainly decrease preload: nitrates (glyceryl trinitrate, isosorbide dinitrate and isosorbide mononitrate).

(b) Mainly decrease afterload: hydralazine.

(c) Decrease preload and afterload: converting enzyme inhibitors (captopril, enalapril, lisinopril, etc.), α_1-antagonists (prazosin) and sodium nitroprusside.

Diuretics

These drugs are first-line treatment for patients with heart failure. In mild failure a thiazide (Chapter 8, Section 8.1) may suffice. Moderate or severe failure requires a loop diuretic.

Loop diuretics: frusemide, bumetanide

Mechanism

Loop diuretics inhibit active chloride reabsorption and also Na^+/K^+ ATPase in the ascending limb of the loop of Henle, resulting in increased salt and water loss. The increased delivery of sodium to the distal tubule encourages Na^+/K^+ exchange, with a tendency to hypokalaemic alkalosis.

Pharmacokinetics

Both drugs are well absorbed following oral administration and are also available in intravenous formulations. Elimination is largely by renal excretion, with a small contribution by liver metabolism. These drugs have a rapid onset and short duration of action.

Adverse effects

Salt and water depletion can occur; regular monitoring of serum potassium is required and additional potassium supplementation is advisable. Glucose intolerance and urate retention can occur, as with thiazides. Rapid intravenous injection of large doses can produce deafness.

Drug interactions

These include potentiation of nephrotoxic effects of gentamicin and cephaloridine; hypokalaemia enhances the risk of digoxin toxicity.

Doses

Frusemide: oral, 20 mg each morning up to 1 or 2 g each day in very resistant oedema or cardiac failure; intravenous, 20–40 mg slowly. In resistant cases, up to 1 g can be infused over 2–4 h.

Bumetanide: oral, 0.5–5 mg each day; intravenous, 0.5–2 mg or infusion up to 5 mg slowly.

Potassium supplementation

There are three occasions when supplementation of dietary potassium is likely to be required:

1 Administration of high doses of loop diuretics in treating heart failure.

2 Coadministration of digoxin, since hypokalaemia potentiates digoxin toxicity.

3 Administration of a thiazide diuretic to a patient with a poor potassium intake, e.g. the older patient.

In general, a serum potassium below 3.5 mmol/l is a definite indication for potassium supplements.

Potassium supplements are available as the chloride salt in tablets of 8 or 12 mmol and granules of 20 mmol. The starting dose is 8 mmol two or three times daily.

Potassium sparing diuretics: amiloride, triamterene, spironolactone

As an alternative to giving potassium it is possible to give drugs that decrease potassium secretion. These drugs are all diuretics themselves, but their effect is weak and they are rarely used alone.

Amiloride decreases potassium loss caused by loop diuretics and thiazides.

Spironolactone competitively inhibits the effects of aldosterone. It is, therefore, useful in treating the resistant oedema of conditions associated with excess aldosterone: cirrhosis and refractory heart failure. In addition, it is effective in high doses for the treatment of primary aldosteronism (Conn's syndrome). Recent reports of carcinogenic effects in animals have led to its use being limited to refractory oedema.

The adverse effect common to all these drugs is hyperkalaemia, and is particularly likely in patients with impaired renal function. Potassium supplements should rarely be required with potassium sparing diuretics. If they are used, close monitoring of serum potassium is necessary. Potassium sparing drugs should be avoided in patients taking angiotensin converting enzyme inhibitors as both agents raise potassium and severe hyperkalaemia may occur, especially in the presence of renal failure. Spironolactone commonly causes nausea, gynaecomastia in men and menstrual irregularities in women. It can decrease the renal secretion of digoxin.

Doses

Amiloride: 5–20 mg/day; higher doses in primary aldosteronism.
Triamterene: 100–200 mg/day.
Spironolactone: 100–200 mg/day in divided doses.

Comment

Potassium sparing diuretics are available in proprietary formulations combined with a thiazide or frusemide. Combination tablets are expensive but may improve compliance by reducing the number of tablets to be taken.

Drugs with a positive inotropic effect

Digoxin

The pharmacodynamics and pharmacokinetics of digoxin together with clinical uses and doses are discussed in full in Chapter 6, Section 6.6.

Once considered an indispensable part of antifailure treatment, the role of digoxin has been questioned. Digoxin improves cardiac performance in patients with atrial fibrillation. In patients with sinus rhythm, digoxin has a positive inotropic effect when given acutely but there is controversy as to whether this effect is maintained in long-term therapy in all patients. Recent double blind studies have confirmed the long-term beneficial effect of digoxin in sinus rhythm, an effect best seen in patients with severe heart failure. If digoxin is used, the dose should be adjusted to take account of renal function. Monitoring of plasma drug levels may be useful.

Comment

The controversy relating to digoxin in heart failure with sinus rhythm is not new. During the eighteenth century, Withering, in his writings on what we now know to be digitalis, indicated that its role was mainly in oedematous patients with an irregular heart rhythm.

Adrenoceptor agonists: dopamine and dobutamine

These drugs are currently used only in acute severe heart failure accompanied by hypotension and poor tissue perfusion. They have established short-term effects when given intravenously.

Mechanism

Both drugs produce their inotropic effect by β_1-adrenoceptor stimulation of the myocardium. The effects of dopamine are dose dependent and depend partly on direct action and partly on indirect effects through increased noradrenaline release. Below 5 μg/kg/min the major effect is to increase renal blood flow by stimulation of dopamine receptors. As the dose is increased in the 5–20 μg/kg/min range, both β_1- and α-adrenoceptor stimulant effects are seen with increased cardiac output and a modest rise in blood pressure. Above this dose range α-receptor effects are more marked, with a further rise in blood pressure; this tends to increase afterload and is undesirable. Dobutamine has no renal vasodilator effect, less vasoconstrictor (α-receptor) effect and a similar inotropic effect to dopamine. The search continues for an effective orally active inotropic drug. Amongst the drugs currently under evaluation are β-receptor agonists with and without partial antagonist activity, phosphodiesterase inhibitors and drugs which directly stimulate adenylate cyclase.

Pharmacokinetics

These drugs undergo rapid clearance. Dopamine and dobutamine must be given intravenously.

Adverse effects

Adverse effects are mainly tachyarrhythmias from β_1-receptor stimulation when used in excessive doses.

Doses

Dopamine: 5 μg/kg/min initially, increasing as required by the clinical response.
Dobutamine: 2.5 μg/kg/min initially, increasing as necessary.

Drugs that offload the ventricles by reducing preload and afterload

Many drugs with vasodilator activity have shown beneficial actions in cardiac failure by reducing aortic impedance (afterload) or reducing cardiac venous return (preload). The usefulness of an individual drug depends on the haemodynamic changes in the individual patient and its relative effect on preload and afterload. Venodilators reduce the left ventricular end-diastolic pressure and volume, thus reducing pulmonary congestion and the symptoms of breathlessness. Arteriolar dilators reduce aortic impedance and enhance cardiac output, thereby improving the symptoms of tiredness. When the symptoms of tiredness are prominent, an arteriolar dilator is appropriate. When the main symptom is dyspnoea, then a venodilator is the logical choice. In practice, a mixed agent is often used. Vasodilators are contra-indicated in the presence of obstructive or stenotic valvular lesions, such as mitral or aortic stenosis. There is evidence of improved survival after treatment with angiotensin converting enzyme (ACE) inhibitors and also a combination of hydralazine and nitrates.

Drugs affecting preload

Glyceryl trinitrate

Sublingual nitroglycerin leads to direct relaxation of smooth muscle of the systemic venous system. Subsequent venous pooling in cardiac failure leads to a reduction in left ventricular end-diastolic pressure and volume, reducing pulmonary congestion. There is usually no associated rise in cardiac output.

Intravenous glyceryl trinitrate can be used acutely until oral agents can be introduced.

'Long-acting' preparations of isosorbide dinitrate may have beneficial long-term haemodynamic effects in heart failure.

Similar claims have been made for pentaerythritol tetranitrate and isosorbide mononitrate but remain to be confirmed.

Drugs affecting afterload

Angiotensin converting enzyme (ACE) inhibitors

Captopril and enalapril are the first of many drugs of this class. These drugs prevent the formation of angiotensin II and have been found acutely and chronically to improve cardiac performance and symptoms of chronic heart failure. Reduction in arteriolar resistance is well established but these drugs probably also have venous dilating effects. ACE inhibitors increase serum and total body potassium and should not be used with potassium sparing drugs. Profound hypotension may occur after the first dose in patients on diuretics or with hyponatraemia. Other adverse reactions include postural hypotension, renal dysfunction, hyperkalaemia and cough.

Doses

Captopril: 6.25–50 mg two or three times daily.
Enalapril: 2.5–40 mg once daily.

Hydralazine

This has a direct vasodilator effect confined to the arterial bed. Reduction in systemic vascular resistance leads to a considerable rise in cardiac output. Changes in arterial blood pressure and heart rate are smaller than in patients with hypertension so may be used in combination with nitrates. Doses up to 200 mg daily are used in heart failure.

Drugs affecting preload and afterload

Sodium nitroprusside

This is a mixed venous and arteriolar dilator also used for acute reduction of blood pressure (p. 82). It must be given intravenously by continuous infusion in the dose range 25–125 μg/min. Blood pressure falls rapidly and the effects wear off over 1–2 min after stopping the infusion. This agent is particularly useful in acute cardiac failure following myocardial infarction and in acute valvular insufficiency, such as mitral incompetence following an acute infarct or aortic incompetence in bacterial endocarditis. It should not be used for more than 24–48 h because of accumulation of thiocyanate.

Comment

Vasodilators at present are used in patients with severe cardiac failure with grade III or grade IV (New York Heart Association) symptoms. Further experience is likely to extend their use to milder cases. Choice of drug depends on the profile of symptoms and, when available, the haemodynamic findings in the individual patient. If cardiac output is low and filling pressure is moderate, then an arteriolar dilator is indicated. If the filling pressure is high and cardiac output adequate, then a venous dilator is indicated. If the filling pressure is high and cardiac output low, a mixed dilator is indicated. In most patients, however, a pragmatic view is taken and a drug with mixed effects is given empirically. The first choice is usually an ACE inhibitor. If this is not tolerated, then hydralazine with nitrates is an alternative.

General principles of management

Acute left ventricular failure or pulmonary oedema presents with severe breathlessness, orthopnoea or nocturnal dyspnoea.

1 Sit the patient up.

2 Give 100% oxygen.

3 Establish an intravenous line.

4 Give 5 mg diamorphine or 10 mg morphine i.v. because:

(a) It has a venodilator effect, reducing preload.

(b) It reduces the intense distress of the patient.

5 Give 40 mg frusemide i.v., or more if the patient is already receiving a loop diuretic, because:

(a) It has a rapid offloading effect resulting from venous dilatation.

(b) It has a slower offloading effect resulting from diuresis and natriuresis.

6 If these measures fail to control symptoms, many would give aminophylline 250 mg i.v. slowly (15–20 min) because:

(a) It has a positive inotropic effect.

(b) It has a bronchodilating effect.

(c) It has a modest effect on renal blood flow and may augment the action of the diuretic.

7 In resistant patients, invasive haemodynamic monitoring is indicated to help selection of appropriate vasodilator therapy with intravenous sodium nitroprusside or nitrates together with dobutamine.

Cardiogenic shock consists of hypotension and oliguria with clinical signs of poor tissue perfusion. It is usually caused by recent extensive myocardial infarction.

1 Where possible, monitor both arterial and pulmonary wedge pressure.

2 Give 100% oxygen.

3 Improve cardiac performance with dobutamine or a similar inotropic drug.
4 Low-dose dopamine intravenously may improve renal function.
5 If this fails then, depending on the haemodynamic features, try offloading either instead of or in addition to dobutamine.

Chronic heart failure: long-term management.
1 Modify cardiovascular risk factor profile, e.g. cigarette smoking, obesity.
2 Underlying causes should be treated, e.g. anaemia, hypertension, valvular disease.
3 If this proves inadequate, or when there is no treatable underlying cause, diuretics should be the first stage. The type of diuretic and dose depends on the severity of failure.
4 The next step would be to add an ACE inhibitor followed by digoxin, especially in patients with atrial fibrillation.
5 An improvement in survival in patients with severe and moderately severe heart failure has recently been shown with enalapril, while in less severely ill patients a combination of hydralazine and nitrates has been shown to prolong survival also. Nevertheless, the latter combination is rarely used in practice on account of side effects.

7.2 ANGINA PECTORIS

Aims

The aims are relief of symptoms and, particularly in unstable angina, prevention of progression to myocardial infarction and improved survival.

Relevant pathophysiology

Angina is the symptom experienced when coronary blood supply is insufficient to meet myocardial energy requirements. Angina occurs in two forms:
1 Stable angina: attacks are predictably provoked by exertion or excitement and recede when the increased energy demand is withdrawn. The underlying pathology is usually chronic coronary artery disease.

Treatment is undertaken on the assumption that the coronary obstructive disease is 'fixed', although changes in vascular tone are now believed to be important in some patients. Therefore, the opportunity for therapeutic benefit depends mainly on adjustments in myocardial energy requirements and emphasis falls on drugs that reduce heart rate, contractility, preload and afterload and which thus reduce metabolic demands.
2 Unstable angina: attacks occur with lesser exertion or at rest and are unpredictable. The underlying pathology is usually rupture or dissection of an atheromatous plaque with thrombus formation or extension in the coronary arteries. Spasm may be an additional mechanism or, rarely, the only cause.

Acute changes in coronary artery pathology are presumed and therapeutic attention directed to halting, reversing or bypassing the coronary arterial occlusive process in the hope of avoiding myocardial infarction. At the same time, treatment is aimed at reducing myocardial energy requirements.

Severe unstable angina can progress to myocardial infarction or death. Where medical measures have evidently failed to stabilize or reverse the progress of severe unstable angina, coronary angiography and bypass surgery may be considered on an urgent basis if infarction is to be prevented.

Drugs used in angina

Glyceryl trinitrate

Mechanism

Glyceryl trinitrate is a potent, direct, short-acting smooth muscle relaxant with widespread vasodilator activity. In stable angina its major benefit results not from coronary artery dilatation but probably from a brief drop in preload (venous return) by its action on venules and from a reduced afterload by peripheral arteriolar relaxation.

In unstable angina, all these factors may be relevant but, in addition, direct coronary artery dilatation may also be important, particularly in those instances of variant rest angina in which coronary artery spasm can be demonstrated.

Pharmacokinetics

Glyceryl trinitrate has a virtually 100% first-pass metabolism and is, therefore, given sublingually or transdermally as a 'patch' or paste. It has very rapid clearance by liver metabolism: half-life about 2 min.

Adverse effects

These are dose related and result from vasodilation and reflex adverse effects to hypotension: headache, flushing and postural dizziness. These symptoms can be terminated by swallowing the tablet, spitting it out or by removing the patch.

Clinical use and dose

Glyceryl trinitrate, 0.5 mg tablets, should be taken sublingually by the patient before carrying out a task known to produce angina. The total daily dose may be individually determined as that required to control symptoms.

Isosorbide dinitrate and isosorbide mononitrate

The clinical pharmacology of isosorbide dinitrate is similar to glyceryl trinitrate, but it is also effective orally and has a longer half-life of 40 min. It is used in the management of the acute phase of unstable angina.

Recently, isosorbide mononitrate has been introduced. This is the active metabolite of isosorbide dinitrate and is claimed to have more consistent pharmacokinetics and a longer duration of action. Its usefulness, especially in chronic stable angina, is still controversial, as are advantages over other nitrate preparations.

Doses

Isosorbide dinitrate: 30–120 mg daily in divided doses.
Isosorbide mononitrate: 20–120 mg daily in divided doses.

Comment
The usefulness and effectiveness of 'long-acting nitrates' has been questioned because tolerance may develop after relatively short periods (hours–days). A nitrate-free interval of at least 8 h has been recommended between doses. This is especially relevant to the use of nitrate patches. These should be removed at night to ensure efficacy during the day.

β-Receptor blockers

The detailed clinical pharmacology of these drugs is described in Chapter 8.

Their value in angina depends mainly on decreasing myocardial oxygen consumption by:

1 Limiting the increased heart rate associated with exercise and anxiety in patients whose heart failure is complicated by angina.

2 Limiting the increased force of contraction associated with the same stimuli. In addition, beta-blockers can improve myocardial perfusion by their effects on heart rate, since tachycardia decreases the duration of diastole and, therefore, decreases the time available for effective coronary blood flow. Beta-blockers have been shown to reduce sudden death and reinfarction following a myocardial infarct.

Adverse effects (see pp. 84–5)

Rebound worsening of angina, myocardial infarction or tachycardia have been reported when beta-blockers are suddenly withdrawn. Reduce dose over 24–48 h if beta-blockers are being withdrawn in such patients.

Clinical use

β_1-Selective blocking drugs are currently preferred in stable and unstable angina as they appear to cause fewer respiratory, central or peripheral vascular side effects than non-selective agents.

Doses

See pp. 83, 85 for dose ranges of all beta-blockers.
Atenolol: 50–200 mg daily.
Metoprolol: 100–400 mg daily.
Propranolol: 80–360 mg daily.

These drugs must all be given in an individually titrated dose to control symptoms and attenuate postural and exercise induced tachycardia.

Calcium antagonists

There are two major groups:

1 Dihydropyridines, including nifedipine, nicardipine, nitrendipine, felodipine.

2 Others, including verapamil and diltiazem.

Calcium antagonists are further described in Chapter 8. Their principal action is inhibition of the slow calcium ion channel component of the muscle action potential, leading to:

(a) Decreased tone in vascular smooth muscle cells, including coronary arteries.

(b) Decreased contractility in myocardial cells.

Verapamil and diltiazem also have depressant effects on sinus node and AV node function (Chapter 6) and additional antiarrhythmic activity.

Pharmacokinetics

All drugs are well absorbed following oral administration. They are cleared by liver metabolism. All undergo extensive first-pass metabolism. Active metabolites may contribute to their effects.

Adverse effects

Headache, nausea and flushing and ankle swelling have been reported with nifedipine and other dihydropyridines, and constipation with verapamil.

Drug interactions

Verapamil or diltiazem should not be given routinely with beta-blockers since the combined negative inotropic and dromotropic effects can cause bradyarrhythmias and rarely precipitate heart failure.

Clinical use

They may be used in stable or unstable angina. Verapamil and diltiazem are of established use as single agents in stable angina. Nifedipine and other dihydropyridines are used to best effect in combination with beta-blockers in severe angina.

Doses

Verapamil: 40 mg two or three times daily up to 360 mg daily in divided doses.
Nifedipine: 10–20 mg two or three times daily up to 120 mg daily in divided doses.
Diltiazem: 60 mg two or three times daily up to 48 mg daily in divided doses.

General principles of management

Stable angina

1 Try to modify cardiovascular risk factors, such as cigarette smoking, hypertension and hypercholesterolaemia.

2 Treat any underlying precipitating cause, such as anaemia, arrhythmias.

3 Begin treatment with glyceryl trinitrate, taken before undertaking the effort or activity which provokes pain.

4 If unsuccessful, add a beta-blocker.

5 If unsuccessful, use verapamil or diltiazem instead of, or nifedipine or other dihydropyridine in addition to, a beta-blocker.

6 Prophylactic aspirin is being increasingly used as routine treatment without, as yet, definite proof of efficacy.

Unstable angina

Current aggressive regimens are under evaluation. Aspirin (Chapter 9) is widely used and reduces the frequency of progression to myocardial infarction. Additional management may involve combined treatment with a beta-blocker, isosorbide dinitrate and a calcium antagonist under close supervision in hospital. Patients not responding to this approach are submitted to early coronary arteriography and, if indicated, coronary artery surgery.

Comment

Angina pectoris is a subjective symptom of coronary artery disease. Where possible, objective evidence of coronary disease should be sought using electrocardiography and exercise testing. This provides diagnostic confirmation and, importantly, objective evidence of the severity of the underlying ischaemia, thereby, in addition to symptoms, providing the indication for coronary angiography.

Treatment of angina is symptomatic with nitrates, beta-blockers and/or calcium antagonists. Any underlying cardiac or non-cardiac factors should be treated where possible. Surgery should be considered in those symptoms refractory to medical therapy or with extensive ischaemic changes on an exercise test. In certain subsets, coronary artery bypass graft significantly improves survival (e.g. early positive exercise test, triple vessel disease and impaired left ventricular function).

Chapter 8
Hypertension and Hyperlipidaemia

Comment

Myocardial infarction and stroke are amongst the commonest causes of death in the Western world. Raised blood pressure, elevated plasma cholesterol and cigarette smoking are major predictors of risk. Both hypertension and hyperlipidaemia predispose to atherosclerosis and occlusive disease of the aorta and coronary, cerebral and peripheral arteries. Hypertension also predisposes to haemorrhagic stroke, cardiac failure and progressive renal failure. Reduction of cholesterol by diet and drugs will reduce cardiovascular mortality, and treatment of hypertension will reduce stroke. An integrated approach to the management of these two major factors is indicated in individuals at increased risk.

8.1 HYPERTENSION

Aim

The goal is to reduce blood pressure and improve the risk of cardiovascular disease without inducing adverse effects on the well-being of the patient. A target blood pressure of 90 mmHg or less diastolic is widely accepted, although this may be modified in the very young or the very old. There is increasing evidence that targets for systolic blood pressure should also be considered.

Relevant pathophysiology

Blood pressure is the hydrostatic pressure within the systemic arteries and is determined by cardiac output and total peripheral resistance. There is no evidence of consistent increases in cardiac output or heart rate in hypertension. Total peripheral resistance is increased but the cause is not clear.

Blood pressure is normally or unimodally distributed in the population. There is no clear cut-off between normotensives and hypertensives. Long-term prospective studies indicate that for both systolic and diastolic blood pressure, the higher the pressure the greater the risk of cardiovascular disease. The frequency of hypertension depends on the arbitrary cut-off point selected, and varies with age, sex and the population studied.

Hypertension is either primary or secondary. Even in younger age groups, high blood pressure is primary (idiopathic or essential) with no obvious cause in over 90% of patients. There is a strong polygenic familial trend with superimposed environmental factors, including salt and alcohol consumption.

Less commonly, hypertension is secondary to renal or endocrine disease, including:

1 Acute or chronic renal disease (particularly glomerulonephritis).

2 Renal artery stenosis (atheroma in older age group; fibromuscular hyperplasia in younger group).

3 Hyperaldosteronism.

4 Cushing's syndrome.

5 Acromegaly.

6 Phaeochromocytoma.

7 Drugs: oral contraceptives, oestrogens, steroids, carbenoxolone, sympathomimetics, non-steroidal anti-inflammatory drugs.

Risks of hypertension

Both systolic and diastolic blood pressure predict the likelihood of cardiovascular disease. Increased blood pressure is associated with increased morbidity and mortality from:

1 Cerebrovascular disease, haemorrhagic and thrombotic strokes.

2 Progressive chronic renal failure.

3 Coronary artery disease: angina and myocardial infarction.

4 Hypertensive congestive heart failure.

5 Peripheral vascular disease.

Coronary heart disease is now the major cause of death in hypertensives.

There is a direct relationship between the severity of hypertension and the increase in morbidity. Mild hypertension carries an increased risk of these complications. Moderately raised blood pressure has a higher risk and malignant hypertension (severe hypertension with fibrinoid necrosis causing proteinuria and retinal haemorrhages, soft exudates or papilloedema), if untreated, leads to death from cerebral haemorrhage or renal failure in over 90% of patients within 1 year.

Hypertension is an important risk factor but not the only cardiovascular risk predictor. Other identified risk factors include:

1 Cigarette smoking.

2 Diabetes.

3 Hyperlipidaemia (Chapter 8, Section 8.2).

4 Family history of vascular disease.

These factors have independent additive effects on cardiovascular morbidity.

Benefits of treatment

Antihypertensive treatment reduces stroke and progression of renal and cardiac failure. Treatment has not been shown to improve mortality from coronary artery disease.

The benefits are well established in:

1 Malignant or accelerated hypertension at any age.

2 Severe hypertension (blood pressure >200 mmHg systolic and/or 110 mmHg diastolic).

There is evidence of benefit in moderate hypertension (systolic 160–199 mmHg and/or diastolic 100–109 mmHg) in both young and older (65–80 years) patients.

The benefits of treatment in mild hypertension (systolic 140–159 mmHg and/or diastolic 90–99 mmHg) are more modest. Non-pharmacological approaches should be tried first. Younger patients with other risk factors are likely to benefit most.

Principles of drug treatment

1 Hypertension should be confirmed by several measurements of blood pressure over several days, weeks or months.

2 Hypertension should be treated as a part of a management plan for all identifiable risk factors.

3 Non-pharmacological approaches should always be considered when appropriate:

(a) If obese, weight reduction of 10 kg lowers blood pressure by 20/10 mmHg on average.

(b) If salt intake is very high (> 200 mEq/day), a modest reduction (by avoiding salty foods and table salt) may aid blood pressure control.

4 The patient should be counselled about hypertension and its risks, and the case for long-term treatment should be explained carefully.

5 A simple drug regimen, without unacceptable adverse effects or toxicity, should be established.

6 Regular convenient long-term follow-up should be arranged with blood pressure measurements.

The simplest drug regimens are the most successful. Drugs should be given alone or in rational combinations which do not lead to adverse effects. Patient compliance is improved if drugs are only given once or twice daily. While a step care approach using diuretics or beta-blockers is still widely used, there is now a wider range of first-line drugs available. These include ACE inhibitors and calcium antagonists, as well as beta-blockers or diuretics. An alternative to step care is to select the most appropriate monotherapy from the list above and to evaluate the response to treatment over weeks or months. If the effect is insufficient and side effects not apparent, the dose can be increased. If side effects occur, either an alternative drug can be tried as monotherapy or low doses of two drugs can be used in combination. Individualization and substitution can complement, and may in time replace, step care. Combination treatment with beta-blocker and diuretic is well established. Beta-blockers with dihydropyridine calcium antagonists are also well tolerated and effective, as are diuretics with ACE inhibitors. Calcium antagonists and ACE inhibitors, while effective, are currently an expensive regimen.

Comment

The management of hypertension is a long-term undertaking, often in asymptomatic patients. The simplest, safest regimen should be determined for each individual.

Reduction of blood pressure and control of other risk factors, like smoking and hyperlipidaemia, is undertaken to improve cardiovascular morbidity and mortality, without impairing the quality of life.

Emergency reduction of blood pressure

There are no indications for rapid, uncontrolled (within seconds or minutes) reduction of blood pressure. There remain a few indications for controlled moderate reduction (over minutes and hours). These include:

Hypertensive encephalopathy.

Eclampsia.

Hypertensive acute left ventricular failure.

Malignant or accelerated hypertension.

In most patients treatment can be given orally with the same agents used for long-term therapy: atenolol, 50 or 100 mg orally. Nifedipine, 10 or 20 mg, is an alternative or may be given with atenolol.

Intravenous drug administration is only rarely necessary in patients who are unconscious or vomiting.

Sodium nitroprusside is given as a continuous titrated intravenous infusion. It has a short duration of action (1–2 min) so precipitous and prolonged falls in pressure, which may cause cerebrovascular accidents, can be avoided. The starting dose is 1 μg/kg/min and is increased until the desired effect is obtained. Treatment for longer than 1–2 days may lead to thiocyanate accumulation and poisoning, especially in patients with impaired renal function.

Antihypertensive drugs

β-Adrenoceptor antagonists (beta-blockers)

Mechanism

Beta-blockers antagonize the effects of noradrenaline and adrenaline on β-receptors in:

1 *Heart*. The responses to sympathetic nerve stimulation or circulating catecholamines are mediated by β-receptors.

β_1-Receptors in the SA node have positive chronotropic actions. Blockade leads to bradycardia. Bradyarrhythmias are an adverse effect, especially in the elderly.

β_1-Receptors in the myocardium have a positive inotropic action. Blockade leads to an acute fall in cardiac output, not always maintained during chronic therapy, and a reduction in cardiac work, which may lead to precipitation or exacerbation of cardiac failure.

Acute haemodynamic effects of beta-blockers vary. Beta-blockers without intrinsic sympathomimetic activity (ISA) cause a substantial fall in cardiac output and a small fall in resting heart rate but a large fall in exercise heart rate. Peripheral resistance may be acutely increased. Beta-blockers cause a fall in cardiac work and a reduction in myocardial oxygen demands, which justify their use in angina pectoris (Chapter 7, Section 7.2). Beta-blockers also reduce the incidence of sudden death and reinfarction following a myocardial infarct, although the mechanism is unknown.

2 *Kidney*. β-Receptors control the release of renin from the juxtaglomerular cells of the kidney after renal nerve stimulation. Beta-blockers lower renin release and thus angiotensin II formation and aldosterone release.

3 *Peripheral blood vessels*. β_2-Receptors in peripheral vessels subserve a vasodilator role, especially in muscle beds. Blockade of β_2-receptors may lead to cold hands and feet, Raynaud's phenomenon and worsening of peripheral vascular disease.

4 *Bronchial smooth muscle*. β_2-Receptors cause dilatation of bronchial smooth muscle. Blockade may precipitate an acute attack of bronchospasm in a susceptible person.

5 *Central nervous system*. Blockade of central β-receptors may cause nightmares, vivid dreams and, rarely, hallucinations.

6 *Other tissues*. Uterus: stimulation of β_2-receptors relaxes the gravid uterus and β_2-agonists may be used to delay premature labour. Eye: β_2-receptors control the formation of aqueous humour and beta-blockers applied topically are used in the treatment of glaucoma.

In addition to blockade of β-receptors these drugs may have other pharmacological effects (Table 8.1):

1 ISA or partial agonist activity (oxprenolol, pindolol).

2 Membrane stabilizing activity; quinidine-like or local anaesthetic effect (propranolol, oxprenolol).

3 α-Receptor blockade (labetalol).

4 Cardioselectivity or relatively greater blockade of β_1- than β_2-receptors (atenolol, metoprolol, bisoprolol).

Cardioselectivity may reduce adverse effects resulting from β_2-blockade. Membrane stabilizing activity is unlikely to contribute to the effects of beta-blockers in man. The relevance of intrinsic sympathomimetic activity is controversial. Co-existing α-blockade may be useful in more severe hypertension.

Table 8.1. Pharmacological properties, route of excretion and dose range of some beta-blockers in clinical use

Approved name	Cardio-selectivity	Intrinsic sympathomimetic activity (ISA)	Membrane activity	Major route of elimination	Daily dose range (mg)
Propranolol	–	–	+	Liver	40–320
Pindolol	–	+ +	+	Liver	10–30
Sotalol	–	–	–	Liver	160–600
Labetalol	–	–	+	Liver	300–2400
Atenolol	+ +	–	–	Kidney	50–200
Metoprolol	+ +	–	+	Liver	100–400
Acebutolol	+	+ +	+	Liver	400–1200
Bisoprolol	+ +	–	–	Liver/kidney	10–20

Pharmacokinetics

Beta-blockers are usually given orally except for rapid control of arrhythmias. As a group they show a wide variation of absorption, distribution, metabolism and elimination. The major determinants of these differences are:

1 Hepatic metabolism, first-pass metabolism and systemic clearance.
2 The rôle of the kidneys in elimination.
3 Lipid solubility or ability to cross the blood–brain barrier.

Hepatic metabolism

Several beta-blockers show extensive first-pass metabolism after oral administration and uptake from the portal venous system (propranolol, oxprenolol, labetalol). These drugs are extensively metabolized by the liver. Propranolol is an example of a drug whose elimination depends on hepatic blood flow and is thus flow limited (p. 31). Wide differences in response between individuals are observed with variable bioavailability. There is a relatively wide range of doses required in clinical practice.

Renal elimination

Other beta-blockers (atenolol, nadolol) are eliminated almost entirely unchanged by the kidney. The dose range is relatively narrow, and it should be reduced and/or the frequency of administration adjusted in patients with renal impairment.

Lipid solubility

This determines the distribution of the drug across cell membranes in general, and across the blood–brain barrier in particular.

Propranolol and oxprenolol have a high lipid solubility, penetrate the brain and are present there in large amounts. They often cause nightmares, vivid dreams, etc.

Atenolol and nadolol are both polar (non-lipid-soluble) drugs. They cross the blood–brain barrier less readily and accumulate to a lesser extent in the nervous system.

Half-life

The half-life of most beta-blockers is short (< 4 h) but is longer for atenolol, nadolol and sotalol. The half-life, however, is only one factor contributing to duration of action, which depends on the magnitude and intensity of effect and thus also on the dose given. All beta-blockers given in a large enough dose act for 24 h, but drugs given in large doses may cause adverse effects at early times corresponding to peak drug levels.

Adverse effects

These are often predictable and result from blockade of β-receptors.

1 Tiredness, fatigue and weakness.
2 Bradycardia and heart block.
3 Bronchospasm, especially in asthmatics.
4 Vivid dreams, nightmares and hallucinations.
5 Congestive cardiac failure.

6 Cold hands, Raynaud's phenomenon and worsening claudication.
7 Loss of symptoms of hypoglycaemia in insulin dependent diabetics.
8 Non-selective beta-blockers may reduce high density lipoprotein (HDL) cholesterol and raise triglycerides.
9 Patients with phaeochromocytoma may develop increases in blood pressure owing to unopposed α-receptor mediated vasoconstriction by tumour catecholamines.

Drug interactions

1 Hypertension as a result of unopposed peripheral α-adrenoceptor vasoconstriction.

Beta-blockers may increase the severity of withdrawal hypertension if concurrent clonidine treatment is interrupted.

Sympathomimetic amines such as amphetamine, ergotamine, ephedrine and phenylpropanolamine may cause severe hypertensive reactions. Phenylpropanolamine may be included in 'over the counter' proprietary cold cures.

2 Myocardial depression (prenylamine) or interference with conducting mechanisms (verapamil) causing asystole may complicate combined treatment with beta-blockers.

3 Cimetidine decreases hepatic metabolism of propranolol and may increase bradycardia. However, as the therapeutic range is wide, interactions involving metabolism or protein binding do not often lead to serious clinical consequences.

Clinical use

All beta-blockers lower blood pressure to a similar extent. Most beta-blockers can be given once or at the most twice daily with adequate blood pressure control.

Beta-blockers are widely used alone as first-line treatment in mild or moderate hypertension, or in combination with other drugs (thiazide diuretics, vasodilators) in more severe hypertension.

Cardioselective drugs (atenolol, metoprolol) are preferred. Beta-blockers should be avoided in patients with asthma or peripheral vascular disease. Polar (non-lipid-soluble) drugs such as atenolol are less likely to cause dreams and nightmares.

Beta-blockers are also used to treat the following complaints:
Arrhythmias (Chapter 6, Section 6.3).
Angina pectoris (Chapter 7, Section 7.2).
Anxiety neurosis (Chapter 19, Section 19.1).
Migraine (Chapter 20, Section 20.3).
Thyrotoxicosis
Glaucoma: beta-blockers may be used as eye drops (or systemically) in chronic simple glaucoma to reduce the rate of formation of aqueous humour.

Doses for hypertension

Atenolol: 50–100 mg once daily.
Metoprolol: 100–300 mg once or twice daily.
Propranolol: 40–320 mg once or twice daily.

Comment

A simple once or twice daily regimen with beta-blockers encourages compliance in many patients and is effective and well tolerated. All beta-blockers lower blood pressure if given in an adequate dose. Cardioselective drugs are less likely to cause respiratory, metabolic and peripheral vascular adverse effects.

Diuretics

Mechanism

These agents increase urine volume and sodium excretion by actions on salt and water transport across renal tubular and other cell membranes.

Several groups of diuretic drugs, with different sites of action, have been found to lower blood pressure (Table 8.2). Efficacy as an antihypertensive is not directly related to diuretic potency, and blood pressure lowering may result from an action on vascular smooth muscle.

Thiazides are weak diuretics but useful antihypertensives. Diazoxide, a close structural analogue, causes sodium retention but is a powerful vasodilator anti-hypertensive. Frusemide and loop diuretics are potent diuretics with modest effects on blood pressure.

The hypotensive dose–response curve for thiazides is flat but the diuretic and kaliuretic relation is much steeper. There is little to be gained from the use of large doses of thiazides in hypertension.

Thiazides are the diuretic treatment of choice in uncomplicated hypertension with normal renal function. Loop diuretics and aldosterone antagonists have a role

Table 8.2. Classification and mechanisms of action of diuretics

	Mechanism	Comment
Thiazides		
Bendrofluazide	?Distal tubule	All have an antihypertensive effect. Little evidence that newer agents have any advantages over older established agents
Hydrochlorothiazide		
Chlorthalidone	?Proximal tubule	
Clopamide		
Cyclopenthiazide		
Indapamide		
Polythiazide		
Zipamide		
Loop diuretics		
Frusemide	Ascending limb of loop of Henle	Potent diuretic and saliuretic
Bumetanide		
Potassium sparing diuretics		
Spironolactone	Aldosterone antagonist	May be used in combination with loop diuretics in refractory oedema. Also alone in hyperaldosteronism. May cause hyperkalaemia in renal failure or in the elderly
Triamterene	Distal tubule	
Amiloride	Sodium potassium exchange	

in the treatment of the refractory oedema of heart failure (Chapter 7, Section 7.1) and cirrhosis with ascites.

In hypertensive patients, potent loop diuretics such as frusemide are only indicated in:

1 Chronic renal failure when thiazides are inactive.
2 Hypertension resistant to standard triple therapy including a thiazide.
3 Combination with vasodilators or captopril in severe resistant hypertension.
4 Coexisting refractory congestive cardiac failure.

Potassium sparing diuretics have few advantages in uncomplicated hypertension. In patients with renal impairment they may cause hyperkalaemia and cardiac arrhythmias.

Pharmacokinetics

Thiazides are well absorbed orally, widely distributed and subject to hepatic metabolism. Renal actions depend on excretion of the drug into the tubule. Thus thiazides may be ineffective diuretics in severe renal impairment. The onset of diuretic action may be observed within 60 min and may last for 12 h or more. With repeated dosing the acute diuretic effect may be lost. The antihypertensive effect develops gradually over days, and it may take weeks or months to reach a maximum. The duration of antihypertensive effect is long (> 24 h), permitting once daily dosing.

Adverse effects

Hypokalaemia

Use of low doses of thiazides and concurrent beta-blockers can reduce this problem. Hypokalaemia may precipitate cardiac arrhythmias, especially in patients also on digoxin. Potassium supplements may be necessary (potassium chloride, 1.2 g twice or more times daily) in these patients. Formulations that combine potassium with a diuretic seldom include a large enough supplemental dose. Severe hypokalaemia caused by a thiazide suggests that mineralocorticoid excess, Conn's syndrome, may be the secondary cause for hypertension.

Hyperuricaemia

Inhibition of renal urate excretion raises serum uric acid and may provoke acute gouty arthritis.

Hyperlipidaemia

Increases in total cholesterol and low-density lipoprotein (LDL) cholesterol and a reduction in high-density lipoprotein (HDL) cholesterol have been reported after long-term use of diuretics.

Hyperglycaemia

Long-term diuretic therapy impairs glucose tolerance by inhibiting the release of insulin from the pancreas. Normal glucose tolerance may become diabetic and control is worsened in clinical diabetes.

Hypercalcaemia

This is a rare adverse effect resulting from reduced renal calcium excretion.

Impotence and reduced male sexual activity

This has recently been noted to be common with diuretics. The mechanism is not known. Other adverse effects include skin rash and thrombocytopenia.

Doses

Bendrofluazide: 2.5 or 5 mg twice daily.
Hydrochlorothiazide: 25 or 50 mg once daily.
Chlorthalidone: 12.5 or 25 mg once daily or on alternate days.

Comment

Thiazide diuretics alone or together with a beta-blocker are widely used effective antihypertensives in mild, moderate and severe hypertension. Loop diuretics like frusemide with potassium supplements may be required in the management of resistant hypertension or chronic renal failure. Combinations of thiazides with potassium sparing agents are widely used. Spironolactone should not be used in mild/moderate hypertension.

Vasodilators

Vasodilators such as hydralazine have been widely used in step care with a beta-blocker and a diuretic. Their use alone is limited by reflex increases in sympathetic activity, leading to headache and flushing.

Vasodilators may act preferentially on arterioles (hydralazine) or veins (nitrates) or have a mixed effect (sodium nitroprusside). Vasodilators are also used in the treatment of heart failure and are considered in detail in Chapter 7, Section 7.1.

Hydralazine

Mechanism

This hydrazine derivative has been widely used together with a beta-blocker and a diuretic in hypertension not responding to simpler regimens.

Pharmacokinetics

It is rapidly absorbed and distributed widely. The plasma half-life is short, but persistent binding of the drug to smooth muscle ensures a longer (> 12 h) duration of effect. Hydralazine is metabolized by acetylation in the liver by the same genetically determined enzyme system as isoniazid, procainamide, dapsone, etc. Acetylator phenotype is an important determinant of response to drug (fast acetylators have a poor response) and also of toxicity (drug induced lupus is rare in fast acetylators). Phenotyping may give a guide to the upper limits of dosing: 200 mg in slow acetylators, 400 mg in fast acetylators.

Adverse effects

1 Facial flushing and conjunctival injection: peripheral vasodilation.

2 Weight gain and oedema from salt and water retention: a result of secondary hyperaldosteronism and direct effects on renal function.
3 Headache: throbbing and vascular type (Chapter 20, Section 20.3).
4 Palpitations and tachycardia result from increased reflex drive and may aggravate angina or provoke myocardial infarction.
5 Drug induced lupus syndrome. Fever, arthralgia, malaise and hepatitis associated with positive antinuclear antibody test but normal DNA binding. The syndrome is similar to the connective tissue disease, systemic lupus erythematosus but it is reversible and only rarely has renal or neurological features. Women are more often affected than men and HLA DL4 tissue type has a high prevalence.

Dose

Hydralazine: 25–100 mg twice daily; higher doses may be given in fast acetylators.

Comment

Alternative second- or third-step 'vasodilators' include calcium antagonists, α_1-receptor blockers and ACE inhibitors. Hydralazine is being less widely used in view of toxicity and the need for coadministration of a beta-blocker and diuretic.

Calcium antagonists

Mechanism

These drugs with widely different chemical structures inhibit the slow inward calcium current in smooth muscle and cardiac cells. Calcium antagonists or calcium entry blockers interact with specific receptors on calcium channels on the cell membrane and reduce calcium influx through voltage operated channels (and to a lesser extent receptor operated channels).

Intracellular calcium is an important intracellular messenger in cardiac muscle, smooth muscle and conducting tissue in the heart. Reduction of intracellular calcium by calcium antagonists thus has a vasodilator action with additional potential negative inotropic, chronotropic and dromotropic properties.

Calcium antagonists can be divided into dihydropyridine derivatives (nifedipine, nicardipine, nimodipine, amlodipine, felodipine, etc.) and several other groups with different structures, which include verapamil and diltiazem. Dihydropyridines in man have few, if any, direct cardiac actions and can be considered selective arterial vasodilators. They are widely used in hypertension and angina pectoris (Chapter 7, Section 7.2) either alone or combined with a beta-blocker.

Verapamil and diltiazem to a greater and lesser extent, respectively, have cardiac actions in addition to vascular effects. These agents are used in hypertension and angina pectoris (Chapter 7, Section 7.2) and verapamil also has a role in atrial tachyarrhythmias (Chapter 6, Section 6.5). Beta-blockers are not routinely used with these drugs (see below) but most other groups of antihypertensives can be given in combination.

Calcium antagonists have effects in animals to protect the brain and myocardium from ischaemic damage. Nimodipine has been demonstrated in man to be of benefit when cerebral spasm accompanies subarachnoid haemorrhage.

Pharmacokinetics

Nifedipine, verapamil and diltiazem all have low and variable oral bioavailability and are subject to extensive first-pass metabolism. The vascular, cardiac and adverse effects are closely related to the levels of the drug in plasma. The currently available drugs all have short half-lives after acute dosing. In the case of verapamil, the half-life increases with chronic administration. The development of slow- or sustained-release formulations has permitted verapamil and nifedipine to be given as once or twice daily doses.

Adverse effects

Dihydropyridines frequently cause early symptoms of reflex sympathetic activation, headache, flushing and palpitations. These symptoms usually disappear with continued treatment but may necessitate dose reduction or withdrawal of treatment. Oedema of the ankles and hands occurs with longer-term dihydropyridine treatment. This is not simple fluid retention and appears to be due to a disturbance of local microcirculatory dynamics.

Verapamil and diltiazem are less likely to cause early reflex activation or late oedema. Constipation is a not infrequent complaint with verapamil.

Drug interactions

Nifedipine and other dihydropyridines can be combined usefully with a beta-blocker to enhance efficacy and reduce early side effects in both hypertension and angina pectoris.

Verapamil when given with beta-blockers has been reported to cause profound conduction defects and cardiac failure. This combination should be avoided in routine practice.

Nifedipine and verapamil have been reported to alter the pharmacokinetics and effects of digoxin.

Verapamil may affect the disposition of the anti-epileptic drug carbamazepine and also modify the tissue uptake and toxicity of some cytotoxic drugs.

Doses

Nifedipine: (as tablets) 10–60 mg twice daily.
Verapamil: 80–480 mg once or twice daily in divided doses.
Diltiazem: 60–180 mg twice daily in divided doses.

α-Receptors and blood pressure

α-Receptors have been divided into two types: α_1 and α_2. Both influence blood pressure.

Stimulation of α_1-receptors on peripheral vascular smooth muscle increases vascular resistance and blood pressure. α_1-Receptor blockers thus lower blood pressure.

Stimulation of α_2-receptors in the brain stem lowers blood pressure by reducing central sympathetic outflow. α_2-Agonists or stimulants will thus lower blood pressure.

α-Adrenoceptor antagonists

Prazosin is a selective competitive blocker of classical (α_1) receptors on both arteries and veins.

α-Receptor blockers can be used alone in mild hypertension or in combination with beta-blockers or diuretics. α_1-Receptor blockers may lower LDL cholesterol.

Adverse effects

Postural hypotension with syncope may occur after the first dose or with dose increments. Other side effects and toxicity are rare.

Dose

Prazosin is given at a dose of 1–10 mg twice daily. It is always started cautiously with low doses because orthostatic hypotension and syncope may be severe after the first dose. Terazosin and doxazosin have similar actions but can be given once daily.

α_2-Receptor agonists (centrally-acting antihypertensives)

Methyldopa (via an active metabolite, methylnoradrenaline) and clonidine (directly) act on α_2-receptors in the brain stem to reduce efferent sympathetic tone and blood pressure. They may have other effects on pre- and post-synaptic α_2-receptors in the periphery.

Adverse effects

Both clonidine and methyldopa have other CNS effects, including drowsiness, sedation and depression resulting from actions on other central α_2-receptors. They also cause dry mouth. Interference with sexual activity and impotence in men is not uncommon. Clonidine also causes constipation.

Postural hypotension may occur with methyldopa, especially in the elderly. It causes a positive direct antiglobulin test and rarely haemolytic anaemia. Drug induced hepatitis with fever may occur within the first few weeks of methyldopa treatment or on rechallenge.

If clonidine treatment is interrupted or stopped suddenly, a hypertensive reaction with sweating, anxiety and tremor may occur within 24–36 h.

Doses

Methyldopa: 250–1000 mg twice daily.
Clonidine: 100–400 mg twice daily.

Comment

Centrally acting drugs are not widely used as there are alternative agents of comparable efficacy with fewer adverse effects.

ACE inhibitors

Mechanism

ACE inhibitors prevent the formation of the active octapeptide angiotensin II from inactive angiotensin I by competitive inhibition of the converting enzyme (also termed kininase II) in the blood and other tissues, including the kidney, heart, blood vessels, adrenal gland and brain. Angiotensin II is a potent vasoconstrictor and it also promotes aldosterone release and facilitates sympathetic activity both centrally and peripherally. Although the fall in blood pressure is greatest when the renin–angiotensin system is stimulated (sodium depletion, renal artery stenosis and malignant hypertension), ACE inhibitors also lower blood pressure in essential hypertensives with normal or low plasma renin. The fall in blood pressure is not associated with a reflex tachycardia. ACE inhibitors are now widely used in mild, moderate or severe hypertension alone or in combination with other drugs, especially diuretics. They should be used with care in patients with renal vascular disease where renal failure may result from intrarenal ACE blockade in the stenotic kidney (or kidneys). ACE inhibitors also improve symptoms and prolong life in cardiac failure (Chapter 7, Section 7.1).

In addition to earlier drugs, such as captopril and enalapril, several other agents are now available, including lisinopril, quinapril, perindopril and ramipril. At present there are no clear differences in dynamics between these agents that cannot be attributed to differences in pharmacokinetics.

Pharmacokinetics

All ACE inhibitors reveal tissue and plasma protein binding which causes a characteristic concentration–time profile with long-lasting slow elimination but little evidence of accumulation on chronic dosing.

Captopril is rapidly absorbed, it has a short duration of effect and is usually given two or three times daily. Enalapril is an inactive prodrug which is hydrolysed to the active acid enalaprilat *in vivo*. Enalaprilat, like its analogue lisinopril, is a potent long-acting ACE inhibitor suitable for once daily dosing. All three agents are eliminated largely unchanged by renal excretion. Impairment of renal function by parenchymal renal disease or ageing will result in drug accumulation and enhanced effects. The dose or dose frequency should be reduced in renal failure and the elderly.

The dose–response relationship is steep initially, with therapeutic doses appearing flat because they are on the top of the sigmoid curve. In general, dose increases do not increase the intensity of effect (on blood pressure or plasma ACE) but will prolong the duration of action.

Adverse effects

Profound hypotension may complicate the first dose of ACE inhibitors, especially in patients with an activated renin–angiotensin system due to sodium depletion or diuretic therapy. First-dose hypotension is more common in patients with cardiac failure (Chapter 7, Section 7.1) and is of longer duration with long-acting drugs like enalapril.

Serious side effects, such as leucopenia and proteinuria, reported with captopril in the early days have been rare in the larger recent long-term experience with lower doses in patients with essential hypertension.

Captopril does cause taste disturbance and skin rashes. Enalapril is associated with angioneurotic oedema.

All ACE inhibitors may cause a troublesome dry cough.

Drug interactions

As ACE inhibitors have potassium sparing antialdosterone effects, it is unwise to combine ACE inhibitors with potassium supplements or potassium sparing diuretics. Hyperkalaemia may result, especially if there is any pre-existing renal impairment.

The antihypertensive effect of ACE inhibitors can be reversed by non-steroidal anti-inflammatory drugs and these drugs should be avoided if possible.

Doses

Captopril: 12.5–50 mg two or three times daily.
Enalapril: 5–20 mg once or twice daily.
Lisinopril: 5–20 mg once daily.

It is advisable to use lower doses when starting therapy in cardiac failure or the elderly.

8.2 HYPERLIPIDAEMIA

Aim

The overall aim is to prevent the development of atherosclerosis or the progression of cardiovascular diseases by reducing the levels of atherogenic lipids and liproproteins in blood.

Relevant pathophysiology

Cholesterol is a major component of lipid-containing atherosclerotic plaques. Raised plasma levels of cholesterol have been identified as a major risk factor (along with smoking and hypertension) for ischaemic heart disease and stroke. Cholesterol is derived both from the diet and by synthesis in the liver. It is a component of cell membranes and is a precursor of steroid hormones, bile salts and glycoproteins and quinones.

The biochemistry and metabolism of cholesterol is complex. Cholesterol and other lipids are transported in blood in association with lipoproteins of different densities. In addition to total cholesterol, increase in the LDL fraction of cholesterol has been linked to accelerated atheroma and coronary artery disease. LDL is cleared from the circulation by specific receptors on the surface of cells. The function of these receptors plays an important role in determining plasma levels of LDL cholesterol and thus cardiovascular risk. In contrast, HDL cholesterol appears to have a protective antiatherogenic effect. HDL appears to be involved in the mobilization of cholesterol in the tissues and its 'reverse' transport back to the liver. At present it is not clear whether increases in other lipid fractions, such as triglycerides and very low-density lipoproteins (VLDL), are independent risk factors. VLDL is the major precursor of LDL and is degraded to LDL mainly by the action of lipoprotein lipase.

Very high levels of LDL cholesterol occur in familial hypercholesterolaemia, which is a rare genetic disease of expression of LDL receptors. It is inherited as an autosomal dominant. Heterozygotes have 50% of the LDL receptors of normals and homozygotes have none. LDL cholesterol is very high, especially in the homozygotes who develop premature atheroma. Drug therapy which acts by up-regulation of LDL receptors will be ineffective in homozygotes. In these patients, diet and drugs may need to be supplemented with physical approaches to removal, such as apheresis using LDL affinity columns.

Moderate (6.0–8.5 mM) increases in LDL cholesterol are very common (25–50% of some Western populations). They are likely to be the result of unidentified polygenic genetic influences acting together with environmental factors, such as diet, alcohol, smoking and other diseases. In these individuals, down-regulation of LDL receptors is also the mechanism of hyperlipidaemia. Although the influence of raised cholesterol on coronary artery disease has been well recognized for some time, it is only recently that clear evidence has emerged that modification of plasma cholesterol by diet and/or drugs will alter prognosis.

Large scale primary prevention studies have shown a reduction in myocardial infarction and sudden death in those with moderate/severe hyperlipidaemia when diet is used with cholestyramine or gemfibrozil. However, these studies have not shown a reduction in total mortality and in a further study with clofibrate, mortality due to hepatobiliary disease was increased. Although further trials must be undertaken before exposing large numbers of asymptomatic people with 'mild' hyperlipidaemia (cholesterol 5.2–6.5 mM) to life-long drug treatment, modification of diet and lifestyle appears justifiable at present. Thus hyperlipidaemia, like hypertension, is a risk factor for cardiovascular disease for which dietary or pharmacological modification can be justified.

General principles of management

Primary and secondary hyperlipidaemia

Diagnosis of hyperlipidaemia requires accurate measurement of cholesterol and it is also useful to measure HDL cholesterol to give an indication of the proportions of HDL and LDL fractions. Non-fasting blood can be assayed for total cholesterol. For measurement of triglycerides the blood must be collected in the fasting state.

Secondary causes of hyperlipidaemia, for which specific treatment or management is indicated, should be excluded. These include renal or hepatic disease, hypothyroidism, diabetes, alcohol abuse, obesity or drugs. Thiazide diuretics may increase LDL cholesterol and some beta-blockers will reduce HDL cholesterol and increase triglycerides.

The principal aims of treatment are to reduce LDL cholesterol by diet and/or drugs and to increase HDL cholesterol with diet and physical exercise.

Diet

The cornerstone of management of hyperlipidaemia is diet. Dietary advice should include:

1 Reduction of intake of saturated fats.
2 Reduction in carbohydrate and total calories if obese.
3 Reduction of intake of cholesterol.

4 Increase of polyunsaturated and mono-unsaturated fats.
5 Increase in fibre intake.

The end result of these dietary changes is the attainment of an ideal body weight and up-regulation of LDL receptors.

The diet should be planned in discussion with the spouse and family and should take some account of social, cultural and economic conditions of the patient. Diet alone can reduce total cholesterol by 10–15% in compliant motivated persons but many fail to respond or relapse. Diet should be combined with advice to increase physical exercise and stop smoking.

Diet alone is currently advised in those with milder hypercholesterolaemia (5.2–6.5 mM). Moderate elevation (6.5–8.0 mM) may require diet with drug therapy. In those with marked elevation (> 8.0 mM), diet combined with one or more drugs will usually be required.

Drug treatment strategies available at present to lower LDL cholesterol include:

1 Resins or sequestrants, which bind bile acids in the gastrointestinal tract and interrupt the enterohepatic circulation of cholesterol derived bile acids.
2 Fibrates, which activate lipoprotein lipase and enhance degradation of lipoprotein particles.
3 3-Hydroxy-3-methoxyglutaryl coenzyme A (HMGCoA) reductase inhibitors, which inhibit hepatic cholesterol synthesis.
4 Other treatments, which include nicotinic acid, probucol and fish oils.

The effects of these agents on lipoproteins and triglycerides are summarized in Table 8.3.

Table 8.3. Summary of the actions of lipid lowering drugs

Drug	LDL	HDL	Triglycerides
Cholestyramine	↓	→	→
Gemfibrozil	↓	↑	↓
Clofibrate	→	↑	↓
HMGCoA reductase inhibitors	↓↓	↑	→
Nicotinic acid	↓	↑	↓
Probucol	↓	↓	→

Drug approaches may be used alone or in combination. Their success in lowering cholesterol appears to depend at least in part on the up-regulation of LDL receptors and increased clearance of LDL cholesterol from the circulation. Some agents have preferential actions on VLDL and are indicated if hypertriglyceridaemia is present. Strategies to raise HDL cholesterol can be used concurrently, although their value is more controversial.

Lipid lowering drugs

Bile acid sequestrants: cholestyramine, colestipol

Cholestyramine and colestipol are resins which bind bile salts in the gut and thus interrupt the enterohepatic circulation. They increase hepatic cholesterol synthesis and promote receptor mediated uptake of LDL cholesterol from plasma. The resins lower LDL cholesterol, with less marked increases in HDL and no effect on triglycerides. They are not significantly absorbed but can interfere with absorption of fat-soluble vitamins (especially vitamin K) and to a lesser extent fats. Folic acid deficiency may occur and impaired absorption of other drugs, such as digoxin, may occur. Gastrointestinal side effects are not uncommon and compliance may be poor. Cholestyramine is unpalatable and must be given in large (20–30 g) daily doses.

Fibrates: gemfibrozil, bezafibrate, clofibrate

Gemfibrozil and bezafibrate lower LDL cholesterol by 10–20% by activation of lipoprotein lipase and may also inhibit HMGCoA reductase. They also raise HDL cholesterol. Clofibrate has less effect on LDL but reduces triglycerides by promoting lipolysis of triglyceride-rich particles. Long-term clofibrate therapy has been associated with an increase in hepatobiliary diseases, particularly cholesterol cholelithiasis. Gallstones result from increased cholesterol saturation of the bile. Fibrates as a group are completely absorbed and largely excreted unchanged by the kidney. Extensive plasma protein binding to albumin is one mechanism of drug interactions with these drugs. Gemfibrozil and clofibrate may potentiate the effects of oral anticoagulants.

Fibrates may be used alone or combined with resins or other agents.

3-Hydroxy-3-methoxyglutaryl coenzyme A (HMGCoA) reductase inhibitors: lovastatin, simvastatin, pravastatin

HMGCoA reductase is a rate limiting step in the hepatic synthesis of cholesterol. Blockade of this enzyme leads to increases in LDL cholesterol uptake by the liver. Lovastatin, simvastatin and pravastatin are available in the USA and Europe. Substantial falls (30–40%) in LDL cholesterol may occur, especially if the drug is combined with a resin. Lovastatin is well tolerated. It can be taken once or twice daily and side effects are rare. However, long-term experience with HMGCoA reductase inhibitors is limited and large scale postmarketing surveillance data are not yet available. There have not been any controlled trials to date confirming that reduction of cholesterol by this means reduces cardiovascular mortality.

Other lipid lowering drugs

Probucol lowers LDL cholesterol by 10–20% but also inhibits the production of HDL cholesterol. The implications of the latter finding are not clear.

Nicotinic acid or niacin is a B vitamin which is a potent inhibitor of LDL and VLDL formation. Nicotinic acid and its derivative nicofuranose lower LDL and raise HDL cholesterol. Unfortunately nicotinic acid is not well tolerated. Severe facial flushing is a common dose limiting effect. This is prostaglandin mediated and may be alleviated in part by the coadministration of aspirin.

Fish oils high in unsaturated fatty acids such as eicosapentaenoic and docosahexaenoic acid may be used particularly to reduce high triglycerides. These preparations are not very palatable.

Comment

Raised cholesterol, specifically LDL cholesterol, is an important determinant of cardiovascular risk. While diet is the main stratagem in mild hypercholesterolaemia, diet combined with drug therapy is indicated in moderate and severe hypercholesterolaemia. Treatment of raised cholesterol should be part of an overall plan in the individual patient for prevention of cardiovascular disease. This plan should include advice to stop smoking and control of elevated blood pressure.

Chapter 9
Thrombosis and Coagulation

9.1 RELEVANT PATHOPHYSIOLOGY

Vascular disease is a major cause of morbidity and mortality in developed countries. The development of atheroma may be insidious, but local plaque complications may lead to the acute formation of thrombus. This results in a reduction in blood flow, which may be partial or total, and leads to a wide variation in clinical presentation. The development of thrombus depends on three factors:

1 The formation of a thrombogenic surface, such as damaged vascular endothelium.

2 Platelet activation with resulting adhesion and aggregation, with subsequent release of vasoactive compounds which promote further aggregation and vasoconstriction.

3 Activation of the clotting cascade with generation of thrombin and stimulation of fibrin formation (Fig. 9.1).

Under normal conditions, the activities of the coagulation and natural fibrinolytic systems are balanced. Thrombin initiated fibrin formation is in equilibrium with plasmin degradation of fibrin with production of fibrin degradation products.

Antithrombotic therapy may include compounds which inhibit platelet activity (antiplatelet agents), anticoagulant therapy or the use of agents with fibrinolytic, i.e. thrombolytic, activity. In the arterial circulation with rapid blood flow, 'white' thrombus is formed. This is composed mainly of platelets. In the setting of low flow, as in the venous circulation, 'red' thrombus with a high proportion of red blood cells forms. In general, platelet inhibiting compounds are indicated in clinical syndromes associated with arterial thrombi, such as transient ischaemic attacks in the cerebral circulation or unstable angina and acute myocardial infarction, whereas anticoagulants are indicated in the prophylaxis and/or treatment of venous thrombosis or in the prevention of thrombus development in dilated cardiac chambers. Fibrinolytic or thrombolytic compounds have an increasing clinical role in the treatment of acute myocardial infarction, as well as in peripheral artery thrombosis and in the treatment of pulmonary emboli.

9.2 ANTIPLATELET DRUGS

Observations from pathological studies suggest that platelets play a major role in the initiation of thrombus formation in atherosclerotic arteries. Increased platelet aggregation has been demonstrated in patients with angina pectoris.

Platelet-active drugs affect the synthesis of prostaglandins and other eicosanoids and through this mechanism may affect the balance of vasoactivity and

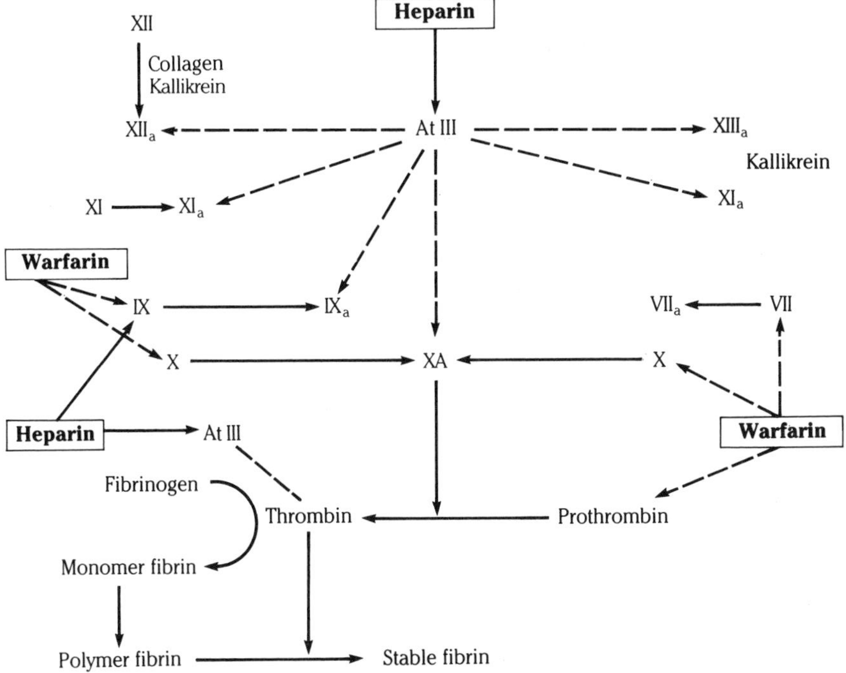

Fig. 9.1. Congulation pathways and sites of action of anticoagulant drugs.

platelet aggregation in the arterial circulation. Thromboxane A_2 may be released in the coronary circulation following endothelial damage. It stimulates platelet aggregation and is a local vasoconstrictor leading to increased coronary arterial tone or spasm, which in turn may promote further platelet aggregation. Vascular endothelium produces prostacyclin (PGI_2), which inhibits platelet aggregation and may be a local vasodilator. The ideal prostaglandin synthetase inhibitor in ischaemic syndromes would reduce thromboxane A_2 production while maintaining prostacyclin generation.

Aspirin

Mechanism

Salicylates inhibit the biosynthesis of prostaglandins by binding covalently and irreversibly to the enzyme cyclo-oxygenase. Acetyl salicylic acid (aspirin) has potent inhibitory effects on platelet adhesion and aggregation. Experimental observations have suggested that very low doses of aspirin may selectively block thromboxane synthesis without affecting prostacyclin production. It may be, however, that both cyclo-oxygenase systems are affected equally but that regeneration may occur within 36 h in endothelial cells, whereas platelets are affected throughout their lifetime and are incapable of such enzyme regeneration. By extending the dosing intervals of aspirin, thromboxane A_2 may be inhibited without affecting prostacyclin production.

Pharmacokinetics

Salicylates are rapidly absorbed, with therapeutic levels being observed within 30 min, a peak at 2 h and then a gradual fall. Gastrointestinal absorption depends on the gastric pH and on the release characteristics of the tablet formulation. A variable hepatic first-pass metabolism is recognized. Its predominant metabolic product is salicyluric acid. Renal excretion is influenced by urinary pH; alkaline urine enhances renal excretion of this acidic drug. To reduce gastrointestinal side effects during oral administration, many formulations have been developed, including buffered preparations or enteric coated tablets.

Adverse effects

Aspirin has significant side effects but in most cases these are dose related and are relatively rare when low doses are used:

1 Gastric erosions with gastrointestinal bleeding.

2 Prolongation of the bleeding time may occur secondary to the action on platelet cyclo-oxygenase.

3 Hypersensitivity reactions with skin rashes may occur, and asthma may be provoked in some individuals.

Relative or absolute contra-indications include:

1 Known aspirin intolerance.

2 Blood dyscrasias or bleeding tendency, such as haemophilia.

3 History of gastrointestinal bleeding or peptic ulcer.

4 Severe renal failure or hepatic cirrhosis.

Clinical use and dose

Although soluble aspirin may be given for rheumatic diseases (Chapter 12) in doses up to 6–9 g daily, when used as an antiplatelet compound the dosage becomes 300–1300 mg daily. This is now regarded as high-dose aspirin. Lower doses are now being advocated, using 75 mg daily or even every second or third day. Evidence for clinical efficacy has been limited to dosage schedules of at least 150–300 mg daily.

Clinical indications for aspirin that have been established include the treatment of unstable angina, using dosage schedules of 300–1300 mg daily. Clinical benefit also has been shown with 300 mg aspirin daily in patients with transient ischaemic attacks and minor ischaemic strokes. Recent information suggests myocardial infarction also may be reduced, and there is increasing evidence that reinfarction may be reduced in patients treated with aspirin as secondary prevention. The ISIS II study has confirmed an additive role of aspirin in combination with streptokinase in reducing mortality following myocardial infarction. The doses used were 150 or 160 mg daily. Other clinical indications include the prevention of graft occlusion following coronary artery bypass surgery. Aspirin also has been used to prevent emboli from artificial heart valves, to reduce thrombosis in arteriovenous shunts and following percutaneous transluminal coronary angioplasty.

In combination with dipyridamole

Dipyridamole has several actions inhibiting platelet aggregation. Its main action is as an adenosine uptake inhibitor, allowing more adenosine to be available extracellularly, thereby increasing platelet inhibitory effects via cyclic AMP and also allowing more vasodilatation. At high concentration it acts as a phosphodiesterase inhibitor, raising the intracellular cyclic AMP concentration. Dipyridamole potentiates the effects of prostacyclin and reduces platelet adhesion to damaged endothelium.

In *in vitro* studies, dipyridamole and aspirin have different and additive effects on platelet function. Although the combination has theoretical advantages, clinical trials have not confirmed that the combination is better than aspirin alone.

The side effects of dipyridamole include: gastrointestinal irritation, vasodilation and hypotensive effects such as dizziness, flushing or even syncope.

9.3 ANTICOAGULANT DRUGS

There are many clinical indications for anticoagulant therapy. These include the prophylactic use of low-dose subcutaneous heparin to prevent venous thrombosis, its intravenous administration for systemic anticoagulation and chronic long-term oral anticoagulant therapy which is generally undertaken using warfarin. The coagulation cascade is shown in Fig. 9.1. This demonstrates the activation of proenzymes to active moieties like a domino effect with amplification and the active production of thrombin and fibrin. The sites of action of the anticoagulant drugs are shown.

Heparin

Mechanism

Heparin is a mucopolysaccharide or glycosaminoglycan which has a strongly acidic charge. Heparin binds to and greatly accelerates the anticoagulating effects of antithrombin III, which neutralizes the effect of thrombin and several other clotting factors. If given in low concentration, heparin increases antithrombin III activity, particularly against factor Xa. This is the rationale for the use of low-dose heparin by the subcutaneous route to prevent deep venous thrombosis following surgery or acute myocardial infarction.

Pharmacokinetics

Heparin is given parenterally, either subcutaneously for low-dose therapy or as an intravenous bolus or constant infusion. It follows first-order kinetics and is metabolized by heparinase to inactive metabolites. The half-life is prolonged in patients with renal failure or hepatic disease.

Adverse effects

Haemorrhage: the use of heparin is contra-indicated in the presence of active bleeding from any site or in coagulopathy such as haemophilia. Other contra-indications include the presence of purpura, thrombocytopenia or cerebrovascular disease. Relative contra-indications include the presence of severe hypertension or evidence of occult neoplasm. Sensitivity reactions may occur and thrombocytopenia may rarely complicate continued therapy (platelet counts should be monitored). Long-term therapy may lead to osteoporosis.

Clinical use and dose

For systemic anticoagulation, heparin is given by a loading dose of 5–10 000 units followed by a continuous infusion of 1–2000 units/h. The rate is determined by the measurement of the activated partial thromboplastin time, which should be increased twofold from control or pretreatment levels. Intermittent intravenous therapy may be given following a loading dose of 5–10 000 units given 4–6 hourly, with haematological screening being performed 1 h before each dose.

Low-dose prophylaxis by the subcutaneous route should be given with 5000 units subcutaneously 2 h before surgical operation, with further dosing 4–12 h thereafter. A similar regimen of twice daily dosing may be given to non-surgical patients at high risk, e.g. following acute myocardial infarction. Recent studies have used twice daily dosing with 12 500 units subcutaneously as an alternative regime to full systemic anticoagulation. If subcutaneous injection is continued for prophylactic use, deep sites should be used to slow absorption and prolong activity. Small gauge needles should be used to reduce the risk of local bleeding. The injectate volume should be small, the site of injection varied and local pressure applied after administration. The duration of heparin therapy is determined by the clinical indication and may be continued until the anticoagulant effect of orally administered agents has become established with an infusion for up to 72 h.

Reversal of therapy

Protamine sulphate, which is a low molecular weight protein with a strongly basic charge, may be given. A 1 mg dose of protamine should be given for every 1000 units of heparin predicted to remain in the circulation. The infusion should be given slowly, as it may be associated with dyspnoea, flushing, bradycardia and hypotension.

Ancrod

This anticoagulant for parenteral use is an enzyme derived from Malayan pit viper venom which has been used for the treatment of deep vein thrombosis and for prophylactic treatment in patients likely to develop deep vein thrombosis.

Dose and administration

An initial slow infusion may be given using 2–3 units/kg over 4–12 h, then by slow infusion 2 units/kg every 12 h. Prophylaxis of deep venous thrombosis may be effected by 280 units immediately after surgery, then 70 units daily for 4–8 days.

Side effects

Some patients may develop resistance. The major complication of ancrod is haemorrhage secondary to the cleavage of fibrin. Ancrod antivenom may be required as an antidote. Occasionally, anaphylactic reactions may occur in response to its administration.

Oral anticoagulants

The coumarin group are the drugs of choice. The phenindione group may be used as an alternative.

Warfarin

Mechanism

Warfarin is the most widely used oral anticoagulant. It is a derivative of 4-hydroxycoumarin and its anticoagulant activity is the result of inhibition of hepatic synthesis of vitamin K dependent clotting factors. Its onset of action is influenced by the half-life of the circulating clotting factors, and therapeutic effects are delayed for at least 8–12 h after oral administration. Warfarin is given usually by a loading dose over a 72 h period, followed by a maintenance dose determined by the one-stage prothrombin activity. Following absorption, warfarin is almost totally bound (99%) to plasma albumin and has a long half-life of some 35 h. The volume of distribution is 11–12% of body weight, and contra-indications to its use are similar to those for heparin or other anticoagulants. The activity of warfarin may be influenced by the presence of physiological and pathological factors, including vitamin K deficiency, congestive cardiac failure and alcoholic or other hepatic disease.

Drug interactions

In view of the high degree of protein binding and hepatic metabolism, there are many potential interactions of warfarin with other drugs. These are detailed in Table 9.1. As warfarin influences haemostasis and is used in severely ill patients, both excessive effect or loss of effect may result in significant morbidity or mortality. Its major adverse effects are related to the development of haemorrhage which may arise at any site, including echymosis or haematoma formation in the skin at sites of venepuncture or other invasive interventions. If the degree of anticoagulation is poorly controlled, haemorrhage may develop at a distant

Table 9.1. Drug interactions with warfarin

Reduce anticoagulant effect	Increase anticoagulant effect
Vitamin K	Antiplatelet drugs
Rifampicin	Several broad spectrum antibiotics
Oral contraceptives	Anabolic steroids and antiandrogens
Griseofulvin	Ketoconazole
Anticonvulsants: barbiturates, phenytoin, carbamazepine	Lipid lowering drugs
	Amiodarone Cimetidine
	Dextropropoxyphene
	Alcohol

site with gastrointestinal, uterine or urinary tract bleeding. In the presence of significant bleeding, warfarin is discontinued and vitamin K administered. In the presence of haemodynamic impairment, 50 mg vitamin K_1 may be given by the intravenous route and fresh frozen plasma may be given, or alternatively the vitamin K dependent clotting factors may be administered. Large doses of vitamin K_1 can be given only if it is not intended to reintroduce anticoagulation.

Clinical use and indications

Long-term anticoagulant management depends on good supervision and patient education. Warfarin is available as 1, 2 and 5 mg tablets with a different colour for each dose. The loading dose may be 20–30 mg over a 3 day period. Thereafter, the individual dose should be determined on the basis of daily estimation of the prothrombin time, reported as the International Normalized Ratio (INR). The currently recommended therapeutic ranges for the INR are 2–2.5 for prophylactic therapy of deep vein thrombosis, 3–4.5 for arterial disease, including following myocardial infarction, arterial grafts and prosthetic heart valves, and 2–3 for treatment of current deep vein thrombosis or pulmonary embolism. Patients should be given detailed instructions, both oral and written, concerning their drug regimen, the importance of compliance and advice concerning modification of their lifestyle if necessary. The possibility of drug interactions should be explained, placing particular emphasis on commonly prescribed drugs with high protein binding, including 'over-the-counter' products such as aspirin. Patients should carry an anticoagulant card at all times or have other proof that they are receiving anticoagulants. Specific modifications of therapy are indicated before elective surgery or in female patients within childbearing years if pregnancy is contemplated. Warfarin should be discontinued before surgery for at least 2 days and serial coagulation screens performed. Where continued prophylactic anticoagulant cover is required, e.g. in the presence of prosthetic valves, subcutaneous heparin may be substituted and continued for 5–7 days postsurgery, at which time warfarin can be reintroduced. In the elderly and patients with uncontrolled hypertension, warfarin may present increased risks. In patients with liver disease, thrombocytopenia or peptic ulcer, warfarin should be avoided.

9.4 THROMBOLYTIC AGENTS

It has been long recognized that natural or spontaneous fibrinolysis may occur in patients with acute thrombotic occlusion. Pharmacological agents with fibrinolytic activity have an established place in the treatment of deep venous thrombosis, pulmonary embolism and peripheral arterial occlusion and are now being assessed in subsets of patients with thrombotic stroke (Fig. 9.2). The early use of streptokinase for the treatment of acute myocardial infarction, although showing promising results, was not accepted widely in clinical practice. This was due to the prolonged and complicated infusion regimens, a continued debate concerning the role of coronary artery thrombus in the initiation of acute myocardial infarction and the introduction of other pharmacological methods to reduce myocardial damage following coronary occlusion. Thrombolytic therapy is now firmly established as standard treatment in acute myocardial infarction. Pathological

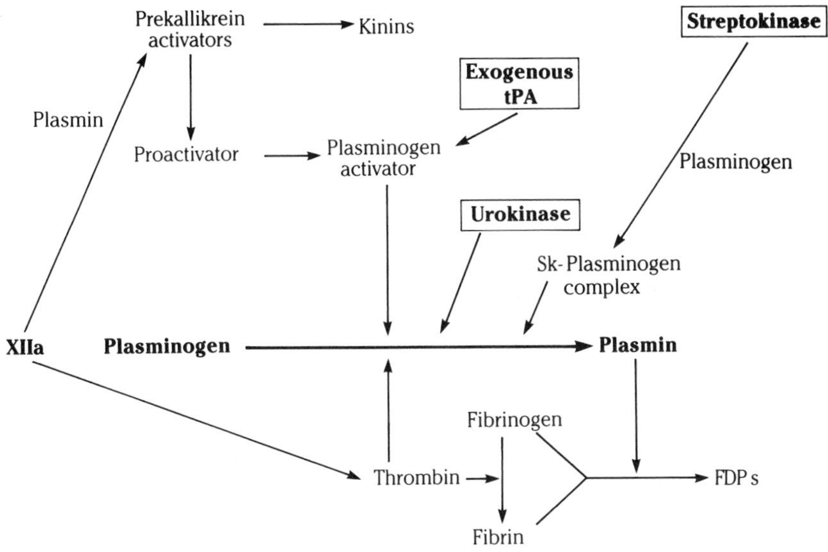

Fig. 9.2. Fibrinolytic mechanisms and sites of action of fibrinolytic drugs.

observations had confirmed coronary artery thrombus in most patients dying from acute myocardial infarction, and clinical observations confirmed that some 90% of patients have total thrombotic occlusion of their coronary artery on angiography during the first 4 h of symptoms. Serial investigations using local intracoronary administration of thrombolytic drugs showed that many of these total occlusions could be cleared and that coronary artery reperfusion could be obtained in up to 80% of patients. This invasive method of administration of therapy had the advantage of allowing visualization of the infarct related vessel, and with local delivery of the thrombolytic compound to the thrombus the total dose of drug could be reduced. The practical limitations from the non-availability of coronary arteriographic facilities limited the widespread use of intracoronary drugs. The development of intravenous infusion regimens has allowed much wider application of thrombolytic therapy. Large scale studies have confirmed the efficacy of these agents in achieving coronary artery patency, reducing left ventricular damage and, most importantly, reducing mortality.

The ideal agent for thrombolytic treatment would possess:

1 A high fibrin affinity with local fibrinolytic activity on the obstructing thrombus, so that a high reperfusion rate may be obtained.

2 Little fibrinogenolytic activity allowing only a modest systemic effect, with a low incidence of bleeding complications.

3 A simple standard intravenous dosage regimen to allow administration to all patients in the early phase of their illness, in order that tissue damage may be minimized.

4 Kinetics which include a rapid onset of action, but with sustained local activity to prevent the reaccumulation of the thrombus.

5 Chemical structures similar or identical to those occurring naturally to prevent antigen stimulation.

Presently available agents include streptokinase, urokinase, the acylated derivative of streptokinase (anistreplase, APSAC) and the recombinant form of the naturally occurring tissue plasminogen activator (rtPA). The urokinase precursor for single chain urokinase is under investigation.

Streptokinase

This is produced from Lancefield group A β-haemolytic streptococci. Previous exposure to streptococcal infection leads to variable amounts of circulating antistreptococcal antibody. Some 250 000 units of streptokinase given intravenously is usually sufficient to neutralize such antibodies and initiate a thrombolytic state. The presence of antibodies may predispose to allergic reactions with hypotension, and in 1–2% of patients this may extend to the development of rash, urticaria, angioneurotic oedema, bronchospasm and even anaphylactoid reaction. Pretreatment with intravenous hydrocortisone and an antihistamine is often used. Further treatment with streptokinase is contra-indicated for at least 12 months.

Mechanism

Streptokinase forms an intermediate one-to-one complex with plasminogen or plasmin following administration and generates active plasmin. It activates both plasma (soluble phase) and fibrin-bound (gel phase) plasminogen. This leads to systemic hyperplasminaemia, which predisposes to haemorrhagic complication. Streptokinase has an initial distribution half-life of 16 min, associated with antibody complexing and removal, and an elimination half-life of some 80 min, reflecting the biological half-life of the protein. Fibrin and fibrinogen degradation fragments following fibrinolysis have an additional anticoagulant effect by limiting the ability of platelets to aggregate and by causing a partial degradation of factors V and VIII.

Clinical use and dose

The dosage schedule for the treatment of pulmonary embolism or deep venous thrombosis involves a loading dose of 250 000 units with an hourly infusion of 100 000 units for 48–72 h. In the treatment of acute myocardial infarction, a brief high-dose infusion of 1.5×10^6 units of streptokinase over 1 h has been advocated and been shown to be effective in achieving coronary artery reperfusion in 50–70% of patients, resulting in improved left ventricular function and a reduction in mortality. Localized intra-arterial infusions of streptokinase can be used in the treatment of peripheral arterial occlusion.

Contra-indications to the use of thrombolytic compounds are similar to those for the use of anticoagulants, and include:

1 Bleeding diathesis.
2 Active peptic ulceration or other cause for gastrointestinal bleeding.
3 Severe hypertension.
4 Recent cerebrovascular accident.
5 Proliferative diabetic retinopathy.
6 Recent operation.

Urokinase

This active protease has a two-chain molecular structure and is isolated from urine or from human fetal renal cell culture. It directly cleaves plasminogen to plasmin and has a half-life of 146 min. Advantages over streptokinase include non-antigenicity, potentially greater fibrin affinity and specificity causing potentially less systemic lytic effects. It is much more expensive, and this has limited its application.

Acylated streptokinase (anistreplase, APSAC)

Anistreplase is an acylated plasminogen–streptokinase complex which evades the normal plasmin inhibitors by acylation of its active serine site. It has a high fibrin binding specificity and, following binding, deacylation occurs with the generation of plasminogen activator locally following hydrolysis. It has a deacylation half-life of 40 min and a plasma half-life of some 60–70 min, extended to 90 min in patients with myocardial infarction. Anistreplase can be given by rapid intravenous bolus injection over 5 min, and a standard dose of 30 mg has been widely used. Serial investigations have confirmed a high reperfusion rate following intravenous use, and recent studies have shown a reduction in mortality after acute myocardial infarction. It has a systemic fibrinogenolytic effect similar to conventional streptokinase. Its method of administration by bolus may make it applicable to the community and to non-specialist centres.

Tissue plasminogen activator

Tissue plasminogen activator is a naturally occurring plasminogen activator now produced by genetic techniqnes. Human tissue type activator has been isolated and extracted from various tissue sources. The tPA gene has been cloned and expressed in bacteria. Major studies have been undertaken using rtPA by the intravenous route. rtPA seems more effective than streptokinase in obtaining early coronary reperfusion, it has no problems of antigen formation or associated allergic reactions and repeat therapy may be given. Following its intravenous use in myocardial infarction, high reperfusion rates are obtained, left ventricular function is maintained and mortality is reduced.

Comment

Comparison of individual thrombolytic agents in the treatment of acute myocardial infarction has shown similar efficacy in reducing mortality. However, the more fibrin-specific compounds anistreplase and rtPA may be associated with a higher incidence of haemorrhagic stroke secondary to dissolution of protective haemostatic plugs. In addition, streptokinase is substantially less expensive than other agents.

Chapter 10
Antimicrobial Therapy

Aim

The aim is to control infection without damage to the patient.

10.1 PRINCIPLES OF DRUG TREATMENT

One of the greatest of all therapeutic advances was the introduction of drugs that eradicated bacterial infections in man. The introduction of sulphonamides in 1936 and penicillin in 1941 dramatically reduced mortality from infections. During the decades since then there has been a vast increase in the number of antimicrobials available for clinical use. This ready availability of drugs has enhanced the likelihood that a suitable agent can be found for a particular infection, but it has also resulted in a confusing range of choice and a readiness to prescribe antimicrobials even when the presence of bacterial infection is poorly documented. The newer antibiotics are expensive and not necessarily better than established agents: they should be prescribed only after careful consideration.

Table 10.1. General principles of antimicrobial therapy

Patient	Organism	Drug
Document infection	Culture	Absorption
Factors altering kinetics: age; renal/hepatic function	Identification	Tissue distribution
	Typing	Route of elimination
Previous drug sensitivity	Sensitivity	Adverse reactions
General health (resistance to infection)		Drug interactions
Pregnancy		

The patient

Documentation of infection

Whenever possible the clinical suspicion of infection should be supported by laboratory diagnosis. Relevant samples, e.g. sputum, urine, pus, blood, etc., should be obtained before treatment is commenced.

Age

Drug kinetics are influenced by age dependent changes in pathways of elimination (Chapter 4). Clinically important examples involving antimicrobials include:

1 Relative deficiency of hepatic glucuronyl transferase in neonates, leading to an accumulation of chloramphenicol with a likelihood of cardiovascular collapse if serum concentration exceeds 25 mg/l.

2 Physiological decrease in renal function with age, leading to an accumulation of aminoglycosides in the elderly with a likelihood of toxicity: dose modification is necessary.

Other antimicrobials contraindicated in specific age groups are:

3 Sulphonamides in the neonate (displacement of bilirubin, leading to kernicterus).

4 Tetracyclines in growing children (tooth discoloration).

Renal and hepatic function (Chapter 3, Section 3.2)

Many commonly used antimicrobials are eliminated by the kidney while a few undergo hepatic metabolism. Dose modification is likely to be necessary if renal function is moderately or severely impaired (Table 10.2). Drug level monitoring is mandatory for antimicrobials with concentration related toxicity.

Table 10.2. Antimicrobials for which dose modification is required in mild, moderate or severe renal failure and in liver disease

Renal failure			
Mild	Moderate	Severe	Liver disease
Aminoglycosides	Metronidazole	Co-trimoxazole	Clindamycin
Amphotericin B	Ticarcillin	Penicillins	Isoniazid
Cephalosporins		Acyclovir	Rifampicin
Ethambutol			Avoid: erythromycin estolate, pyrazinamide, talampicillin
Flucytosine			
Vancomycin			
Avoid: cephalothin, cephaloridine, nalidixic acid, nitrofurantoin, talampicillin, tetracyclines			

Drug sensitivity

Always ask about previous exposure to drugs. Penicillins and cephalosporins are the antimicrobials most frequently associated with sensitivity reactions and there is a 5–10% cross-sensitivity between these two drug groups because they both contain the β-lactam ring. Sulphonamides also frequently cause allergic reactions.

Diminished resistance to infection

Patients with malignant disease or who are receiving cytotoxic or immunosuppressant drugs are susceptible to severe infections often with less common organisms, e.g. commensal bacteria, some viruses, yeasts, fungi and protozoa. In particular, granulocytopaenia of less than 500×10^6/l is accompanied by a high risk of septicaemia. Fever in such patients must be assumed to have an infective aetiology and should be treated aggressively before definitive bacteriological information is available.

Pregnancy (Chapter 5, Section 5.1)

Penicillins and cephalosporins are not harmful to the fetus. Fetal damage has been associated definitely with streptomycin and the tetracyclines. Possible adverse fetal effects have been ascribed to gentamicin, kanamycin and co-trimoxazole.

Comment

The patient's age, sex and general state of health must be considered when choosing both the drug and its dose.

The organism

Bacteria

Sensitivity

Bactericidal drugs destroy the organisms against which they are effective. Bacteriostatic drugs do not kill the organism but destroy its ability to replicate. Use of a bacteriostatic drug assumes that body defences can destroy the organisms whose replication has been prevented. *In vitro* testing is available for most antibacterial drugs. Application of *in vitro* findings to the patient assumes that adequate drug concentrations are achieved at the site of infection.

Resistance

Some bacteria have always been resistant to the effects of certain drugs, while others have developed resistance in the course of repeated exposure to antimicrobials. The two major mechanisms by which resistance is produced are gene mutation and exchange of DNA between bacteria. Resistance may take three main forms:

1 An alteration in the bacterial component on which the drug acts, e.g. changes in the 30S ribosomal subunit in organisms developing resistance to aminoglycosides.

2 The drug might be destroyed by the organisms, as in the case of penicillins which are inactivated by β-lactamases produced by resistant bacteria.

3 Cell membrane permeability to drugs is reduced, as in resistance to tetracyclines.

The development of resistance can be reduced if antimicrobials are not given indiscriminately. Additionally, the use of drug combinations should limit the appearance of resistant organisms in conditions such as tuberculosis where prolonged treatment is necessary.

Viruses and fungi

The range of effective drugs is limited and in many cases treatment is still experimental. Consequently, information about sensitivity or resistance to treatment is far less complete than for bacteria. Organisms are considered individually under specific agents.

Comment
Antimicrobial treatment must take account of the organism's susceptibility to drugs and the patient's intrinsic ability to combat infection.

The drug

Absorption

Certain antimicrobials, e.g. the aminoglycosides, can only be given parenterally because absorption from the gastrointestinal tract is negligible. Where a choice exists between oral and parenteral drug formulations, the decision must rest on the severity of the illness and the need to achieve high tissue concentration.

Tissue distribution

The principles determining drug distribution are described in Chapter 1, Section 1.2. In addition to these general considerations of blood concentration, protein binding, lipid solubility, etc., a further factor influencing antimicrobial distribution is the presence of inflammation, which tends to improve tissue penetration. However, it must not be assumed that the presence of inflammation greatly transforms the penetration of drugs. For example, gentamicin and cephalosporins cross poorly into the cerebrospinal fluid (CSF) even in the presence of meningitis. Table 10.3 indicates those agents with high penetration to CSF, bile and urine.

Table 10.3. Antimicrobials for which high concentrations are achieved

CSF	Bile	Urine
Chloramphenicol	Penicillins	Penicillins
Erythromycin	Cephalosporins	Cephalosporins
Isoniazid	Erythromycin	Aminoglycosides
Pyrazinamide		Sulphonamides
Rifampicin		Nitrofurantoin
Flucytosine		Nalidixic acid
		Ethambutol
		Flucytosine

Route of elimination

This is usually renal or hepatic metabolism (or rarely biliary excretion). See Chapter 3 and the section above on renal and hepatic function.

Adverse effects

These are of two general types:

1 Hypersensitivity reactions which are either immediate or delayed. The former produce anaphylaxis while the latter manifest themselves in various ways, the most common being rashes. Hypersensitivity reactions usually occur with no prior warning and are most commonly seen with penicillins, cephalosporins and sulphonamides.

2 The other type of adverse reaction is usually predictable in being concentration related; aminoglycoside ototoxicity is an example. Fortunately, the toxic concentrations of most antimicrobials in common use greatly exceed the required therapeutic concentrations. Where this is not the case, e.g. gentamicin, drug level monitoring is mandatory. Adverse reactions to antimicrobials are summarized in Table 10.4 and discussed in more detail under specific agents.

Table 10.4. Major adverse reactions of antimicrobial drugs

Organ system	Drug	Comment
Kidney	Aminoglycosides	Concentration related
	Cephalosporins	Mainly earlier drugs of this group
	Sulphonamides	
	Methicillin	Other penicillins rarely
	Amphotericin B	
	Polymyxins	Limits use
Bone marrow suppression	Antiviral agents	
	Amphotericin B	
	Flucytosine	
	Chloramphenicol	
	Sulphonamides	Rare
Haemolytic anaemia	Sulphonamides	Two distinct mechanisms: immune and glucose-6-phosphate deficiency
	Nitrofurantoin	
	4-Aminoquinolones	
	Penicillins	Rare
	Cephalosporins	Rare
Thrombocytopaenia	Sulphonamides	Rare
	Cephalosporins	Rare
	Latamoxef	Dose dependent
	Rifampicin	Intermittent therapy
Neutropaenia	Penicillins	Rare: mainly ampicillin, carbenicillin
	Cephalosporins	Rare
	Sulphonamides	Rare
	Chloramphenicol	
Neurological		
Eighth nerve	Aminoglycosides	Concentration related
	Vancomycin	
Optic nerve	Ethambutol	
Peripheral neuropathy	Isoniazid	Prevented by pyridoxine
	Metronidazole	Prolonged treatment
	Nitrofurantoin	
Convulsions	Penicillins	Large intrathecal or massive intravenous doses
	Cephalosporins	Large intrathecal doses
	4-Aminoquinolones	Large doses

Table 10.4. (cont.)

Organ system	Drug	Comment
Benign intracranial hypertension	Tetracyclines	
	Penicillins	
	Nalidixic acid	
Neuromuscular blockade	Aminoglycosides	
Gastrointestinal system		
Liver	Isoniazid	More often rapid acetylators
	Rifampicin	Usually mild—worse in alcoholics/preceding damage
	Tetracyclines	Massive doses
	Erythromycin estolate	
	Nitrofurantoin	
Transient rise in transaminases	Penicillins	
	Cephalosporins	
Diarrhoea	Penicillins	Specially ampicillin
	Tetracyclines	
	Clindamycin	Pseudomembranous colitis (*Clostridium difficile*)
Other adverse reactions		
Hypersensitivity	Penicillins	10% cross-sensitivity
	Sulphonamides	
Stevens–Johnson syndrome	Sulphonamides	
	Penicillins	
Bone development/ tooth staining	Tetracyclines	Contra-indicated in childhood and pregnancy
Pulmonary fibrosis	Nitrofurantoin	
Rashes	Commonly penicillins and sulphonamides but virtually any drug can cause rashes	

Drug interactions

These can be either kinetic, e.g. enzyme induction or inhibition, or dynamic, e.g. two drugs adversely affecting the same organ. Examples include:

1 Aminoglycosides and frusemide have an additive nephrotoxic effect.

2 Rifampicin induces the same enzymes that metabolize the contraceptive pill and can cause failure of contraception.

3 Sulphonamides inhibit the enzymes that metabolize phenytoin and can cause phenytoin toxicity.

4 Tetracyclines form insoluble complexes in the gut lumen with both antacids and iron, leading to treatment failure.

Antimicrobial prophylaxis

Antimicrobials are sometimes given to people who do not have an infection but who are considered to be at risk from a specific organism. Examples include the use of minocycline or rifampicin in close contacts of patients with meningococcal meningitis, the administration of penicillin before and following dental procedures in people at risk of endocarditis and the long-term use of co-trimoxazole in children with repeated urinary tract infections and evidence of vesicoureteric reflux. Perioperative prophylaxis in certain types of surgery where the risk of infection is high (e.g. colorectal) or the consequences of infection are life-threatening (e.g. open heart) is now standard practice.

Comment

An antimicrobial might be quite ineffective, or even dangerous, unless its clinical pharmacology is viewed in relation to the whole clinical situation. The drug chosen must reach the site of infection, in an effective concentration, without producing toxicity or adversely influencing any concurrent therapy.

10.2 ANTIBACTERIAL DRUGS

Penicillins

Mechanism

Penicillins have a bactericidal action. They inhibit cell wall synthesis by preventing the formation of peptidoglycan cross-bridges.

Pharmacokinetics

Oral absorption

Not absorbed: carbenicillin, ticarcillin, mecillinam.
Moderately absorbed: benzylpenicillin (penicillin G), ampicillin, cloxacillin.
Well absorbed: phenoxypenicillin, amoxycillin, bacampicillin, pivampicillin, talampicillin, ciclacillin, flucloxicillin, pivmecillinam.

Even relatively well absorbed penicillins are destroyed to some extent by gastric acid and should, therefore, be given at least 30 min before meals.

Distribution

The penicillins have good penetration to most tissues but poor entry to CSF. This is compensated for in treating meningitis by giving large doses intravenously.

Elimination

Penicillins undergo enterohepatic circulation: drug is excreted via bile and re-absorbed. The major route of elimination after reabsorption is active secretion in the renal tubules. This tubular secretion can be blocked by probenecid with doubling of penicillin blood levels. Dose modification is necessary in severe renal failure.

Adverse effects

Immediate hypersensitivity

This occurs in 0.05% of patients with manifestations ranging from urticaria or wheezing to a life-threatening anaphylactic response.

Delayed hypersensitivity

This occurs in <5% of patients, mainly as rashes. Rare manifestations are haemolytic anaemia, leukopenia, interstitial nephritis (mainly reported with methicillin). Cross-sensitivity with cephalosporins occurs in around 10% of patients.

Toxicity

Convulsions follow large (>15 mg) intrathecal or very high (100 g/day) intravenous doses of penicillin. Patients with renal insufficiency can develop cation overload following large doses of potassium penicillin or sodium carbenicillin. Diarrhoea is commonly reported, particularly with ampicillin (20%).

Ampicillin has a unique adverse effect comprising a rash in up to 90% of patients with mononucleosis or chronic lymphocytic leukaemia.

Drug interactions

Ampicillin can lead to oral contraceptive failure. This is probably because of diminished enterohepatic circulation. The anticoagulant effect of warfarin is potentiated.

Antibacterial spectrum

The major factor limiting efficacy is the production by certain organisms of enzymes (β-lactamases) which destroy the β-lactam ring of the penicillin molecule. This structure is essential to the antibacterial action of penicillins. Several synthetic penicillins incorporate side chains which protect the β-lactam ring against these enzymes. However, this also has the effect of protecting bacteria from the β-lactam ring. These types of β-lactamase resistant drugs, therefore, are generally less effective than their β-lactamase sensitive counterparts and are indicated only for the treatment of infection caused by β-lactamase-producing staphylococci. An alternative approach has been to combine amoxycillin with clavulanic acid, which itself has no antibacterial activity but inhibits β-lactamase.

Penicillinase-sensitive penicillins

Benzylpenicillin and phenoxypenicillins are active against streptococci, pneumococci, gonococci and meningococci, *Treponema pallidum*, *Actinomyces israelii* and many anaerobic organisms, but not *Bacteroides fragilis*.

Ampicillin has a broader spectrum and is effective against some strains of *Escherichia coli*, *Proteus mirabilis*, *Shigella*, *Salmonella*, *Haemophilus influenzae* and various enterococci. Several derivatives of ampicillin are better absorbed but have the same antibacterial spectrum: amoxycillin, bacampicillin, ciclacillin, pivampicillin and talampicillin. The main indications are acute exacerbations of chronic bronchitis, urinary tract infection, cholecystitis and, parenterally (ampicillin), *H. influenzae* meningitis (depending on the sensitivity of the organism).

Carbenicillin and ticarcillin are active against *Pseudomonas aeruginosa* and *Proteus* species. At least *in vitro*, ticarcillin is more effective than carbenicillin and azlocillin is more effective than ticarcillin against *Ps. aeruginosa*. All three drugs must be given parenterally. The phenyl ester of carbenicillin (carfecillin) achieves antibacterial concentrations in the urine when given orally. Bacterial resistance is encountered in some strains. Mecillinam and its orally active ester pivmecillinam are effective against *Salmonella* species.

Penicillinase-resistant penicillins

Cloxacillin, flucloxacillin and methicillin are indicated only in the treatment of infections caused by penicillinase-producing staphylococci. Flucloxacillin is better absorbed from the gut than cloxacillin. More cases of interstitial nephritis have been reported following methicillin therapy than with any other penicillin.

Co-amoxiclav

The amoxycillin/clavulanic acid combination is mainly used in treating urinary tract infections caused by β-lactamase-producing coliforms.

Doses

Benzylpenicillin: intramuscular 300–600 mg 2–4 times daily (children 10–20 mg/kg daily); intravenous up to 24 g daily; intrathecal 6–12 mg daily.
Phenoxymethylpenicillin: oral dose 250–500 mg 6 hourly (children, 125–250 mg 6 hourly).
Ampicillin: oral dose 250–1000 mg 6 hourly; intravenous or intramuscular 500–1000 mg 6 hourly (children, half doses).
Amoxycillin: oral 250–500 mg 8 hourly (children, half dose).
Bacampicillin: 400 mg 8–12 hourly.
Ciclacillin: 250–500 mg 6 hourly.
Pivampicillin: 500 mg 12 hourly.
Talampicillin: oral 250–500 mg 8 hourly.
Carbenicillin: intravenous (rapid infusion) 5 g 4–6 hourly (children, 250–400 mg/kg daily divided doses); intramuscular 2 g 6 hourly (children, 50–100 mg/kg divided doses).
Ticarcillin: intravenous infusion (rapid) or intramuscular 15–20 g daily divided doses.
Azlocillin: 2 g 8 hourly by intravenous injection; up to 5 g 8 hourly by infusion.
Carfecillin: 0.5–1 g 8 hourly.
Mecillinam: slow intravenous injection or intramuscular 5–15 mg/kg 6 hourly.
Pivmecillinam: oral 1.2–2.4 g daily in salmonellosis.
Cloxacillin: intramuscular 500 mg 6 hourly; intravenous 500–1000 mg 6 hourly (children, quarter to half dose).
Flucloxacillin: oral 250 mg 6 hourly.

Co-amoxiclav: oral 1–2 tablets (of 250 mg amoxycillin, 125 mg clavulanic acid) 8 hourly.

Cephalosporins

Mechanism

Cephalosporins are bactericidal. They contain a β-lactam ring and their mechanism of action is similar to penicillins.

Pharmacokinetics

Six cephalosporins are effective orally: cephalexin, cephradine, cefaclor, cefixime, cefadroxil and cefuroxime. They distribute widely. Cefuroxime and cefotaxime are used in meningitis. Cephaloridine does not cross the blood–brain barrier. The drugs are eliminated renally, partly by glomerular filtration and partly by tubular secretion, with the contribution of each route varying with individual cephalosporins.

Adverse effects

Hypersensitivity is the main adverse effect, with around a 10% cross-reactivity with penicillin-sensitive patients. Cephaloridine can cause renal tubular necrosis, particularly when given in doses above 6 g/day. A positive Coombs' test occurs in about 5% of patients receiving cephalothin but haemolytic anaemia is rare. Cephalosporins, particularly latamoxef, can reduce prothrombin concentration and bleeding has been described. Several cephalosporins, including those commonly used orally, cause false positive urinalysis tests for glucose, as measured by reducing substances.

Drug interactions

The nephrotoxicity of cephaloridine is potentiated by loop diuretics and aminoglycoside antibiotics.

Antibacterial spectrum

The early cephalosporins were broad spectrum but with limited activity against Gram-negative organisms. Cephamandole and cefuroxime are more resistant to β-lactamases and are effective against a number of Gram-negative bacilli. Cefotaxime is more effective than cephamandole or cefuroxime against Gram-negative bacilli but less effective against Gram-positive organisms. Cefsulodin and ceftazidime are active against *Ps. aeruginosa*. Cefoxitin is closely related to the basic cephalosporin structure and is active against Gram-negative and anaerobic bacteria.

Doses

Oral

Cephalexin and cephradine: 250–500 mg 6 hourly (children, 25–50 mg/kg daily in divided doses).
Cefaclor: 250 mg 8 hourly (children, 20–40 mg/kg daily in divided doses).
Cefadroxil: 0.5–1 g 12 hourly.

Intravenous
Cephradine: 500–1000 mg 6 hourly (children, 50–100 mg/kg daily in 6 hourly doses).
Ceftazidime: 1–2 g 8–12 hourly.
Cephazolin: 500–1000 mg 6 hourly (children, 125–250 mg 8 hourly).
Cefuroxime: 1.5 g 6 hourly (children, 30–100 mg/kg daily in divided doses).
Cephamandole: 500–2000 mg 6 hourly (children, 50–100 mg/kg daily in divided doses).
Cefsulodin: 1–4 g daily in divided doses (children, 20–50 mg/kg daily).
Cefotaxime: 1 g 12 hourly to 3 g 6 hourly, depending on severity (children, 100–200 mg/kg daily in divided doses).
Cefoxitin: 1–2 g 8 hourly (children, 80–160 mg/kg daily in divided doses).

Comment
The cephalosporins are used extensively but, in most infections for which a cephalosporin might be considered, another antibiotic is usually at least as effective, at least as safe and almost certainly much less expensive.

Aminoglycosides

Mechanism

Aminoglycosides are bactericidal. They bind to the 30S subunit of bacterial ribosomes, leading to misreading of m-RNA codons.

Pharmacokinetics

Oral absorption is negligible. They have poor penetration into CSF and only moderate penetration to bile. Otherwise, there is good entry to inflamed tissue. Elimination is mainly by glomerular filtration.

Adverse effects

There are two major adverse reactions, both concentration related: nephrotoxicity and ototoxicity. The renal lesion consists of tubular destruction. Eighth nerve damage can be mainly vestibular (streptomycin, gentamicin) or mainly auditory (kanamycin).

The severity of these reactions is related to aminoglycoside serum concentration, which in turn is related to dose and rate of elimination. Accumulation of drug occurs when glomerular filtration is decreased by renal disease or at the extremes of age. Doses must be modified in these situations and drug concentration monitoring is mandatory. Aminoglycosides cross the placenta and can cause eighth nerve damage in the fetus. An uncommon effect of aminoglycosides is neuromuscular blockade occurring after rapid intravenous injection; this is marked in patients with myasthenia gravis.

Drug interactions

Nephrotoxicity is enhanced by co-administration with cephaloridine or polymyxins. Similarly, ototoxicity is enhanced by loop diuretics. The neuromuscular blockade of curare-like drugs can be prolonged by aminoglycosides.

Antibacterial spectrum

Gentamicin is the most widely used aminoglycoside and is active against all aerobic Gram-negative rods, including pseudomonas and proteus, and also against staphylococci. Most streptococci are resistant because gentamicin cannot penetrate the cell. However, penicillin and aminoglycosides have synergistic effect against some streptococci. Anaerobic organisms are all resistant. Tobramycin is 2–4 times more active against pseudomonas but is otherwise very similar to gentamicin. Amikacin is resistant to most of the bacterial enzymes which inactivate gentamicin and is only indicated for infections caused by aerobic Gram-negative rods against which gentamicin is no longer effective. Netilmicin has a similar antibacterial spectrum to gentamicin, but is claimed to be less ototoxic: confirmatory evidence is limited.

Neomycin is given orally to decrease the bacterial content of the colon in liver failure or before bowel surgery. If there is severe liver or renal failure or inflammatory bowel disease, sufficient neomycin can be absorbed to cause ototoxicity.

Streptomycin is effective against tubercle bacilli and is discussed later.

Doses

Gentamicin: if renal function is normal, the intramuscular dose is 2–5 mg/kg daily given at 8 hourly intervals. Various nomograms and formulae are widely available for calculating dose modifications in renal impairment. A rough guide, based on creatinine clearance, is: >70 ml/min 8 hourly; 30–70 ml/min 12 hourly; 10–30 ml/min 24 hourly; 5–10 ml/min 48 hourly. It must be emphasized that rules of thumb are not a substitute for drug level monitoring.

Tobramycin: 3–5 mg/kg daily given in divided doses 8 hourly. Modify dose in renal failure.

Amikacin: 15 mg/kg daily in 12 hourly doses. Modify dose in renal failure.

Netilmicin: 4–6 mg/kg daily in divided doses.

Comment

The major role of aminoglycosides is the parenteral treatment of serious infection caused by sensitive organisms. These drugs are popular for the initial management of life-threatening septicaemia of uncertain aetiology. In this situation an aminoglycoside is usually combined with metronidazole and/or an extended spectrum penicillin.

Sulphonamide–trimethoprim combinations

Mechanism

These drugs are bactericidal. Co-trimoxazole contains a sulphonamide, sulphamethoxazole, and trimethoprim in the ratio 5:1. The basis of the action of sulphonamides is that bacterial cells are impermeable to folic acid so must synthesize their own from *p*-aminobenzoic acid, with which sulphonamides have a strong similarity. Thus, competitive inhibition of folic acid synthesis occurs. Trimethoprim blocks the next synthetic step, from folic acid to tetrahydrofolate, by inhibiting the enzyme dihydrofolate reductase.

Pharmacokinetics

Co-trimoxazole is well absorbed following oral administration and is also available for intravenous use. There is wide tissue distribution and elimination is by renal excretion.

Adverse effects

The sulphonamide component can cause rashes and, much less commonly, Stevens–Johnson syndrome, renal failure and blood dyscrasias. Trimethoprim can also cause rashes and impaired haemopoiesis and can produce gastro-intestinal symptoms. The trimethoprim component has been implicated in terato-genesis. In the newborn, sulphonamides can displace bilirubin from protein binding sites and cause kernicterus.

Drug interactions

The sulphonamide component competes for hepatic enzyme binding sites and can decrease the clearance of phenytoin, tolbutamide and warfarin sufficiently to produce phenytoin toxicity, hypoglycaemia and enhanced anticoagulation, respectively. Displacement of methotrexate from protein binding sites can also lead to toxicity.

Antibacterial spectrum

These drugs have a broad spectrum, including Gram-positive cocci, *Neisseria gonorrheae*, *Haemophilus influenzae*, *E. coli*, *Proteus mirabilis*, *Shigella* species, *Salmonella* species, *Pneumocystis carinii* and *Brucella* species.

Dose

Co-trimoxazole: 960 mg (two tablets of 400 mg sulphamethoxazole, 80 mg trimethoprim) 12 hourly for oral or intravenous administration (children, 120–480 mg 12 hourly, depending on age).

Comment

The combination of sulphonamide and trimethoprim is the treatment of first choice in urinary tract infections but is also a good alternative regimen in several other conditions, including typhoid fever, exacerbation of chronic bronchitis and gonorrhoea in penicillin-sensitive patients.

Trimethoprim alone is also used in treating urinary tract and respiratory infections. Dose: 300 mg daily or 100 mg daily for prophylaxis.

Tetracyclines

Mechanism

Tetracyclines are bacteriostatic, binding to the 30S ribosomal subunit with consequent misreading of information for protein synthesis.

Pharmacokinetics

Tetracyclines are adequately absorbed following oral administration. Tissue distribution is good and the drugs are eliminated mainly unmetabolized by biliary excretion.

Adverse effects

Tetracyclines bind to calcium in bones and teeth, leading to impaired bone growth and discoloration of teeth during active mineralization (up to 7 years). Tetracyclines cross the placenta and are contra-indicated in pregnancy. Following large doses, both hepatic necrosis and renal failure have been reported. Except for doxycycline and minocycline, these drugs are contra-indicated in renal failure because they impair protein synthesis and so enhance the effects of catabolism. Many patients develop diarrhoea on tetracycline therapy.

Drug interactions

Milk, antacids, calcium, magnesium and iron form insoluble complexes with tetracyclines in the gut lumen, leading to treatment failure, the exception being minocycline.

Antibacterial spectrum

The tetracyclines are effective against a wide range of bacteria but resistance is increasing, and they should no longer be considered useful broad spectrum antibiotics. The importance of tetracyclines is based on their efficacy against chlamydia (e.g. non-specific urethritis, psittacosis), rickettsia (e.g. Q fever, typhus, Rocky Mountain spotted fever), mycoplasma, brucella and cholera. In these infections, tetracyclines are the drugs of first choice. Tetracyclines are also useful adjuncts to the treatment of acne by preventing the growth of *Propionibacterium acnes* in the pustules. The other specific indication for a tetracycline is the use of minocycline for meningococcal prophylaxis.

Dose

Tetracycline and oxytetracycline: 250–500 mg 6 hourly.
Minocycline: 200 mg then 100 mg 12 hourly.

Other antibacterial drugs

Metronidazole

Metronidazole is initially used in protozoal infections, but later found to be very effective against anaerobic bacteria, including *Bacteroides fragilis*. It is currently popular in treating serious anaerobic infections. In addition, metronidazole is often combined with gentamicin in treating serious mixed infections or septicaemia of uncertain aetiology. The other major uses are in treating trichomonal vaginitis, amoebiasis and giardiasis. The only major adverse effects are peripheral neuropathy following prolonged therapy and seizures following high doses.

Dose

For severe infections, intravenous infusion of metronidazole is given at the rate of 500 mg every 8 hours in adults and 7.5 mg/kg 12 hourly in children for 7 days.

Oral: 200 mg 8 hourly for 7 days for trichomoniasis and 2 g daily for 3 days in amoebiasis and giardiasis. If appropriate, suppositories can be used in circumstances where intravenous infusion might be considered: similar blood levels but much cheaper. Dose: 1 g 8 hourly.

Erythromycin

Erythromycin has an antibacterial spectrum similar to penicillin and is a suitable second-line drug for patients allergic to penicillin. It is currently the drug of choice for *Legionella pneumophilia*, it is of some value in whooping cough prophylaxis and is effective against *Mycoplasma*. It is also used in chlamydial non-specific urethritis and campylobacter enteritis. The only major adverse effect is cholestatic jaundice associated primarily with the estolate formulation. This formulation is therefore contra-indicated in liver disease.

Dose

Oral: 250–500 mg 6 hourly for adults, 125–250 mg 6 hourly for children.
Intravenous: 300 mg by infusion 6 hourly, children, 30–50 mg/kg daily in divided doses 6 hourly.

Chloramphenicol

Chloramphenicol is a very effective broad spectrum bacteriostatic antibiotic but use is restricted because of bone marrow suppression, which occurs as a rare complication of treatment. Chloramphenicol is indicated in life-threatening infections for which other agents are unsuitable because of bacterial resistance or patient allergy. The drug is particularly useful in *H. influenzae* meningitis and typhoid fever. Chloramphenicol is contra-indicated in neonates because of cardiovascular collapse (Chapter 4).

Dose

Intravenous: 1 g 6 hourly in adults. Children require 50–100 mg/kg daily, divided into 6 hourly doses.

Fusidic acid

This drug has a narrow spectrum and is indicated in combination with another antistaphylococcal drug only in serious penicillin-resistant staphylococcal infections, e.g. those of bone.

Dose

Fusidic acid is given at a dose of 500 mg 8 hourly by intravenous infusion or orally.

Clindamycin

Clindamycin is effective against penicillin-resistant staphylococci and many anaerobic organisms. However, a major adverse effect is pseudomembranous colitis caused by a toxin produced by *Clostridium difficile*, and clindamycin is indicated only in serious conditions where other agents are contra-indicated, or ineffective, notably staphylococcal bone and joint infections.

Dose

0.6–2.7 g clindamycin daily are given in divided doses by slow intravenous infusion; children, 15–40 mg/kg daily in divided doses.

Nitrofurantoin

Nitrofurantoin, an orally administered drug which achieves antibacterial concentrations only in urine, is effective against many organisms infecting the urinary tract. However, it is a second-line drug for this indication because of frequent adverse effects, including gastrointestinal symptoms and rashes. It precipitates haemolytic anaemia in glucose-6-phosphate deficiency and can cause peripheral neuropathy and pulmonary fibrosis.

Vancomycin

Vancomycin is effective against *Cl. difficile* and is given orally to treat pseudomembranous colitis. It is also used intravenously in the prophylaxis and treatment of endocarditis caused by Gram-positive cocci.

Quinolones

Nalidixic acid, the first quinolone, has been available for 30 years. Administered orally, it achieves low tissue concentrations and its use is restricted to the treatment of uncomplicated urinary tract infections. Chemical modifications have produced a series of improved drugs and the most recent are the 4-fluoroquinolones; ciprofloxacin is the first agent in this group available in the UK.

Ciprofloxacin

Mechanism

Bactericidal in action, ciprofloxacin inhibits DNA-gyrase activity by binding to chromosomal DNA strands. This interferes with DNA replication and prevents supercoiling within the chromosome.

Pharmacokinetics

It is well absorbed after oral administration and is distributed rapidly into body tissues. Most of the drug is eliminated unaltered by the kidneys; the remainder is excreted by hepatic metabolism or unchanged in the faeces.

Adverse effects

The most frequently reported side effects are minor gastrointestinal upsets, and severe systemic adverse reactions are rare. However, CNS disturbances such as insomnia, confusion and convulsions have been reported. Since it can cause damage to cartilage in young animals, ciprofloxacin is contra-indicated in children and growing adolescents.

Drug interactions

Its absorption is reduced significantly by the coadministration of aluminium and magnesium antacids. It interferes with the metabolism of theophylline, caffeine and warfarin so that the toxic effects of these drugs may be encountered if they are given along with ciprofloxacin.

Antibacterial spectrum

It is active against a broad spectrum of both aerobic Gram-negative bacteria, including *Ps. aeruginosa*, and Gram-positive bacteria: staphylococci are more sensitive than streptococci. Anaerobes, in general, are resistant. Ciproflaxacin is particularly useful for pseudomonas infections where oral therapy is preferred, such as urinary tract infection or respiratory tract infection in patients with cystic fibrosis. It is very effective in gastrointestinal infections ranging from traveller's diarrhoea to typhoid fever.

Dose

Oral: 250–750 mg 12 hourly; intravenous: 100–200 mg 12 hourly.

Comments

Ciprofloxacin is an important new drug but there is no reason why it should replace established, effective and much less expensive antibiotics for the majority of urinary and respiratory infections.

10.3 ANTITUBERCULOUS DRUGS

Isoniazid

Mechanism

The precise mechanism is unknown, but it is bactericidal.

Pharmacokinetics

Isoniazid is well absorbed following oral administration and is widely distributed, including the CSF where concentrations equal those in blood. Isoniazid is inactivated in the liver by pathways including genetically dependent acetylation. The same metabolic pathway is involved in the acetylation of hydralazine, procainamide and dapsone (Chapter 1, Section 1.3). About 50% of European and USA population are slow acetylators but the proportion varies widely in other populations, and slow acetylation is very common in orientals.

Adverse effects

Peripheral neuropathy occurs mainly in slow acetylators and can be prevented by coadministration of pyridoxine (20 mg/day). Hepatotoxicity occasionally occurs and is more frequent in the elderly and those with a large alcohol intake. Very high doses of isoniazid can lead to psychosis, convulsions or coma.

Drug interactions

Isoniazid inhibits enzymes which metabolize phenytoin and warfarin, so phenytoin concentrations and anticoagulation level should be carefully monitored.

Dose

Oral: 3 mg/kg adults or 6 mg/kg daily in children, i.e. children require more on a weight basis. For tuberculous meningitis, 10 mg/kg daily. Also available for parenteral use.

Rifampicin

Mechanism

It is bactericidal, and inhibits the DNA dependent RNA polymerase of mycobacteria.

Pharmacokinetics

Rifampicin is well absorbed following oral administration and widely distributed, including the CSF. It is deacetylated in the liver and eliminated by biliary excretion.

Adverse effects

There is often a transient elevation of liver enzymes but serious hepatotoxicity is uncommon. The risk of liver damage is increased by alcoholism and pre-existing liver disease. Intermittent treatment is associated with more frequent and serious adverse effects, including renal failure and thrombocytopaenia. Rifampicin causes red urine, tears and sputum.

Drug interactions

Rifampicin induces hepatic enzymes and, because of increased clearance, can cause treatment failure with oral contraceptives, sulphonylureas, warfarin, steroids and barbiturates.

Dose

Rifampicin is given at a dose of 10 mg/kg daily before breakfast.

Ethambutol

Mechanism

The mechanism is uncertain but bacteriostatic.

Pharmacokinetics

Ethambutol is well absorbed following oral administration. It has poor penetration to CSF but otherwise is adequately distributed. Excretion of unchanged drug is mainly renal.

Adverse effects

The most important reaction is retrobulbar neuritis with loss of visual acuity and colour vision. This is largely preventable by using doses below 25 mg/kg daily. The visual defect usually reverses over several months after stopping the drug.

Drug interactions

Aluminium hydroxide can decrease absorption.

Dose

A 15–25 mg/kg daily dose is given.

Pyrazinamide

Mechanism

Pyrazinamide is bactericidal.

Pharmacokinetics

It is well absorbed following oral administration and has good penetration to CSF. It is eliminated by renal excretion.

Adverse effects

Pyrazinamide causes hepatotoxicity and arthralgia. Dose modification is required in patients with renal impairment.

Dose

A 20–30 mg/kg daily dose is given up to a maximum of 3 g.

Second-line drugs

Streptomycin is now infrequently used. It is an aminoglycoside which is eliminated by the kidneys. Ototoxicity is the main adverse reaction. Streptomycin could particularly be considered for use in patients with liver disease. Several other agents are available for use in situations of bacterial resistance or adverse reactions to first-line drugs, e.g. capreomycin, cycloserine, ethionamide and *p*-aminosalicylic acid.

Comment
Mycobacterium tuberculosis multiplies slowly and the long periods of treatment required encourage the emergence of resistant strains. Combination chemotherapy is thus the basis of treatment. Initially, isoniazid, rifampicin and either ethambutol or pyrazinamide are administered for 8 weeks. Subsequently, isoniazid and rifampicin are given. Six months of treatment with this regimen is adequate for pulmonary TB. If other drugs are used, 9 months of therapy is necessary. If TB occurs elsewhere, or if intermittent therapy is used, 12–18 months is required.

10.4 ANTIFUNGAL DRUGS

Amphotericin B

Mechanism

Amphotericin B combines with sterols in the plasma membrane, with a resulting increase in permeability and cell death.

Pharmacokinetics

Absorption is negligible following oral administration. In practice it is usually given intravenously. It is highly protein bound with apparently poor penetration to tissues and body fluids. It is not removed by haemodialysis. The mode of elimination is unknown but it is not influenced by renal function.

Adverse effects

These are very common. Most patients develop fever, chills and nausea. Nephrotoxicity (distal tubular destruction and calcification) usually occurs during prolonged treatment at or above 1 mg/kg daily and manifests as hypokalaemia, loss of concentrating ability and renal tubular acidosis; nephrotoxicity reverses if detected early.

Drug interaction

It is additive with other nephrotoxic drugs. Concurrent digoxin therapy can become toxic if hypokalaemia develops.

Antifungal spectrum

It is currently the drug of choice for most systemic mycoses: active against *Cryptococcus*, *Candida* and other yeasts, *Aspergillus*, *Coccidioides* and other fungi. Resistance has not been reported.

Dose

A 1 mg test dose is given, then 250 μg/kg daily, increasing to 1–1.5 mg daily depending on disease severity and appearance of nephrotoxicity. Hydrocortisone can reduce febrile reactions and chlorpromazine can reduce nausea.

Comment

Amphotericin B is an example of risks and benefits of treatment having to be carefully weighed. It is highly toxic but untreated systemic mycoses are invariably fatal.

Flucytosine

Mechanism

It is deaminated inside the fungal cell to 5-fluorouracil, which inhibits nucleic acid synthesis with cell death.

Pharmacokinetics

It is well absorbed following oral administration and is widely distributed, including the CSF. Elimination is mainly renal. Clearance is decreased in patients with renal impairment.

Adverse effects

Concentration related bone marrow suppression is the only major problem. This can usually be avoided by drug level monitoring.

Antifungal spectrum

It is only active against yeasts; efficacy is limited by rapid emergence of resistance.

Dose

150–200 mg flucytosine are given daily in divided doses.

Comment

Although much less toxic than amphotericin, flucytosine is of limited value because of its narrow spectrum and the existence of resistant organisms. It is usually administered together with amphotericin B.

Imidazoles and related compounds

Mechanism

Imidazoles increase permeability by preventing ergosterol formation in cell membranes. They also produce cell necrosis by inhibiting peroxidative enzymes.

Miconazole, clotrimazole, econazole

Pharmacokinetics

These drugs are poorly absorbed following oral administration and are usually restricted for topical use.

Antifungal spectrum

They are active against a wide range of yeasts and fungi. Their main use is topical, e.g. athlete's foot or vaginal candidiasis.

Fluconazole, itraconazole, ketoconazole

Pharmacokinetics

Following oral administration these drugs are widely distributed; adequate CSF levels are obtained with the exception of ketoconazole. Fluconazole is eliminated by the kidneys; itraconazole and ketoconazole are metabolized by the liver.

Antifungal spectrum

They are active against a wide range of yeasts and fungi; fluconazole is particularly effective against yeasts and itraconazole against filamentous fungi, e.g. *Aspergillus*.

Adverse effects

Hepatotoxicity is particularly associated with ketoconazole, which requires monitoring of liver function.

Doses

Fluconazole: 100–400 mg orally or by intravenous infusion, daily single dose.
Itraconazole: 100–200 mg orally, daily single dose.
Ketoconazole: 200–400 mg orally, daily single dose.

Nystatin

Nystatin is used topically in the treatment of yeast infections of the skin and mucous membranes. It is not used parenterally because of high toxicity.

Griseofulvin

Griseofulvin is active only against dermatophytes and is given orally in the treatment of skin or nail infections. It is fungistatic so must be given for weeks or months. It diminishes the anticoagulant effect by enzyme induction. Barbiturates lead to griseofulvin treatment failure by enzyme induction. Griseofulvin can precipitate porphyria.

10.5 ANTIVIRAL DRUGS

These are the least developed as a group of antimicrobial agents: viruses use the biochemical system of their host cells, and it is therefore difficult to prevent viral multiplication without seriously damaging the patient. However, effective therapy is now available for a number of virus infections of clinical importance.

Acyclovir

Mechanism

The pharmacological effect of acyclovir depends on its conversion to an active metabolite by a herpes simplex coded enzyme, thymidine kinase. It is only phosphorylated in herpes infected cells and normal cellular processes are unaffected. The resulting acyclovir triphosphate inhibits herpes-specified DNA polymerase, preventing further viral DNA synethesis. The herpes genome in latently (non-replicating) infected cells is not altered during antiviral therapy. Varicella zoster virus is also susceptible to acyclovir but its action is not thymidine kinase dependent.

Pharmacokinetics

Acyclovir is adequately absorbed orally in patients with normal gut function. It is eliminated by renal clearance involving glomerular filtration and tubular secretion. Acyclovir penetrates the blood–brain barrier passively to enter CSF.

Adverse effects

Renal impairment occasionally follows intravenous administration.

Drug interactions

No clinically important interactions have been observed yet.

Clinical use

Acyclovir is indicated for herpes simplex and varicella/zoster infections of the skin and mucous membranes, the brain and in lung disease and in prophylaxis against herpes infections in immunocompromised hosts. An intravenous route is required for serious disease manifestions and in immunocompromised patients.

Dose

For herpes simplex: oral, 200 mg five times per day for 5 days; intravenous,

5 mg/kg over 1 h, repeated every 8 h (10 mg/kg in herpes encephalitis). A dose modification is necessary in renal failure.

For varicella zoster: oral, 800 mg five times per day for 7 days; intravenous, 10 mg/kg 8 hourly.

Idoxuridine

Idoxuridine is a thymidine analogue which inhibits DNA synthesis. It is highly toxic when given systemically and is therefore only used topically in the treatment of herpes simplex infections of the eye, as an aqueous solution, and in dimethyl sulphoxide for skin eruptions. Shingles can be treated similarly.

Vidarabine

Vidarabine inhibits DNA but does not target a specific virus. It has been used systemically in the treatment of chicken pox or herpes zoster infections in immunocompromised hosts but has been largely superseded by acyclovir owing to the low toxicity of acyclovir. It has been shown to decrease the early mortality in herpes simplex encephalitis. The major adverse reactions are suppression of bone marrow and a wide range of neurological effects.

Amantadine

Amantadine (including its analogue, rimantadine) prevents entry of influenza A to host cells and is used predominantly in prophylaxis but also in the treatment of infections caused by this virus. Influenza B virus is not susceptible. Amantadine can produce neurological side effects but usually only if high concentrations are achieved, e.g. in renal failure.

Ribavirin

Ribavirin inhibits a number of DNA and RNA viruses. Its antiviral action has been demonstrated *in vitro* and *in vivo* against a number of important viruses, including respiratory syncytial virus (RSV), influenza A and B viruses, parainfluenza 1 and 3 and Lassa fever virus. The mechanism of action is not completely understood but involves the action of ribavirin triphosphate interfering with the binding of viral messenger RNA to ribosomes. It is predominantly used in the form of a nebulized aerosol in the treatment of bronchitis in infancy due to RSV infection.

Zidovudine (azidothymidine, AZT)

Mechanism

AZT is phosphorylated in both infected and uninfected cells by thymidine kinase and subsequently by other kinases to triphosphate, which is a chain terminator in DNA synthesis. Human immunodeficiency virus (HIV) is not eradicated during or following treatment.

Pharmacokinetics

It is well absorbed from the gut; CSF levels are 50% of plasma levels. It is eliminated by glucuronidation.

Adverse effects

There is serious haematological toxicity: anaemia and neutropaenia are seen in up to one-third of patients treated with AZT.

Clinical use

AZT is indicated in:

1 Serious manifestations of HIV infections in patients with acquired immunodeficiency syndrome or AIDS-related complex. It has been shown to prolong life in this group of patients.

2 Early symptomatic or asymptomatic HIV infection, with markers indicating risk of disease progression.

Dose

200 mg AZT 4 hourly for symptomatic disease.
500 mg AZT daily for asymptomatic patients.
Dose modification is required in anaemia, myelosuppression, renal and hepatic impairment, pregnancy and the elderly.

Ganciclovir

Mechanism

Ganciclovir is an acyclic analogue structurally related to acyclovir. It acts as a substrate for viral DNA polymerase and as a chain terminator aborting virus replication.

Pharmacokinetics

It is excreted primarily unchanged in the kidneys and is largely unbound in plasma. Renal impairment leads to altered kinetics.

Adverse effects

Neutropenia occurs in 40% of patients but is usually reversible. It occurs after 1 week of induction therapy. There is occasional rash, nausea and vomiting.

Drug interactions

No drug interactions have been observed as yet.

Clinical use

Ganciclovir is indicated for life-threatening cytomegalovirus (CMV) infections in immunocompromised individuals, particularly with AIDS or transplanted organs, and in the treatment and prevention of CMV retinitis in these patients.

Dose

Intravenous: 5 mg/kg over 1 h every 12 h for 14 days.
Dose reduction is required in patients with impaired renal function.

Chapter 11
Drugs and Respiratory Disease

11.1 DRUGS AND AIRFLOW OBSTRUCTION

Aims

The aim of treatment in airflow obstruction is to increase ventilation by reducing bronchial smooth muscle tone with specific agonist and antagonist drugs and by blocking the mechanisms of inflammatory and allergic responses.

Relevant pathophysiology

The autonomic nervous system is an important regulator of smooth muscle tone in the airways and this is the main factor which determines airflow resistance. Bronchial smooth muscle tone depends on a complex balance between different bronchoconstrictor and bronchodilator influences.

Bronchoconstrictor influences

1 Cholinergic efferent vagal nerves release acetylcholine at muscarinic receptors in airway smooth muscle. This is the main motor nerve supply to the airways.

2 Non-cholinergic excitatory nerves are thought to release tachykinins such as substance P. The importance of these nerves in man is unknown.

3 Humoral factors such as histamine, leukotrienes and platelet activating factor which may be involved in inflammatory and allergic responses.

Bronchodilator influences

1 Circulating catecholamines which stimulate β_2-adrenoceptors.

2 Sympathetic nerve supply to the airway smooth muscle is sparse but these nerves may reduce airway tone via an inhibitory effect on presynaptic cholinergic efferent vagal nerves.

3 Non-adrenergic non-cholinergic (NANC) inhibitory nerves; the neurotransmitter is unknown but may be nitric oxide.

In normal man there is a degree of resting airway tone due to cholinergic vagal nerve input. In airway diseases abnormalities in the neural control of the airways may contribute to the increase in airflow resistance.

Asthma

Asthma is characterized by airflow obstruction which is reversible either spontaneously or as a result of treatment. The increase in airflow resistance is due to bronchospasm, mucosal oedema and increased airway secretions. In some asthmatic patients attacks can be provoked by specific triggers, such as allergens, some occupational agents or non-steroidal anti-inflammatory drugs. Other non-specific triggers, such as exercise, irritants or cold air, will produce asthma in most, if not all, asthmatic patients.

Asthma developing in childhood is usually associated with increased levels of allergen-specific IgE antibodies and there is often a family or personal history of hay fever or eczema. This type of asthma is often termed extrinsic or early onset asthma.

Late onset asthma characteristically develops in adults, usually after the age of 30 years, and symptoms tend to be persistent. Allergen-specific IgE levels are usually not raised. This type of asthma is often termed intrinsic asthma.

Chronic airflow obstruction

Chronic obstructive airways disease is usually associated with cigarette smoking and is characterized by a progressive decline in airways calibre over many years. The airways obstruction is predominantly irreversible.

This classification is not exclusive and many patients do not readily fit into a single category. Of more importance is the functional assessment of the response which can be obtained to bronchodilator drugs by measuring their effect on peak flow rate or spirometric measurements. In difficult cases a trial of steroids (prednisolone, 30–40 mg/day for 10–14 days) may be necessary to assess the full degree of reversibility of airflow obstruction.

Drugs used in the treatment of airways obstruction

The main groups of drugs used in the treatment of airflow obstruction are:

1 β-Adrenoceptor agonists, which increase cyclic AMP in bronchial muscle cells and mast cells.

2 Theophylline and related methylxanthines, which may also increase intra-cellular cyclic AMP.

3 Anticholinergic (muscarinic) drugs, which reduce cholinergic bronchocon-striction.

4 Anti-allergy drugs, which inhibit mediator release or antagonize mediator effects.

5 Corticosteroids, which may improve pulmonary function in all obstructive airways disease by unidentified mechanisms.

β_2-Adrenoceptor agonists

Salbutamol, terbutaline, salmeterol

Mechanism

These selective β_2-adrenoceptor stimulants act on the bronchi and small airways. They have less β_1-effect than adrenaline or isoprenaline, which are non-selective and can be regarded as obsolete. Relaxation of bronchial smooth muscle is mediated by increased intracellular cyclic AMP. β_2-Stimulants are best given by inhalation as this delivers the drug directly to the site of action, maximizes the selective bronchodilator effect and minimizes generalized systemic effects. The total dose required by aerosol is very much lower than that required by mouth or intravenously, further limiting dose related adverse effects. Duration of action is: short-acting β_2-agonists (salbutamol, terbutaline) 4–6 h; long-acting β_2-agonist (salmeterol) 8–12 h.

Adverse effects

These agents may cause tremor by stimulating skeletal muscle β_2-receptors and hypokalaemia by stimulating cell membrane β_2-receptors, which in turn stimulate the Na^+/K^+ pump on skeletal muscle. Other dose dependent adverse effects result from β_1 activity and include tachycardia. These effects are rare, however, with the higher degree of selectivity afforded by the aerosol route of administration.

Clinical use and dose

Short-acting β_2-agonists (salbutamol, terbutaline) are used in asthma and chronic airflow obstruction, as long-term prophylactic or maintenance therapy (pressurized aerosol or oral tablets) or in acute attacks by nebulizer. Typical recommended dosage is: by pressurized aerosol inhalation, 0.1–0.2 mg four to six times daily; by nebulizer, 2 ml of a 0.5% solution four times daily or 1–2 mg/h. These should be regarded as starting doses, which may require to be increased to achieve maximum effect in an individual patient.

Long-acting β_2-agonist salmeterol is used in patients with asthma in whom control of symptoms is poor in spite of high-dose inhaled corticosteroid treatments. It can be given by pressurized aerosol inhalation or by a dry powder device in a dose of 50–100 mg twice daily. Although there have been claims that salmeterol may additionally improve symptoms by an anti-inflammatory effect, there are also concerns that its slow onset of effect may have disadvantages in the acutely ill asthmatic.

Other selective β_2-stimulants

A number of other β_2-agonists are available, including isoetharine, rimiterol, reproterol and pirbuterol. These agents are either less selective or shorter acting and have no clear advantages.

Comment

β_2-Adrenoceptor agonists given by aerosol inhalation relieve bronchospasm with minimal adverse cardiac effects in patients with reversible airways obstruction. Response depends on the patient using the pressurized aerosol correctly.

By the aerosol route only about 10% of the dose reaches the airways, although this amount is usually sufficient to produce significant bronchodilation.

Many patients experience difficulties in using pressurized aerosol inhalers correctly. For those patients who after instruction are still unable to use a pressurized aerosol inhaler correctly there are a variety of devices which are often helpful. These include dry powder inhalers, spacing devices attached to a metered dose inhaler or nebulizers.

Theophylline

Mechanism

Theophylline is 1,3-dimethyl xanthine. The alkyl group at the 3-position is responsible for its bronchodilator effect; that at the 1-position (which it shares with caffeine and theobromine) produces CNS stimulation and weak diuretic effects. The exact mechanism of action is not clear. It was proposed that it was due to inhibition of phosphodiesterase isoenzymes, leading to increased intracellular cAMP concentrations. Alternative proposals include antagonism of adenosine receptors or actions on transmembrane calcium.

Pharmacokinetics

Theophylline is nearly totally absorbed from the gut. It is extensively metabolized by the liver and differences in hepatic metabolism are the principal reason for the wide variability in pharmacokinetics, both between individuals and within the same individual during the course of an illness (Chapters 1 and 2). There is a well defined relationship between concentration and effect, but response varies from individual to individual. The maximum response may be limited by structural damage to the lungs or by adverse effects at plasma concentrations in excess of about 25 mg/l. The average elimination half-life in adults is about 8–12 h. Theophylline is usually given two or three times daily by mouth and there is great advantage in using slow-release preparations to minimize the differences between peak and trough concentrations. The exact dosage schedule depends on the assessment of clearance in individual patients (see example, Chapter 2, Section 2.4). In children and young adults, theophylline clearance is relatively high, necessitating higher daily doses than those used in elderly patients, particularly those with congestive cardiac failure or respiratory failure where theophylline clearance may be significantly reduced (Chapters 2 and 3).

Adverse effects

Tachycardia, palpitations, nausea, vomiting and convulsions are associated with plasma levels above 25–30 mg/l. Nausea may occur at therapeutic plasma levels.

Clinical use and dose

Theophylline is used orally in the long-term treatment of asthma and chronic airflow obstruction in those patients who show a response to it. Several slow-release tablet formulations are available. The dose should be adjusted using therapeutic response, adverse effects and, if available, pharmacokinetic information based on plasma level measurements. The dose ranges from 200 to 600 mg two or three times daily. Theophylline is rapidly absorbed as a suppository although this method of administration is not now recommended.

Aminophylline contains theophylline and ethylenediamine (2:1); only the theophylline has a therapeutic effect. It can be given orally (450–1250 mg/day in divided doses) or by suppository. Aminophylline is occasionally used intravenously in the treatment of:

1 Severe acute attacks of asthma (status asthmaticus).

2 Exacerbations of chronic airflow obstruction.

A loading dose of 5 mg/kg (250–500 mg) is given over 15–20 min intravenously. Intravenous infusion (0.5–0.9 mg/kg/h) may be continued, but it is advisable to seek clinical pharmacokinetic advice if the infusion has to be maintained for more than 4–6 hours. Aminophylline treatment should be considered only in patients not previously taking oral xanthine preparations because of problems with toxicity.

Comment

Oral theophylline preparations are useful as second-line bronchodilators in the long-term treatment of asthma and the reversible component of chronic airflow obstruction. A useful bronchodilator response can often be achieved within the therapeutic range and adverse effects can be minimized with the aid of plasma level measurements.

Anti-allergy drugs

Sodium cromoglycate, nedocromil sodium and ketotifen

Mechanism

These drugs are not bronchodilators. Their mechanism of action in the treatment of asthma is unclear. They stabilize sensitized mast cells and inhibit the release of bronchoconstrictor mediators such as histamine and prostaglandins. Sodium cromoglycate and nedocromil sodium may also inhibit some neural reflexes in the lung, as well as having inhibitory effects on neutrophils and eosinophils. Ketotifen has H_1-receptor antagonist properties.

Clinical use and dose

These drugs are used in the prophylaxis of asthma. They are of no value in patients with chronic airflow obstruction. They have no effect in the treatment of acute attacks as their effect develops only on repeated, regular administration.

Sodium cromoglycate is useful in extrinsic (allergic) asthma, particularly in children and young adults, and can prevent exercise induced asthma. Response in late-onset asthma is usually disappointing.

Sodium cromoglycate can be administered to the lungs by inhalation from a spinhaler as a powder (20 mg four times daily) or from a metered dose pressurized inhaler as an aerosol (10 mg/2 puffs) four times daily. There is also a nebulizer solution (10 mg/ml).

Nedocromil sodium can inhibit exercise induced asthma and may have a role in the treatment of adult patients with asthma in whom symptoms are not controlled with inhaled bronchodilators alone. It is less effective than inhaled corticosteroids.

Nedocromil sodium is administered from a metered dose inhaler (4 mg/2 puffs) two to four times daily.

Ketotifen is given orally as tablets or capsules, 1–2 mg daily. Its usefulness is controversial. Sedation and dry mouth may result from additional antihistaminic effects.

Corticosteroids

The actions of corticosteroids on the bronchi are not fully understood, but they may contribute to:

1 Anti-inflammatory activity.

2 Reduction of mucosal oedema.

3 Modification of immune responses.

4 Increased β-adrenoceptor responsiveness to agonists. The actions of corticosteroids and their adverse effects are discussed in Chapter 14, Section 14.1.

In the management of airways obstruction, corticosteroids can be given by the following routes:

Inhalation.
Orally.
Intravenously.

Inhalation

Topical steroid aerosols represent a significant advance in the management of bronchospasm because generalized adverse effects associated with systemic routes of administration are minimized. Beclomethasone, betamethasone and budesonide are administered by regular aerosol inhalation, the dose depending on the particular drug.

Adverse effects of inhaled steroids include infection of the pharynx and larynx with candidiasis and laxity of the vocal cords causing hoarseness. High doses of inhaled steroids (beclomethasone dipropionate, 1.5 mg/day, and budesonide, 1.6 mg/day) may cause minor degrees of adrenal suppression.

Intravenous corticosteroids

In acute severe asthma with respiratory failure hydrocortisone is given intravenously (100–200 mg or more). The dose can be repeated 4 hourly but it is important to note that there is a delay of up to 6 h in the onset of any steroid induced bronchodilator effect and other measures should be pursued aggressively at the same time, i.e. nebulized bronchodilators and supplementary oxygen.

Oral corticosteroids

Patients with severe exacerbations of asthma require high doses of prednisolone by mouth after intravenous hydrocortisone.

Steroids are started at 40 mg/day and continued at this dose until asthma symptoms are controlled; it often takes 5–7 days but sometimes longer. Thereafter, the steroid dose can be discontinued or it can be tailed down until the minimal dose required to control symptoms has been reached. Other anti-asthma treatment must be reviewed to assess whether any alterations are required, e.g. increase in dose of inhaled steroid therapy.

Comment

Aerosol inhalation of corticosteroids should replace long-term oral corticosteroid therapy whenever possible as the benefits of drug treatment can be obtained without the adverse consequences of long-term systemic steroid treatment.

Anticholinergic drugs

Ipratropium bromide, oxitropium bromide

Mechanism

The parasympathetic cholinergic bronchoconstrictor effect can be blocked by atropine-like drugs. Usually the effect of anticholinergics on airway resistance is less than that of the sympathetic agents, being restricted to abolishing the bronchoconstrictor effect of vagal tone. Ipratropium bromide is a synthetic derivative of atropine which has very few adverse effects when administered by inhalation. Oxitropium bromide is a quaternary ammonium compound derived from scopolamine.

Clinical use and dose

Ipratropium is given as 40–80 μg three or four times daily by pressurized aerosol or from a nebulizer (500 μg four times daily). Oxitropium is given in a dose of 200 μg (2 puffs) two to three times daily by pressurized aerosol.

The management of airways obstruction

Chronic asthma

1 Patients with extrinsic asthma should avoid known allergens, e.g. house dust mite, animals. This is usually difficult and often proves to be of little therapeutic value.

2 Remember occupational causes of asthma, e.g. isocyanates and flour. These are an important but relatively uncommon cause of asthma.

3 All asthmatic patients should avoid β-adrenoceptor antagonists. Aspirin-sensitive asthmatics (approximately 5% of all cases of asthma) should avoid all non-steroidal anti-inflammatory drugs.

4 Drug treatment includes an inhaled β_2-receptor agonist with the early use of inhaled prophylactic therapy, i.e. inhaled steroids, sodium cromoglycate or nedocromil sodium. Inhaled steroids are the most effective of these prophylactic agents. If symptoms persist, a long-acting β_2-agonist or an oral xanthine may be required. Despite the use of the above drugs, a small percentage of patients with severe chronic asthma will require in addition a daily maintenance dose of oral prednisolone.

5 Short courses of oral prednisolone (see section on oral corticosteroids) should be given for exacerbations of asthma which are not severe enough to require emergency hospital admission.

6 Serial peak expiratory flow rate measurements are helpful in the assessment of the adequacy of asthma control.

7 Remember to check inhaler technique; 20–40% of patients cannot use a metered dose inhaler correctly. If there is a problem, one of the inhaler devices should be used.

8 Patients' education about asthma is essential, and this should include written instructions on what the patients should do if their asthma control deteriorates.

Comment
Asthma is a common condition affecting 10% of children and 5% of the adult population. Recent surveys indicate that it is frequently underdiagnosed and undertreated.

Acute severe asthma (status asthmaticus)

1 Clinical assessment may be misleading. Repeated blood gas measurements and peak expiratory flow rate should be used to assess the severity of the attack and the response to treatment.
2 High concentration oxygen therapy is indicated since hypoxia is acute.
3 Aerosol β_2-agonist is best administered from a nebulizer in the oxygen flow. This route is probably preferable to the intravenous route. The combination of nebulized ipratropium bromide and a β_2-receptor agonist may be more effective than a β_2-agonist alone.
4 Intravenous aminophylline as a loading dose, followed by an intravenous infusion, may be used.
5 Intravenous hydrocortisone as a loading dose, followed by a course of high-dose oral steroids, may be required.
6 Exacerbations are rarely due to bacterial infections and so antibiotics should not be routinely given.
7 Intravenous fluids may be given as dehydration can contribute to the clinical features of status asthmaticus.
8 Sedatives, anxiolytics, opiate analgesics and hypnotics should not be used as central depression of ventilation may worsen respiratory failure.
9 Artificial ventilation may be required if respiratory failure, exhaustion of the respiratory muscles or circulatory collapse occur.

Comment
An asthma attack is a serious condition. Severity is difficult to assess clinically. Asthma may be life-threatening. Failure to respond to the patient's usual treatment is an indication for aggressive intervention with careful monitoring of ventilatory function.

Chronic airflow obstruction

1 Patients should stop smoking.
2 Patients with predominantly irreversible airflow obstruction should not be denied the use of an inhaled bronchodilator (β_2-receptor agonist or anticholinergic drug) since they are likely to obtain some symptomatic benefit from this type of drug.
3 In patients who can be shown to respond to it, oral slow-release theophylline with therapeutic monitoring of plasma levels should be used alone or together with the agents above.
4 Intercurrent chest infections are associated with acute exacerbations and should be treated with a broad spectrum antibiotic.
5 If heart failure (cor pulmonale) develops diuretic therapy is indicated.

Venesection may be indicated for the secondary polycythaemia which is often associated.

6 Patients with severe chronic airflow obstruction who develop respiratory failure with right ventricular failure should be considered for oxygen therapy at low concentration continuously for at least 15 h each day, administered by an oxygen concentrator.

11.2 OXYGEN

The efficiency of carbon dioxide and oxygen exchange in the alveoli of the lungs depends on many factors, including:

1 Alveolar ventilation.
2 Pulmonary blood flow.
3 The matching of ventilation and perfusion.
4 The quantity of haemoglobin in the blood and its affinity for oxygen.

Alveolar ventilation is centrally regulated by a complex mechanism which responds powerfully to oxygen deprivation or carbon dioxide accumulation. When oxygen is given to supplement the amount normally present in inspired air it should be regarded as a drug. Oxygen is given either in as high a concentration as possible or in low (24–28%) controlled concentrations.

High oxygen concentrations

High oxygen concentrations should be given to all hypoxic patients except those with established or potential CO_2 narcosis. Any apparatus which provides an oxygen flow to the oronasal area at a rate of 5 l/min or more is effective in supplying a high concentration of oxygen in the inspired gas. Masks with a dead space volume under 100 ml do not cause carbon dioxide rebreathing; nasal cannulae cause none at all.

Indications for high oxygen concentrations include:

1 Pneumonia.
2 Acute pulmonary oedema.
3 Pulmonary thromboembolism.
4 Fibrosing alveolitis.
5 Acute severe asthma.
6 Acute respiratory failure or arrest (e.g. due to drug overdose).
7 Acute circulatory failure.
8 Severe anaemia.
9 Cyanide and carbon monoxide poisoning.
10 Adult respiratory distress syndrome.

Low (controlled) oxygen concentrations

Low concentration oxygen therapy is reserved for patients with exacerbations of chronic airflow obstruction with respiratory failure. Ventilation is then so ineffective that carbon dioxide excretion is not maintained in spite of a raised arterial $P\text{CO}_2$. The increased $P\text{CO}_2$ leads to a loss of sensitivity of the respiratory centre to CO_2 and a dependence on low arterial $P\text{O}_2$ to drive ventilation. High concentration oxygen administration leads to a further suppression of ventilation by removing the hypoxic drive. Further carbon dioxide accumulation then rapidly produces narcosis and death.

Low concentrations may be administered by masks using the entrainment principle to supply a calibrated inspired oxygen concentration of 24 or 28%. Higher oxygen concentrations can be obtained with similar masks but in these circumstances there is little need for such precision.

Chapter 12
Drugs and Rheumatic Disease

Aims

In inflammatory joint disease, the aims are:

1 To reduce pain.

2 To reduce stiffness and improve mobility.

3 To prevent chronic deformity by minimizing the inflammation which results in synovial membrane proliferation and bone erosions.

Relevant pathophysiology

Anti-inflammatory analgesic drugs are used to relieve the painful symptoms of joint diseases, including:

Rheumatoid arthritis.
Osteoarthritis.
Psoriatic arthritis.
Ankylosing spondylitis.
Gout.
Reactive arthritis (including Reiter's syndrome).
Arthritis associated with systemic lupus erythematosus.

The aetiology of these diseases is varied and in most cases not entirely clear, but with the exception of gout and possibly osteoarthritis there seems to be a disturbance in immune responses. In rheumatoid arthritis, for example, immune complexes composed of immunoglobulins of the IgM type activate complement and release factors which are chemotactic to neutrophil polymorphs. Released lysosomal enzymes damage cartilage while prostaglandins promote synovial vasodilatation and exacerbate pain. Thus there are a number of areas where an anti-inflammatory drug might be effective:

1 Immunosuppression.

2 Inhibition of cell migration.

3 Inhibition of enzyme release.

4 Inhibition of prostaglandin synthesis.

The most potent agents used in rheumatoid arthritis are gold, *n*-penicillamine, sulphasalazine and corticosteroids, but they have major problems associated with their long-term use and are therefore reserved for second-or third-line treatment. Other potent agents are methotrexate, azathioprine, cyclophosphamide and cyclosporin. Initially, symptoms are treated with non-steroidal anti-inflammatory drugs.

12.1 PRINCIPLES OF DRUG TREATMENT

While drugs are an important part of the treatment of patients with inflammatory joint disease, such as rheumatoid arthritis, other aspects demand careful consideration. These include rest, exercise and psychological management.

Rest

Rheumatoid arthritis is typically a disease of exacerbation and remission. During an acute attack it may be necessary to recommend bed rest, with local support and splinting of the affected joints.

Exercise

After an acute attack, carefully graded exercises are required to ensure an early return to normal activities. Either excessive rest or excessive exercise can be harmful.

Psychological management

The patients should be sympathetically introduced to the view that the disease has no ultimate cure. Acute onset and early remission are favourable signs, while an insidious onset or gradual deterioration with no remission over a year herald an unfavourable prognosis.

Various physical aids are available to make domestic life easier for the more severely affected patient. Some forms of physical and hydrotherapy may be helpful.

12.2 SIMPLE ANALGESICS AND NON-STEROIDAL ANTI-INFLAMMATORY DRUGS

Simple analgesics

Simple analgesics such as paracetamol may be used to supplement other therapy, but they are relatively ineffective when used singly in rheumatoid arthritis. They do nothing to retard the progress of the disease and cannot provide adequate pain relief. They may be adequate in the management of some patients with osteoarthritis.

Non-steroidal anti-inflammatory drugs (NSAIDs)

The mechanism of action of NSAIDs is unknown. Many effects have been found *in vitro*, but their correlation with clinical efficacy is poor. All are inhibitors of prostaglandin synthesis, either cyclo-oxygenase or lipoxygenase inhibitors.

Lysosome stabilizing effects and inhibition of cellular migration have also been demonstrated but, again, the clinical significance of this observation is unclear.

Aspirin and related compounds

Aspirin is the longest established and most traditional of the anti-inflammatory drugs and is relatively cheap. However, in the UK its role has been supplanted by other NSAIDs.

Pharmacokinetics

The pharmacokinetics of aspirin are complex and when used in relatively high doses for long periods of time plasma levels should be monitored. Aspirin is readily absorbed from the gastrointestinal tract and is given orally. Elimination normally follows first-order kinetics, but after very large doses the enzymes that metabolize aspirin become saturated.

Adverse effects

1 Gastrointestinal effects. Nausea and vomiting follow high doses of aspirin. Dyspepsia, gastric irritation and occult or frank blood loss are common adverse effects, particularly when aspirin is associated with alcohol ingestion. Blood loss results from superficial gastric erosions or peptic ulceration. Inhibition of prostaglandin synthesis is probably responsible because some prostaglandins increase gastric mucosal blood flow and have other protective effects. Gastrointestinal blood loss occurs even with parenteral aspirin or aspirin by suppository. However, fewer erosions and ulcers are found with these and more recent enteric coated formulations. Newer NSAIDs have been claimed to cause less gastric irritation. These comparisons have not usually been made with enteric coated aspirin. At present there appears to be a dose dependent relationship between anti-inflammatory analgesic effect, prostaglandin synthetase inhibition and the frequency of gastric irritation. Less active analgesics cause less gastric irritation.

2 Prolonged bleeding time may result from the inhibition of thromboxane synthesis and impaired platelet aggregation (Chapter 9) or reduced hepatic clotting factor synthesis.

3 Bronchospasm, urticaria or hay fever may rarely occur in sensitive individuals and appear to result from release of immune mediators secondary to prostaglandin synthesis inhibition.

4 Tinnitus, dizziness and deafness are dose and plasma level related adverse effects. Vomiting and tachypnoea may also occur.

5 In overdose, confusion, convulsions and hyperpyrexia are seen. Forced diuresis may speed elimination of aspirin in cases of poisoning (Chapter 21, Section 21.2)

Dose

Aspirin tablets of 300–900 mg are given 4–6 hourly. In rheumatoid arthritis, up to 4.2 g/day may be required in divided doses.

Phenylbutazone

Phenylbutazone is a potent anti-inflammatory agent which causes marrow depression. It is now limited to ankylosing spondylitis and is available on hospital prescription only.

Azapropazone

Azapropazone is chemically related to phenylbutazone but it does not apparently give rise to the marrow depression which led to the severe restrictions on the use of phenylbutazone. As well as acting as a non-steroidal anti-inflammatory agent, it also has a uricosuric effect and is used in the treatment of gout. In the treatment of osteoarthritis, rheumatoid arthritis and ankylosing spondylitis, dosage in elderly patients with a creatinine clearance of less than 60 ml/min should not exceed 300 mg twice daily. If creatinine clearance in these patients is greater than 60 ml/min, dosage may be increased to 900 mg daily. In younger patients who have normal renal function, the standard dose is 1200 mg daily.

Drug interactions

Azapropazone increases plasma concentrations of phenytoin and combined use should be avoided. It also potentiates the action of warfarin and should not be used with this anticoagulant. It should be used with great caution, if at all, with any other oral anticoagulants. Combination with oral hypoglycaemics may result in excessively low blood sugars and, again, concurrent use should be avoided if at all possible.

Adverse effects

Skin rashes, fluid retention, angioneurotic oedema, dyspepsia and gastrointestinal bleeding have been reported.

Indomethacin and related drugs

Indomethacin has been widely used in inflammatory joint disease for years. It is given by mouth and by suppository. Gastric adverse effects are a predictable problem, but headache, mental confusion and dizziness may also present problems. Salt and water retention with oedema may aggravate cardiac failure or hypertension and reduce the efficacy of antihypertensive drugs. Rectal administration may be associated with pruritus, discomfort and bleeding.

Dose

Oral: 25–50 mg two to three times daily.
Rectal suppository: 100 mg at night; this may be repeated in the morning.

Propionic acid derivatives

A large number of agents from this group of drugs have been marketed recently. They are well absorbed orally and have fewer gastric adverse effects than plain aspirin. This has led some rheumatologists to favour them as first-line therapy.

This group consists of the following drugs:
Ibuprofen.
Fenoprofen.
Ketoprofen.
Naproxen.
Flurbiprofen.
Fenbufen.

Note that fenbufen is a prodrug with no direct effect on the stomach. None of these propionic acid derivatives have been shown to interact significantly with oral anticoagulants, and if a patient must also receive warfarin this group of drugs is preferable.

Phenylacetic acid derivatives

Diclofenac and fenclofenac are very similar to the propionic acid derivatives.

Fenclofenac has a high incidence of drug rash which appears early in the course of treatment and disappears rapidly when the drug is stopped. This and other adverse effects have led to its withdrawal from clinical use.

Diclofenac is less liable to produce a rash, but it may sometimes cause hepatitis with elevated alkaline phosphatase and transaminase levels.

Fenamates

The long-established mefenamic acid and flufenamic acid are effective in inflammatory joint disease, but they share the problems of salicylates to which they are chemically related. Thus, they share the gastric adverse effects of other anti-inflammatory drugs but, in addition, they cause diarrhoea, a dose related phenomenon the basis for which is not clear.

Piroxicam

This is an anti-inflammatory agent that is chemically unrelated to other drugs. It does, however, share their propensity to cause gastrointestinal adverse effects, and potentiates the effect of oral anticoagulants. It is also contraindicated in asthmatic patients who cannot tolerate aspirin. It may cause fluid retention, a particular hazard in the elderly. Tenoxicam is now available and is reported to have less gastric toxicity.

Comment

This group of drugs forms the first-line and mainstay of treatment of inflammatory arthritis. There is now a bewildering array of strongly promoted agents. Despite this, no drug has been shown to be clearly superior to the remainder in terms of symptomatic relief, disease suppression or toxic effects. It is important that a constant vigilance is maintained for side effects and drug interactions, particularly in elderly patients. It is advisable to become familiar with a few drugs and restrict use to them. Unfortunately, individual response to a particular drug is unpredictable and the choice of drug is inescapably empirical. A list of the principal NSAIDs and their doses is presented in Table 12.1.

12.3 SECOND- AND THIRD-LINE DRUGS IN ARTHRITIS

These antirheumatic agents comprise a group of widely different chemical entities, including gold, penicillamine, chloroquine and, more recently, sulphasalazine. Corticosteroids and immunosuppressant cytotoxic drugs are used as third-line therapy.

Mechanisms of action of second-line drugs are not clear. There is a lag between starting therapy and observing an effect. It is usual to continue with conventional anti-inflammatory drugs. These drugs, unlike most NSAIDs, may influence the underlying disease process. Haemoglobin may rise and the erythrocyte sedimentation rate (ESR) and rheumatoid factor titre may fall in patients who respond.

Table 12.1. Examples of the principal groups of non-steroidal anti-inflammatory drugs

Drug	Dose* (mg)	Dosage interval (h)
Salicylates		
Aspirin	900	4†
Diflunisal	500	12
Benorylate	4g	12
Pyrazoles		
Azapropazone	300	6
Indoles		
Indomethacin	50	8
Sulindac	200	12
Fenamates		
Mefenamic acid	500	8
Flufenamic acid	200	8
Propionates		
Ibuprofen	400	8
Naproxen	250	8
Ketoprofen	50	6
Phenylacetates		
Diclofenac	50	8
Other		
Piroxicam	20	Daily
Tenoxicam	20	Daily

* These doses are near the upper limit and therapy should be commenced with approximately half doses.

† Adjust according to serum concentration.

Gold salts

These have been used for over 40 years in the management of rheumatoid arthritis. Gold salts reduce macrophage activity. One-third of patients derive considerable benefit, one-third have only a modest response and one-third have adverse effects and require interruption of treatment.

Adverse effects

1 Pruritic rashes are common and present in many forms, including mouth ulcers.

2 Proteinuria secondary to a membranous glomerulonephritis occurs in 10% of patients but it resolves on stopping gold treatment.

3 Vasodilatation with orthostatic hypotension may acutely follow drug dosing.

4 Aplastic anaemia is extremely rare now; gold treatment is closely supervised with haematological checks before each dose. Neutropenia and thrombocytopenia may occur suddenly or develop slowly. Recovery is usually assured provided no more gold is given.

Clinical use and dose

An intramuscular injection of sodium aurothiomalate is given initially as a 10 mg test dose followed by 50 mg weekly for up to 3 months or until a response or toxic effects are observed. Dose frequency may be reduced to monthly and continued for years. Gold is indicated commonly in rheumatoid arthritis and occasionally in psoriatic arthropathy.

n-Penicillamine

First introduced as a copper chelating agent in Wilson's disease, *n*-penicillamine modifies the formation of immunoglobulin. It has a similar action to gold salts but relapse may occur with continuing therapy.

Adverse effects

These are similar to those with gold. Cross-toxicity with gold has been reported but is disputed. It is likely that both gold and penicillamine toxicity are associated with the same HLA tissue type (DR3).

1 Skin rashes are common.

2 Taste disturbance (dysgeusia).

3 Proteinuria, as with gold.

4 Marrow toxicity is similar to gold, consisting of thrombocytopenia and neutropenia. As these changes develop gradually, routine weekly haematological monitoring is essential during the initial stages of therapy.

5 Immunological effects. Up to 50% of patients develop positive antinuclear factor tests. Rarely, systemic lupus erythematosus or myasthenia gravis may be precipitated.

Clinical use and dose

Penicillamine is given as a 125 mg dose initially followed by monthly increments of 125 mg to a maximum of 500 mg daily unless good response is achieved at a lower dosage.

Chloroquine and hydroxychloroquine

In rheumatoid arthritis, the mechanisms of action of these preparations, originally developed as antimalarials, may be by reducing the 'T-helper' lymphocyte population and lysosome stabilization.

They are well absorbed orally, taken up by many tissues and then very slowly excreted in the urine. The most disturbing toxic effects are ophthalmological. An early keratitis is reversible but gradual accumulation of the drug in the retina can lead to irreversible retinal damage with permanent blindness after 1 year. Rashes and marrow toxicity are rarely seen. Neuropathies and myopathies have been reported.

Clinical use

Chloroquine is often given in interrupted courses with drug-free periods of 2–3 months each year. Chloroquine may be used in systemic lupus erythematosus as well as rheumatoid arthritis. Ophthalmological checks are advised every 6 months. Hydroxychloroquine is the treatment of choice. Provided that the dosage is kept below 6.5 mm/kg, the risk of retinal toxicity is low.

Sulphasalazine

Sulphasalazine, more commonly thought of as a useful agent in the management of inflammatory bowel disease (Chapter 16), was originally introduced for the treatment of rheumatoid arthritis and is now gaining reputation as a drug that does, indeed, suppress the inflammatory response associated with rheumatoid arthritis.

Adverse effects

These include skin rashes, nausea, headache and occasional leucopenia, neutropenia and thrombocytopenia. The blood abnormalities usually occur early on in the course of treatment (within 6 months) and reverse if the drug is stopped. Other side effects are mentioned in Chapter 16.

Clinical use and dose

Sulphasalazine is administered under expert supervision which takes account of the severity of the disease and individual susceptibility. The oral dose is initially 50 mg daily, usually increased by 500 mg at 1 week intervals to a maximum of 2–3 g daily.

Corticosteroids

Corticosteroids have potent immunosuppressant activity (Chapter 13, Section 13.2) and a range of other effects (Chapter 14). They are the most powerful anti-inflammatory drugs available.

In rheumatoid arthritis there is little evidence that high doses are more effective than low doses. For chronic use not more than 7.5 mg prednisolone per day (or on alternate days) or the equivalent can be given without the development of adverse effects (Chapter 14, Section 14.1). Steroids are particularly useful in systemic lupus erythematosus and are essential in polymyalgia rheumatica and cranial arteritis.

Where one or two joints are particularly troublesome in an otherwise reasonably controlled patient, an intra-articular injection of corticosteroid is widely used.

Cytotoxic drugs

Methotrexate, azathioprine, cyclophosphamide and chlorambucil have been the most widely used. Their use as immunosuppressants is discussed in Chapter 13, Section 13.2. Methotrexate is now used as the first 'second-line' cytotoxic drug in a dosage of 5–15 mg per week. The onset of action is more rapid (6–8 weeks) compared with other cytotoxics.

Comment

No hard and fast rules can be laid down about the use of antirheumatic drugs. The most logical approach is to work through the sequence of first-, second- and third-line drugs, moving from one category to the next only when there is convincing clinical evidence of therapeutic failure. Second- and third-line drugs carry a much greater risk of serious toxicity and this must be weighed against their benefits in terms of pain relief and minimization of joint destruction and deformity. Inflammatory joint disease remains an important and difficult therapeutic challenge.

12.4 DRUGS USED IN GOUT

It is important to distinguish:

1 Management of the acute attack.

2 Long-term management.

Management of the acute attack

An acute attack of gout is extremely painful and effective anti-inflammatory drugs should be given at once. The drugs used are:

1 Non-steroidal anti-inflammatory agents such as indomethacin or naproxen in large doses for 24–48 h.

2 Colchicine: this drug can still be used in acute gout (orally or intravenously) or in the early months of treatment with allopurinol. Adverse effects—nausea, vomiting, abdominal pain and diarrhoea—can be less common with low-dose regimens.

Long-term management

As the underlying mechanism in gout involves excess production of uric acid and its deposition in joints and in the kidney, long-term management aims at reducing uric acid in the body in two ways:

1 Inhibition of uric acid formation from purines by xanthine oxidase inhibition.

2 Promotion of urate excretion in the urine.

Xanthine oxidase inhibition

Allopurinol

Pharmacokinetics

Allopurinol is well absorbed from the gastrointestinal tract and is rapidly cleared from the plasma with a half-life of 2–3 h. It is converted to alloxanthine and this metabolite in turn inhibits the metabolism of the parent drug. Alloxathine is also a xanthine oxidase inhibitor.

Adverse effects

These are not common. Hypersensitivity reactions, which subside on withdrawing the drug, consist of a skin rash accompanied by fever, malaise and muscle pain. Rarely, leucopenia or leukocytosis with eosinophilia occur.

Drug interactions

Drugs depending on xanthine oxidase for their metabolic conversion should be given with caution in association with allopurinol. This applies to 6-mercaptopurine and azathioprine. Inhibition of warfarin metabolism may also occur: anticoagulant control should be monitored closely in circumstances such as these.

Clinical use and dose

Allopurinol must not be used in an acute attack of gout because this will be prolonged. Initially, 100 mg allopurinol are given daily as a single dose, increasing to about 300 mg daily depending on serum uric acid levels. Colchicine or indomethacin may be given over the first few months to prevent acute gout.

Uricosuric drugs

Probenecid

Probenecid inhibits the transport of organic acids across lipid membranes, including the renal tubule. Whereas this leads to an increase in the plasma concentration of a number of acidic drugs, the uric acid concentration falls because its reabsorption from tubular fluid is inhibited.

Pharmacokinetics

Probenecid is well absorbed from the gastrointestinal tract and peak concentrations are achieved in 2–4 h. Metabolism and renal excretion result in a half-life of about 9 h; a large proportion of the parent drug is actively secreted by the proximal tubules.

Adverse effects

About 25% of patients experience dyspepsia and this limits its use in peptic ulceration. Hypersensitivity reactions occur occasionally as skin rashes. Drug induced nephrotic syndrome has been reported.

Drug interactions

The uricosuric effect of probenecld may be inhibited by large doses of salicylates. Aspirin should therefore be avoided in patients receiving probenecid.

Dose

A 250 mg dose of probenecid is given twice daily initially, increasing to a maximum of 2 g daily over 2–3 weeks, depending on serum uric acid concentrations.

Sulphinpyrazone

Sulphinpyrazone inhibits the tubular reabsorption of uric acid when given in sufficient dose. Like probenecid, it reduces the renal tubular secretion of many other organic acids.

Pharmacokinetics

Sulphinpyrazone is well absorbed from the gastrointestinal tract. It is strongly bound (98–99%) to plasma albumin; 90% is excreted unchanged in the urine; 10% is metabolized to the *N-p*-hydroxyphenyl metabolite, itself a potent uricosuric.

Adverse effects

Ten to fifteen per cent of patients receiving sulphinpyrazone develop gastrointestinal symptoms and as a rule it should be avoided in patients with a history of peptic ulceration. Rarely, it causes skin rashes and fever.

Drug interactions

As with probenecid, salicylates inhibit the uricosuric effect of sulphinpyrazone and more than occasional doses of aspirin should be avoided. Decreased excretion of oral hypoglycaemic agents may lead to hypoglycaemia and sulphinpyrazone may enhance the effect of warfarin.

Dose

A 100–200 mg dose of sulphinpyrazone is given daily, increasing over 2–3 weeks to about 600–800 mg daily, depending on serum uric acid concentrations.

Azapropazone

Azapropazone has a uricosuric effect and is used in acute attacks of gout and in long-term prophylaxis.

Dose

During the first 24 h of an acute attack, 2400 mg azapropazone are given in divided doses, then 1800 mg daily until acute symptoms subside followed by 1200 mg daily until symptoms have disappeared. In chronic gout, 600 mg twice daily are given unless the patient is elderly (over 65 years of age: see above).

Comment

The management of gout aims to reduce uric acid formation prophylactically by xanthine oxidase inhibition with allopurinol and thus prevent arthritis and renal damage. If acute arthritis occurs it should be managed symptomatically with high doses of NSAIDs and allopurinol therapy begun after symptoms subside. The uricosuric drugs are now used less commonly.

Chapter 13
Cytotoxic Drugs and Immunopharmacology

13.1 CYTOTOXIC DRUGS AND CANCER CHEMOTHERAPY

Aims

Drug therapy in cancer may be employed to:

1 Eradicate the disease.

2 Induce a remission.

3 Control symptoms.

In recent years increasing use has been made of drugs that modify the growth of cells and tissue. Such drugs are indicated in the treatment of cancer, in the control of the immune responses in organ transplantation and in the management of autoimmune diseases.

Relevant pathophysiology

Chemotherapy or use of drugs in the management of cancer was introduced in the 1890s with non-specific cell poisons. More specific agents became available with the discovery in the 1940s of nitrogen mustard, an alkylating agent, and methotrexate, an antimetabolite. There are now 30–40 drugs used in the management of a variety of different forms of cancer.

Initially treatment was restricted to patients with leukaemia and lymphomas, but drugs are now used in patients with solid tumours, including adults as well as children. Formerly, most cytotoxic drugs were used in patients with advanced or metastatic disease. Considerable progress has been made towards curative treatment of some of the childhood cancers and rarer solid tumours. Nevertheless, there are still many forms of cancer which are difficult to treat with chemotherapy.

To obtain maximum therapeutic benefit it is important to define the aims of therapy at the start of treatment, as this often dictates the choice, duration and potential adverse effects of the drugs used.

Chemotherapy is only one aspect of cancer management. Although surgery and radiotherapy are of considerable value, increasing use is made of 'combined modality therapy', or the integration of several different approaches to cancer treatment.

Cytotoxic drugs may be used:

1 As potentially curative therapy either before or after surgery or radiotherapy for the primary tumour (neoadjuvant or adjuvant chemotherapy). The aim is to eradicate micrometastatic disease (Table 13.1).

Table 13.1. Chemotherapy as part of combined modality treatment of primary tumours

Breast	Colon	Osteogenic and Ewing's sarcoma	Bladder, cervix, head and neck
Premenopausal axillary nodes positive for cancer	Stage Duke's C	Preoperative	Locally advanced disease (trial only)

Table 13.2. Chemotherapy for the management of metastatic cancer

Curative	Prolongs survival	Useful palliation	Benefit unlikely
Testis	Ovary	Breast	Pancreas
Lymphoma	Small cell lung	Bladder, cervix	Renal
Acute leukaemia	Chronic leukaemia	Head and neck	Brain
Certain childhood cancers	Myeloma	(Colon, gastric)* (Non-small cell lung)	
Choriocarcinoma			

* Lower overall prospect of response.

2 In the treatment of metastatic disease. In rare cases this may be curative; in others, life may be significantly prolonged. Commonly, disease control rather than cure is the aim, and symptomatic benefit is an important consideration (Table 13.2).

Principles of drug treatment

Formerly patients were treated with only one cytotoxic drug. Now it is more common to use a combination of two to six drugs given simultaneously, or closely related in time. With a few important exceptions, combinations of drugs are more effective than single agents. This is achieved by:

1 Combining drugs which are active when used alone.
2 Combining drugs with different mechanisms of action.
3 Combining drugs with different toxicities.
4 Using drugs at doses close to the maximum tolerated levels.

Most drug combinations have been developed empirically. As the number of drugs used increases so the potential toxicity also increases.

The availability of supportive measures, such as platelet transfusions together with therapeutic drug monitoring, has allowed much larger and more effective doses of some drugs to be used. High-dose methotrexate treatment is a good example of this. Methotrexate is a potent but reversible inhibitor of the enzyme dihydrofolate reductase, a key enzyme for DNA synthesis. Enzyme inhibition and the toxic effects of methotrexate can be reversed by the subsequent administration of folinic acid. It is possible therefore to give methotrexate at doses of 100–1000 times that used previously, using folinic acid 'rescue' with minimal effects. This method of treatment may be of considerable therapeutic value in some situations. In addition to methotrexate, high doses of drugs such as cyclophosphamide, melphalan, etoposide and carboplatin have also been tried. When these are employed it is essential that adequate services are available to deal with marrow failure, infection and bleeding. Very high doses of some drugs are used in the hope of eliminating the tumour completely. This has been used in association with bone marrow transplantation in the management of leukaemias and experimentally in some solid tumours.

It is common practice to administer cytotoxic drug regimens intermittently. Pulses of drug or drug combination are given at 3–4 weekly intervals, increasing the effectiveness and reducing the toxicity of the combination.

In the future, the co-administration of haemapoietic growth factors now available for clinical use may be important in allowing drugs to be given more frequently or at higher doses.

In addition to oral or intravenous dosing, cytotoxics may be given:

1 Intrathecally to achieve effective concentration in the CSF, particularly for drugs that do not readily cross the blood–brain barrier.

2 Intra-arterially into a limb, the head and neck or the liver.

3 Intraperitoneally or intrapleurally to increase the local concentration of drug, particularly where rapidly accumulating ascites or pleural effusions present clinical problems.

4 Topically onto lesions of the skin, vagina or buccal mucosa.

If a drug requires metabolic activation by the liver, e.g. cyclophosphamide or azathioprine, it is of little value to administer it locally, intraperitoneally or intrathecally.

Drugs used in cancer chemotherapy

Cytotoxic drugs

Mechanisms

Cytotoxic drugs can be classified as follows:

1 Alkylating agents, including drugs such as nitrogen mustard, cyclophosphamide, chlorambucil and melphalan. These are highly reactive molecules when activated and bind irreversibly to macromolecules in the cell, notably DNA, RNA and proteins.

2 Antimetabolites, which are closely related analogues of the normal components of intermediary metabolism or DNA synthesis. Methotrexate inhibits folic acid metabolism and the nucleotides (5-fluorouracil, cytosine arabinoside, 6-mercaptopurine) inhibit DNA synthesis.

3 Natural products. A wide range of drugs has been developed from plants, bacteria, yeasts and fungi. These act by inhibiting cell division (by preventing spindle formation) or by inhibiting DNA synthesis through intercalation into the helix or through binding to nuclear topoisomerase. They include:

(a) Mitosis inhibitors: vincristine, vinblastine and vindesine.

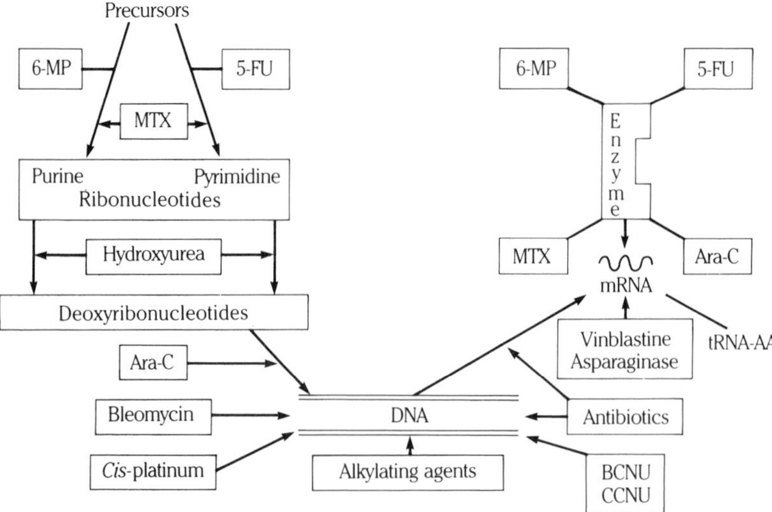

Fig. 13.1. Mechanism of action of cytotoxic drugs.

(b) Antibiotics: such as actinomycin D, bleomycin, doxorubicin and mitomycin.
(c) Podophyllotoxins: etoposide and teneposide.

4 Others: several drugs have been identified, often by random synthesis and screening, whose mechanism of action is not fully established but are thought to interact with DNA synthesis or replication. They include nitrosoureas, hydroxyurea, dacarbazine, procarbazine, cisplatin and its analogue carboplatin.

5 Steroid hormones: these are widely used in cancer management, particularly for the treatment of symptoms such as anorexia and hypercalcaemia. The drug most commonly used is prednisolone.

For clinical purposes, cytotoxic drugs are generally grouped according to their mechanism of action as above, but they may also be classified according to their effect on the cell cycle, as demonstrated in tissue culture. Actively dividing cells pass through several phases. Mitosis is followed by a gap or delay (G1), then a synthetic phase (S), a second gap (G2) and mitosis again. Cells may cycle continuously or enter a quiescent phase. Some drugs act at all phases of the cell cycle, others exert effects specifically at certain of these phases.

Class I drugs are non-specific and act on cells whether or not they are actively dividing, e.g. nitrogen mustard. Class II drugs act only at specific phases of the cell cycle, e.g. vincristine, methotrexate, cystosine arabinoside. Class III drugs act on cells in division and at all phases of the cycle, e.g. cyclophosphamide, actinomycin D, nitrosoureas. Most cytotoxic drugs act by interfering with the synthesis and replication of DNA. The molecular basis of action of some widely used agents is shown in Fig. 13.1.

Pharmacokinetics

Pharmacokinetic aspects of cytotoxic drugs include drug-specific problems and general problems. Some cytotoxic drugs are metabolized in the liver (methotrexate and cyclophosphamide) while others are excreted unchanged by the kidney (cisplatin). Adriamycin and vincristine are examples of drugs which are predominantly excreted via the biliary tract. In patients with renal impairment, dose modification of drugs such as cisplatin and methotrexate is important and similarly in the presence of hepatic impairment, dose reduction of drugs such as adriamycin may be necessary.

Methotrexate is well absorbed when given by mouth at low dose, but variably absorbed at high doses. Plasma level monitoring may help in optimizing the dose and in reducing toxicity. Cyclophosphamide is converted to an active metabolite in the liver. Similarly, inactive azathioprine is converted to the antimetabolite 6-mercaptopurine in the liver.

There are some further clinical pharmacokinetic problems with cytotoxic drugs:

1 The problem of the 'third space'. Many patients with cancer have pleural effusions or ascites. Administration of a cytotoxic drug to such a patient may result in the sequestration of the drug into this compartment with slow release back into the circulation. This may aggravate toxicity.

2 Sanctuary sites. For many purposes, cancer can be considered to be a systemic disease. It is essential, therefore, that the administered drug reaches all parts of the body. Some of the drugs used do not cross the blood–brain barrier and do not, therefore, act on tumour cells in the brain. Another important sanctuary site appears to be the testes, and tumour relapse may occur there. Clinically, perhaps the most important sanctuary site is the large tumour with a poor blood supply into which the drug cannot adequately penetrate. For this reason, new (bioreductive) drugs which may be selectively activated in hypoxic areas within tumours might prove particularly valuable.

Adverse effects

Reactions to chemotherapy are secondary to cell death both in the tumour and in other rapidly dividing cells of bone marrow, gastrointestinal tract, germinal epithelium, etc. These can be divided into:

1 General adverse reactions to chemotherapy.

2 Specific adverse reactions to individual agents.

General adverse reactions

1 Nausea and vomiting may be severe with some drugs, such as cisplatin, and is related to the direct actions of cytotoxic drugs on the chemoreceptor trigger zone (Chapter 16, Section 16.3). Anticipatory vomiting can be a major problem in patients after repeated treatments. High doses of metoclopromide in combination with dexamethasone have proved reasonably effective in controlling vomiting in a proportion of cases. However, dystonic reactions are quite common, particularly in young patients. The mechanism of action of high-dose metoclopramide is considered to be antagonism of 5HT3 receptor-mediated pathways. New selective 5HT3 receptor antagonists are at least as effective as metoclopramide, and they have the advantage of being devoid of side effects due to unwanted dopamine antagonism.

2 Alopecia is a common adverse effect of some, but not all, cytotoxic drugs. Hair regrows after the drugs are withdrawn.

3 Hyperuricaemia. Very high levels of plasma uric acid with precipitation of clinical gout or renal failure may complicate treatment of leukaemias and lymphomas. Allopurinol, the xanthine oxidase inhibitor, may be used to prevent gout but care should be taken when azathioprine or mercaptopurine are being given at the same time (see drug interactions below).

4 Mucositis can occur with some drugs, causing ulceration in the mouth. When there is coexistent neutropenia there is increased risk of opportunistic infections.

5 Opportunistic infections occur as a result of neutropenia and immunosuppressant therapy which interfere with humoral and cell-mediated responses. Unusual infection with fungi and protozoa, in addition to more common pathogenic bacteria and viruses, occur.

6 Bone marrow depression. The bone marrow is particularly sensitive to some cytotoxic drugs (Chapter 17, Section 17.2). Neutropenia or thrombocytopenia are common. They result in an increased risk of infection and haemorrhage, respectively.

Specific adverse reactions

Specific effects of some of the more widely used cytotoxic drugs are shown in Table 13.3.

Drug interactions

With many cytotoxic drugs in use, often in combination, it is not surprising that adverse interactions occur. More important, however, are the interactions noted between cytotoxic drugs and non-cytotoxic agents.

Table 13.3. Effects of cytotoxic drugs

Drug	Mechanism	Specific adverse effects	Indications
Cyclophosphamide	Alkylating agent	Haematuria, cystitis	Haematological malignancy, solid tumour
Doxorubicin	Antibiotic	Alopecia, cardiac arrhythmias, local tissue necrosis	Wide range of haematological and solid tumours
Cisplatin	Interacts with DNA	Neurotoxicity Nephrotoxicity Vomiting	Wide range of solid tumours, including lung, ovarian and testicular carcinoma
Bleomycin	Antibiotic	Pulmonary fibrosis, skin rashes	Lymphomas, testicular teratoma, squamous cell carcinoma
Methotrexate	Antimetabolite	Mucositis	Leukaemia

Methotrexate and salicylates

As methotrexate is highly protein bound it is readily displaced from the binding site by aspirin and other salicylates. This may increase the risk of adverse effects of methotrexate. Other acidic drugs which are highly protein bound may show similar effects.

6-Mercaptopurine and allopurinol

These two drugs are frequently used together. Allopurinol is a competitive inhibitor of xanthine oxidase (Chapter 12, Section 12.4) and also inhibits the breakdown of 6-mercaptopurine. The dose of 6-mercaptopurine must be halved at least or toxicity ensues. Azathioprine, which is metabolized to 6-mercaptopurine, should also be given in lower doses if used with allopurinol.

Procarbazine and alcohol

Hot flushing may occur and patients should be warned of this before treatment. Procarbazine is a monoamine oxidase inhibitor and tyramine-containing foods should be avoided (Chapter 19, Section 19.3).

Comment

Cytotoxic drugs should be given by physicians who have experience and facilities for managing malignant disease and the problems associated with chemotherapy. Haemorrhage and opportunistic infections secondary to marrow and immune suppression may shorten life rather than prolong it if they are not aggressively managed.

Hormones and antihormones

Oestrogens and progestogens

Surgical removal of endocrine organs, such as the ovaries, testes, adrenals and pituitary gland, has been used for many years in the treatment of breast and prostatic cancer. Treatment with hormones and antihormones aims to achieve the same effect of changing the hormonal milieu. Hormonal effects are mediated by receptors on the cell surface or within the cells. These receptors, notably oestrogen receptors, can be identified within tumours and allow a prediction of the response to endocrine manipulation in breast cancer. Patients whose breast cancer contains receptors are likely to respond while those without oestrogen receptors are unlikely to respond to anti-oestrogen therapy. The synthetic anti-oestrogen, tamoxifen, is now widely used in breast cancer and has very few adverse effects. Second-line therapy includes aminoglutethimide, which inhibits adrenal steroid synthesis and this has replaced surgical adrenalectomy.

In cancer of the prostate, treatment aimed at reducing testosterone levels may be very effective. This includes the use of stilboestrol, but this may have cardiovascular side effects and an alternative is the use of synthetic LHRH analogues. These inhibit testosterone release and have an effect equivalent to that of orchidectomy.

Progestogens, like medroxyprogesterone, are effective in endometrial cancer as well as in breast cancer.

Glucocorticoids

The corticosteroids cortisol, hydrocortisone and prednisolone are used in drug combinations in the management of leukaemia and lymphomas. In association with combination chemotherapy they are used in the management of breast cancer. Dexamethasone is used in the management of raised intracranial pressure associated with intracerebral primary or secondary tumours, and is also a useful antiemetic agent, often in combination with other agents.

13.2 IMMUNOPHARMACOLOGY

Relevant pathophysiology

The primary function of the immune system is to protect the host from invasion by foreign antigens, in particular pathogenic bacteria and viruses. It is also responsible for causing autoimmune disease and for rejecting allogenic tissue grafts after transplantation. There are two principal immunological effector systems: humoral and cell-mediated immunity.

B-lymphocytes are activated by an antigen to produce specific immunoglobulins or antibodies for *humoral immunity*.

T-lymphocytes are derived from lymphoid stem cells which differentiate in the thymus and are responsible for *cell-mediated immunity* by production of cytotoxic T-cells and release of lymphokines, which in turn activate macrophages and other non-specific cellular effectors. Cell-mediated immunity is particularly directed against viruses and other intracellular pathogens, e.g. tuberculosis.

There are several situations in which an immune response can cause pathology or illness.

Type I: anaphylactic hypersensitivity

Antigen reacts with antibody (IgE) bound to mast cells and releases mediators: monoamines, kinins, prostaglandins, etc., e.g. allergic asthma, hay fever, acute anaphylaxis.

Type II: antibody-dependent hypersensitivity

Antibodies bind to antigen or cell surfaces and activate cytotoxic responses via complement or other mechanisms. This type of response may be involved in organ-specific autoimmune diseases (e.g. pernicious anaemia, Hashimotos disease) and also in non-organ-specific autoimmune diseases (e.g. rheumatoid arthritis, systemic lupus erythematosus). Alternatively, antibody directed to a cell surface component like a hormone receptor results in activation of a functional cell, e.g. thyroid stimulation in Graves disease. Antibody-mediated cytotoxicity is also responsible for hyperacute (immediate) organ allograft rejection in sensitized transplant recipients who have preformed antidonor antibodies.

Type III: immune complex-mediated hypersensitivity

Antibody–antigen complexes both activate the complement system and induce platelet aggregation with release of vasoactive mediators locally. This is most commonly seen in the renal glomeruli but may also occur in other tissues. There is also a systemic form of the disease in a syndrome known as 'serum sickness'.

Type IV: cell-mediated hypersensitivity

T-lymphocytes release lymphokines or are transformed into cytotoxic T-cells and activate a cell-mediated immune response. This form of hypersensitivity is responsible for causing acute rejection of organ allografts and is also likely to be important in organ-specific autoimmunity.

Drugs can modify immune responses in several ways:

1 Suppression of immune responses; used in autoimmune disease, hypersensitivity or organ transplantation.

2 Suppression of mediator release or reversal of mediator effects; used, for example, in asthma (Chapter 11, Section 11.1) and rheumatoid arthritis (Chapter 12, Section 12.2).

3 Activation or stimulation of immune responses either via cell-mediated or humoral mechanisms; undergoing evaluation at present.

Drugs that suppress immune responses

Cytotoxic drugs

The antimetabolites *azathioprine* and *methotrexate* and the alkylating agent *cyclophosphamide* are widely used as immunosuppressives at lower doses than used in cancer chemotherapy. These drugs have their effects on actively dividing cells and at low doses appear to have a relatively selective action on lymphocytes. If lymphocytes have been exposed to antigen and stimulated to divide, the action of cytotoxic drugs is enhanced.

Azathioprine has a selective effect on T-cell-mediated reactions and is widely used in immunosuppression after transplantation and in autoimmune diseases.

Cyclophosphamide also suppresses immune responses but paradoxically enhances cell-mediated hypersensitivity by depletion of suppressor T-cells.

Cyclosporin

Mechanism

Cyclosporin acts predominantly on T-helper cells. It selectively impairs the production of lymphokines, particularly the T-cell growth factor interleukin-2, and inhibits interleukin-2 receptor expression. This prevents T-cell activation and stops the generation of the cell-mediated immune responses responsible for allograft rejection.

Pharmacokinetics

Cyclosporin is poorly absorbed following oral administration, having a bioavailability of approximately 30%. It is a highly lipophilic compound and is distributed widely in body tissues. High concentrations of the drug are found in adipose tissue, kidney, liver and pancreas. Cyclosporin is almost completely metabolized in the liver and at least 17 metabolites exist. The major route of excretion is via the bile. There is considerable variability between and within patients in cyclosporin pharmacokinetics.

Side effects

Nephrotoxicity is the most serious side effect of cyclosporin. In renal transplant patients, it is often difficult to differentiate between nephrotoxicity and rejection. Other side effects are hypertension, hepatotoxicity, tremor, gingival hyperplasia and hirsutism. Toxicity is usually managed by lowering the dose. Infections may also occur as a result of the immunosuppression.

Drug interactions

Drug interactions with cyclosporin are of two types:

1 Drugs which are nephrotoxic themselves. Examples are the aminoglycosides and amphotericin, which may enhance the nephrotoxicity of cyclosporin.

2 Drugs which alter the pharmacokinetics of cyclosporin. Metoclopramide, for example, increases the absorption of cyclosporin. Drugs which induce the cytochrome P-450 enzyme system, e.g. phenytoin, carbamazepine, phenobarbitone and rifampicin, will reduce cyclosporin concentrations. Similarly, drugs such as erythromycin and ketoconazole which inhibit the cytochrome P-450 system result in increased cyclosporin concentrations.

Calcium antagonists such as diltiazem, verapamil and nicardipine modify tissue distribution to increase plasma levels. They may be useful in reducing the dose of cyclosporin required. The mechanism may involve an interaction with a membrane glycoprotein involved in transport of cyclosporin out of cells.

Clinical use and dose

Cyclosporin is used to prevent graft rejection after organ or bone marrow transplantation and in the prophylaxis and treatment of graft vs. host disease. Protocols for immunosuppression after organ transplantation vary between centres, although most include cyclosporin (Table 13.4). The dose of cyclosporin depends on the other drugs being used. The daily oral dose in the immediate

Table 13.4. Immunosuppressive drugs used to prevent graft rejection

Induction/maintenance of immunosuppression	Treatment of rejection
Cyclosporin monotherapy	High-dose prednisolone
or	or
Cyclosporin + prednisolone	Polyclonal/monoclonal antibody
or	
Cyclosporin + prednisolone + azathioprine (triple therapy)	
or	
Polyclonal/monoclonal antibody + cyclosporin + prednisolone + azathioprine (quadruple therapy)	

post-transplant period is usually about 15 mg/kg and this is gradually reduced to a maintenance dose of 2–6 mg/kg several weeks after transplantation. However, because of the wide variability in absorption and metabolism of the drug, dosage should be based on the results of plama level monitoring of the parent compound or its metabolites, together with clinical assessment of response, toxicity or signs of graft rejection. Cyclosporin is not removed by haemodialysis and in renal transplant patients undergoing haemodialysis, dosage adjustment is not required. Immunosuppression after transplantation must be continued indefinitely, although some centres discontinue cyclosporin after the graft is established to avoid the risk of side effects. Cyclosporin may also have a role in the treatment of various diseases which may have an immunological basis, such as rheumatoid arthritis, ulcerative colitis and psoriasis.

Glucocorticoids

Prednisolone and other glucocorticoids have many actions which influence cell-mediated and humoral immune responses (Chapter 14, Section 14.1). These include effects on:

1 Generation of cytotoxic effector cells.
2 Lymphocyte recirculation.
3 Immunoglobulin production.
4 Suppression of macrophage and monocyte functions.

Steroids are widely used as immunosuppressives but long-term use in high dose is associated with an unacceptable incidence of adverse effects (Chapter 14, Section 14.1), and it is therefore preferable to use low-dose steroids combined with other immunosuppressive therapy (cytotoxic drugs).

ALG and OKT3

ALG (antilymphocyte globulin) is a polyclonal antilymphocyte antibody preparation usually raised in the horse or rabbit. OKT3 is a murine monoclonal anti-T-cell antibody. When given by intravenous infusion they deplete lymphocytes from the circulation and block the function of those remaining. Both are powerful immunosuppressives which may be used in selected patients to increase organ allograft survival. They often produce febrile reactions and increase the risk of opportunistic infection, especially by cytomegalovirus. In the longer term, they may also increase the incidence of tumours, particularly lymphomas.

New immunosuppressive agents in transplantation

Several new immunosuppressive agents have recently been described but their role in clinical transplantation remains to be evaluated. These include the fungal macrolide FK-506, which although structurally unrelated to cyclosporin has a very similar mode of action. Both FK-506 and another macrolide, Rapamycin, act synergistically with cyclosporin. Also in this category are monoclonal antibodies directed against either the interleukin-2 receptor or the CD4 molecule on T-helper cells, both of which show promise in increasing graft survival.

Antihistamines

These block classical histamine (H_1) receptors and interfere with the actions of histamine released in type I immune reactions.

They are used in hay fever, allergic rhinitis, urticaria and other acute allergic reactions. The vascular effects of histamine, including flare, wheal and itch, are prevented. They are of no use in asthma.

Older antihistamines like promethazine and diphenhydramine have sedative and anticholinergic side effects. These are less prominent with cyclizine and chlorpheniramine. New agents like terfenadine cause little or no sedation, have non-reversible antagonist properties and can be given once daily.

Antihistamines are also used to treat motion sickness and vestibular disease (Chapter 16).

Drugs that block mediator release

Drugs that increase intracellular cyclic AMP stabilize the mast cell and prevent degranulation and mediator release. This reduces or attenuates the symptoms of IgE-mediated hypersensitivity reactions.

β_2-Adrenoceptor agonists

Drugs like adrenaline, terbutaline or salbutamol (Chapter 11, Section 11.1) increase intracellular cyclic AMP, reduce mediator release and improve symptoms.

Theophylline derivatives

These block phosphodiesterase, prevent cyclic AMP breakdown, increase local levels and thus reduce mediator release.

Disodium cromoglycate and ketotifen

These agents stabilize the mast cell membrane and reduce mediator release. The precise mechanism is unknown but may be related to inhibition of phosphodiesterase.

Glucocorticoids

In large doses these have non-specific membrane stabilizing properties, which may reduce mediator release and contribute to their overall anti-inflammatory and immunosuppressive activity.

Non-steroidal anti-inflammatory drugs (NSAIDs)

Indomethacin and related agents block the synthesis of eicosanoids, including prostaglandins, and interfere with the formation of mediator prostaglandins in macrophages and also leukotrienes. NSAIDs are useful in the management of some autoimmune diseases, particularly rheumatoid arthritis, but the interference with prostaglandin synthesis may provoke acute asthma in some sensitive individuals.

Drugs that enhance immune responses

Immunostimulatory agents

A number of agents, including Bacillus Calmette–Guérin (BCG), *Corynebacterium parvum* and the antihelminthic levamisole, have been reported to potentiate cell-mediated immunity. The mechanisms responsible are poorly understood and none of these are used commonly as immunostimulants in clinical practice.

Cytokines

Cytokines are soluble peptides which have many important but complex effects, including the regulation of immune and inflammatory responses. Recombinant DNA technology has allowed the large scale production of many cytokines and these are being used increasingly in an attempt to modify the biological response to malignancy and infection. Interferon α has been shown in clinical studies to have beneficial effects in a limited number of malignancies, including renal carcinoma, melanoma, chronic granulolytic leukaemia and the rare hairy cell leukaemia. Interleukin-2 therapy has met with limited success in the treatment of metastatic renal carcinoma and melanoma but results for most other solid tumours have been disappointing. Interferons may be effective in treating some viral diseases, e.g. chronic active hepatitis B infection, and granulocyte colony stimulating factor (G-CSF) may be effective in reversing neutropenia. The use of cytokines as biological response modifiers is at an early stage of development and holds promise for the future.

Comment

The pharmacological modification of immune mechanisms offer opportunities to selectively attenuate or enhance humoral or cell-mediated immunological responses contributing to disease states.

Chapter 14
Corticosteroids

Corticosteroids are usually given for one of three reasons:

1 Suppression of inflammation.
2 Suppression of immune responses.
3 Replacement therapy.

They are hormones normally synthesized from cholesterol by the adrenal cortex and have a wide range of physiological functions. Pharmacologically, they are divided according to the relative potencies of their physiological effects into:

1 Glucocorticoids that principally affect carbohydrate and protein metabolism (type II receptor).
2 Mineralocorticoids that principally affect sodium balance (type I receptor).

Production of the naturally occurring glucocorticoid, cortisol (hydrocortisone), is stimulated by the release of adrenocorticotrophic hormone (ACTH) from the anterior pituitary. Production of the major naturally occurring mineralocorticoid, aldosterone, is controlled by other factors in addition to ACTH, including the activity of the renin–angiotensin system and plasma potassium. Synthetic steroids have largely replaced the natural compounds in therapeutic use as they are usually more potent, may be more specific with regard to mineralocorticoid and glucocorticoid activity and can be given orally. Prednisolone, betamethasone and dexamethasone are widely used as anti-inflammatory and immunosuppressant drugs.

14.1 GLUCOCORTICOIDS

Cortisol and its derivatives

Pharmacological effects

1 Inflammatory responses. Irrespective of the injury or the insult, corticosteroids interfere non-specifically with all components of the inflammatory responses. This includes reduced capillary dilatation and exudation, inhibition of leucocyte migration and phagocytic activity and reduced fibrin deposition with diminution of subsequent scar formation (Chapter 12, Section 12.3). It has been suggested that glucocorticoids induce the production of lipocortins in cells taking part in the inflammatory response. These proteins inhibit phospholipase A2 and hence the production of arachidonic acid and both cyclo-oxygenase and lipo-oxygenase products.

2 Immunological response. In high doses, lymphocyte mass and immunoglobulin production are reduced, as are monocyte and macrophage functions. This results in impaired immunological competence (Chapter 13, Section 13.2).
3 Carbohydrate and protein metabolism. Steroids promote glycogen deposition in the liver and gluconeogenesis, an increase in glucose output by the liver and a decrease in glucose utilization by peripheral tissues. There is a concomitant increase in protein catabolism, with mobilization of amino acids from peripheral tissues.
4 Fluid and electrolyte balance. Even glucocorticoids have some mineralocorticoid activity and can act on type I receptors. The principal effect is of enhanced sodium reabsorption from the distal tubule of the kidney, with an associated increase in the urinary excretion of potassium and hydrogen ions. Oedema is rare but moderate hypertension is not uncommon.
5 Lipid metabolism. Corticosteroids facilitate fat mobilization by adrenaline and redistribution of body fat to 'centripetal' areas: face, neck, shoulders.
6 Mood and behaviour changes. Mild euphoria is quite common with higher doses.
7 Increase in the number of red cells, platelets and polymorphs but a decrease in the number of eosinophils and lymphocytes.
8 Increased production of gastric acid and pepsin.
9 Reduction in bone formation, a decrease in calcium absorption from the intestine and an increase in calcium loss from the kidney. There is also reduced secretion of growth hormone and antagonism of its peripheral effects, so that in children there may be growth retardation.

Adverse effects

The adverse effects of corticosteroids are largely predictable from the wide range of known physiological and pharmacological effects.

Toxicity

1 Metabolic effects. Patients on high-dose steroid therapy quickly develop a characteristic appearance: a rounded plethoric face (moon face), deposits of fat over the supraclavicular and cervical areas (buffalo hump), obesity of the trunk with relatively thin limbs, purple striae typically on the thighs and lower abdomen and a tendency to bruising. Disturbed carbohydrate metabolism leads to hyperglycaemia and glycosuria and rarely proceeds to overt diabetes mellitus. In addition to the loss of protein from skeletal muscle, patients also develop muscular weakness, which particularly affects the thighs and upper arms (proximal myopathy).
2 Fluid retention may be associated with hypokalaemic alkalosis and hypertension.
3 Increased susceptibility to infection.
4 Osteoporosis, which may cause compression fractures of the vertebral bodies and avascular necrosis of the head of the femur.
5 Psychosis. A sense of euphoria frequently accompanies high dosage steroid therapy and this may rarely proceed to overt manic psychosis. The increased sense

of well-being leads to an improved appetite and contributes to weight gain. Steroids may precipitate a depressive illness.

6 Cataract. This is a rare complication, usually in children, reflecting prolonged high dosage therapy.

7 Gastrointestinal symptoms. Dyspepsia frequently accompanies high-dose oral steroid therapy. There is an increased incidence of peptic ulceration and upper gastrointestinal bleeding. Signs of peritonitis, which would complicate a perforated peptic ulcer, may be masked by the anti-inflammatory effect of steroids.

These predictable and serious adverse effects should lead to particular caution in the use of steroid therapy in patients who have pre-existing peptic ulceration, severe hypertension, congestive cardiac failure and osteoporosis.

Adrenal suppression

The administration of exogenous corticosteroids results in negative feedback to the anterior pituitary, with inhibition of ACTH release and the consequent withdrawal of trophic stimulation to the adrenal cortex. In time, the adrenal cortex atrophies and when long-term steroid therapy is finally stopped it may be 6–12 months before normal pituitary–adrenal function recovers. An alternate day steroid regimen may cause less adrenal suppression than daily treatment. Adrenal suppression has two consequences:

1 Impairment of patient's response to 'stress' (illness, injury, surgery) and susceptibility to infection.

2 The withdrawal of corticosteroid therapy must be slow and supervised.

Short-term therapy (4–6 weeks) can be reduced quickly and stopped abruptly without difficulty. Long-term therapy, particularly with more than 5–7 mg prednisolone daily, or equivalent, carries the risk of adrenal and hypothalamic–pituitary suppression. Withdrawal must be undertaken cautiously and gradually. Assuming that there is no flare-up of the systemic disease for which the steroid therapy was originally prescribed, the daily dose should be reduced by 5 mg prednisolone, or equivalent, every 1–2 weeks until the total daily dose is at the physiological replacement level of 5 mg daily. This dosage should be converted to a single morning administration, and at intervals of 2 weeks decrements of 1 mg should be made. The safety of this gradual withdrawal can be monitored by the endogenous plasma cortisol level; full recovery can be verified by a Synacthin (ACTH) test. All these patients require supervision and advice for 6 months after steroid withdrawal.

Patients on long-term steroid therapy, and particularly those undergoing steroid withdrawal, require a temporary increase in dose of steroid during periods of stress because of the inability of the hypothalamic–pituitary–adrenal axis to respond normally with an increased production of endogenous corticosteroid, e.g. in times of intercurrent illness. Similarly, patients on steroid therapy who undergo surgery require an increased steroid dosage to enable them to withstand the stress of the operation. Such patients need to carry a steroid card (or bracelet/necklace) so that they can be identified as steroid dependent in the event of an accident/emergency. They should understand the need for uninterrupted treatment and report any problem (vomiting/diarrhoea) immediately. If travelling to remote areas they should be instructed in the self-administration of intravenous hydrocortisone and given the appropriate equipment and drugs.

Topical therapy

Topically applied steroids are absorbed through the skin and in the case of very potent drugs, such as clobetasol or betamethasone, adrenal suppression and the toxic effects described above can occur. This usually happens only if recommended doses are exceeded, extensive areas of skin are covered or very prolonged administration is used.

Other effects peculiar to topical application are:

1 Worsening of local infections. This is particularly important in the eye, where ulcers caused by herpes simplex (dendritic ulcers) spread dramatically and dangerously following application of steroids.

2 Local thinning of the skin. This slowly resolves on stopping steroids, but some permanent damage may remain.

3 Atrophic striae; these are irreversible.

4 Increased hair growth.

5 The use of high doses of beclomethasone by aerosol inhalation can result in hoarseness or candidiasis of the mouth.

Clinical use and dose

Hydrocortisone

Hydrocortisone is used in three different situations:

1 Replacement therapy, when it is given orally in a dose of 20 mg in the morning and 10 mg in the evening. Body size needs to be taken into consideration (12–15 mg/m^2 surface area).

2 Shock and status asthmaticus, when it is given intravenously up to 200 mg 6 hourly.

3 Topical application: e.g. 1% cream or ointment in eczema; 100 mg dose as enema or foam in treating ulcerative colitis.

Cortisone acetate

Cortisone acetate is metabolized to cortisol, although some patients may be deficient in the relevant enzyme.

Prednisolone

Prednisolone is used orally in three types of condition:

1 Inflammatory diseases, e.g. severe rheumatoid arthritis, ulcerative colitis, chronic active hepatitis.

2 Allergic diseases, e.g. severe asthma, minimal change glomerulonephritis.

3 Acute lymphoblastic leukaemia and non-Hodgkin lymphoma.

It would be usual to start at 20 mg 8 hourly and reduce the dose according to clinical improvement.

It is used topically in ulcerative colitis as a 20 mg enema.

Prednisone

Prednisone is a synthetic steroid that is metabolized to prednisolone in much the same way as cortisone acetate is converted to cortisol.

Beclomethasone

Beclomethasone is a fluorinated, and therefore polar, steroid which passes poorly across membranes. It is used topically in:

1 Asthma, when it is given by metered aerosol doses, each of 50 μg. The usual daily dose is 100 μg 6–8 hourly. About 20% of this reaches the lungs; the rest is swallowed and destroyed by first-pass metabolism.

2 Severe eczema, when it is used as 0.025% cream.

Betamethasone

Betamethasone is used for:

1 Cerebral oedema caused by tumours and trauma; given either orally or intramuscularly in doses up to 4 mg 6 hourly. It is ineffective in cerebral oedema resulting from hypoxia.

2 Severe eczema; given topically as 0.1% cream.

Dexamethasone

Dexamethasone is used in cerebral oedema.

Triamcinolone

Triamcinolone is used for:

1 Local inflammation of joints or soft tissue; given by intra-articular injection in doses up to 40 mg depending on joint size.

2 Severe eczema; given topically as 0.1% cream.

Clobetasol

Clobetasol is used topically in severe resistant eczema and discoid lupus erythematosus.

14.2 MINERALOCORTICOIDS

Aldosterone and derivatives

Pharmacological effects

These drugs produce retention of salt and water by the same mechanism as aldosterone on the distal renal tubule. Their main adverse effect is excessive fluid retention and hypertension.

Clinical use and dose

Fludrocortisone is a fluorinated hydrocortisone with powerful mineralocorticoid activity and very little anti-inflammatory action. It is used in:

1 Replacement therapy in doses of 50–200 μg daily.

2 Congenital adrenal hyperplasia in doses up to 2 mg/day.

3 Idiopathic postural hypotension, 100–200 μg each day.

Comment

Steroids are powerful drugs. Dramatic improvement in certain severe diseases is matched by equally dramatic ill health due to adverse effects when these drugs are used in mild inflammatory disorders for which they are not indicated. Steroids, therefore, should be used only when other less toxic drugs have failed, or when the severity of the condition justifies aggressive treatment with steroids in high doses. Once control of the clinical state has been achieved, steroid dose should be reduced to the minimum necessary to maintain the desired effect and, if possible, stopped altogether.

Chapter 15
Drugs and the Reproductive System

15.1 ORAL CONTRACEPTIVES AND OESTROGENS

Oral contraceptives have revolutionized the place of women in society. Their efficacy, convenience and overall safety have allowed women to decide if and when they will become pregnant and to plan their domestic and business lives accordingly. They are, however, potent pharmacological agents and the use of oral contraceptives presents an unacceptable risk to women with certain medical or social characteristics.

Composition

The contraceptive pill contains either an oestrogen and progestogen combined or a progestogen alone. Both of the naturally occurring steroids, oestradiol and progesterone, are ineffective orally because of extensive first-pass metabolism, thus synthetic compounds are used. At present, the oestrogen is usually ethinyloestradiol or its methoxy derivative, mestranol. The term progestogen is misleading since the progestogens in use as contraceptives are mainly synthetic derivatives of 19-nortestosterone and are often metabolized to oestrogens. Therefore, progestogens can have some androgenic and oestrogenic as well as progestational properties. Those in common use are levonorgestrel, norethisterone, ethynodiol diacetate and desogestrel.

Mechanism

The combined oestrogen and progestogen pill inhibits ovulation. The oestrogen component inhibits the release of follicle stimulating hormone (FSH) while the progestogen prevents luteinizing hormone (LH) release. The abrupt withdrawal of progestogen at the end of each dosing period assures a prompt onset of withdrawal bleeding similar to normal menstruation. The progestogen-only pill contains less steroid than the combination tablets and probably works mainly by altering both cervical mucus and endometrium so as to reduce the opportunity for fertilization and implantation. In addition, ovulation is prevented in about 40% of women.

Pharmacokinetics

The constituents of contraceptive pills are well absorbed and are eliminated after liver metabolism.

Adverse effects

The most important, but not the most common, adverse reactions involve the cardiovascular system.

Venous thromboembolic disease

1 The risk is increased by:
(a) Oestrogen content above 50 μg.
(b) Intercurrent major surgical procedures.
(c) Blood groups A, B, AB.

2 The increased risk is confined to those actually taking the pill:
(a) Develops within first month.
(b) Remains constant during use.
(c) Returns to normal within 1 month of stopping.

3 Pathogenesis:
(a) Decreased antithrombin III.
(b) Decreased plasminogen activator in endothelium.

Myocardial infarction and stroke (including subarachnoid haemorrhage)

1 The risk is increased by:
(a) Age.
(b) Cigarette smoking.
(c) Oestrogen and progestogen content, but mainly oestrogen.

Age and cigarette smoking multiply, rather than add to, the risks of the oral contraceptives with regard to myocardial infarction and stroke. Most cases occur in women aged over 35 who smoke.

It is assumed that the risk is also enhanced by hypertension, diabetes, obesity and hyperlipoproteinaemia but numbers are too small for statistical analysis.

2 The risk is not confined to those currently taking the pill, but persists after stopping.

3 Pathogenesis:
(a) Acceleration of platelet aggregation.
(b) Decreased antithrombin III.
(c) Decreased plasminogen activator.

Hypertension

1 Blood pressure rises by a small amount in all women on the pill. There is a progressive rise with duration of use. In most cases this increase in pressure is small and of little clinical significance. Less frequently there is a rise to levels in which treatment might ordinarily be considered. The best course of action in these cases is to stop the pill and observe for several months. Rarely, malignant hypertension occurs and should be treated as a medical emergency. Blood pressure should be checked at each clinic visit in women receiving an oral contraceptive.

2 Blood pressure usually returns to normal 3–6 months after stopping the contraceptive pill.

Oral contraceptives and cancer

This is a controversial area. Oral contraceptive use appears to protect against endometrial and ovarian carcinoma. Cervical neoplasia has been identified more frequently in pill users than in women using an intra-uterine contraceptive device (IUCD). Interpretation of this finding is difficult because age at first intercourse and number of sexual partners are risk factors for cervical carcinoma and could differ substantially between these two groups. The suggestion that oral contraceptive use at a young age increases the risk of breast cancer remains unproven.

Glucose tolerance and lipid metabolism

There is a small decrease in glucose tolerance. Oestrogens increase, and progestogens decrease, high density lipoproteins. The clinical relevance of these observations is unknown.

Other adverse effects

Additional effects of oral contraceptives frequently include:

1 Irregular bleeding during the first few cycles.
2 Headaches.
3 Mood swings.

Less commonly subjects may present with:

1 Cholestatic jaundice; particularly if a history of jaundice or pruritis in pregnancy.
2 Increased incidence of gallstones.
3 Elevation of thyroid binding globulin (does not affect analysis of free T_4).
4 Precipitation of porphyria.

There is no evidence that oral contraceptives containing low doses of oestrogen either impair established lactation or harm a breast fed infant.

Drug interactions

Oral contraceptive failure with unwanted pregnancy can be precipitated by enzyme induction resulting from the co-administration of drugs that induce hepatic microsomal enzymes (Chapter 1, Section 1.3):

Phenytoin.
Carbamazepine.
Phenobarbitone.
Primidone.
Rifampicin.

If long-term treatment with one of these drugs is necessary (e.g. epilepsy) then 50 μg or more of oestrogen should be used if oral contraception is the method of choice.

Oral contraceptive failure can be precipitated by reduced absorption resulting from altered bowel flora caused by the co-administratlon of broad spectrum antimicrobials. The mechanism depends on the fact that oestrogens undergo conjugation in the liver but hydrolytic enzymes produced by gut bacteria cleave these conjugates and release free hormone, which is then reabsorbed. Broad spectrum antimicrobials prevent this process by altering gut flora, and hormone absorption is decreased. When an antibiotic such as ampicillin is prescribed for a woman who is also taking an oral contraceptive she should be advised to use additional contraception during and for 14 days after the course of antibiotic.

Clinical use and dose

The dose of both oestrogen and progestogen should be kept as low as possible.

1 Combination pill: one tablet daily for 21 days starting on day 1 of the menstrual cycle and repeating after seven pill-free days.

2 Progestogen-only pill: continuous administration of one tablet daily starting on the first day of menstruation and taking the dose at the same time each day. A delay of more than 3 hours risks loss of efficacy.

3 Intramuscular medroxyprogesterone acetate: this is a long-acting (3 months) progesterone derivative.

4 Phased formulations (biphasic or triphasic). These provide varying doses of oestrogen and progestogen during the cycle. Deviations from normal metabolism are small and triphasics are recommended for women aged over 35. They are taken from day 1 with a 7-day interval.

The combination oral contraceptive is the most effective form of contraception currently available: the failure rate is around 1/100 woman years. The efficacy of progestogen-only pills is controversial but is probably equal to that of intra-uterine devices, i.e. a failure rate of about 2/100 woman years.

Contra-indications

These are summarized in Table 15.1.

Patients with established diabetes mellitus may use the combined pill with appropriate adjustment of insulin requirements.

Ideally, nobody with a relative contra-indication should receive an oestrogen-containing oral contraceptive. However, real life is not ideal and pressure of social circumstances sometimes dictates that the risks of an unwanted pregnancy outweigh those accompanying the use of the contraceptive pill; the other forms of contraception are less reliable. The presence of two or more relative contra-indications strengthens the case against using an oestrogen-containing contraceptive.

Table 15.1. Contra-indications to the use of oral contraceptives

Absolute	Relative
History of thromboembolism	Diabetes
Moderate–severe hypertension	Cigarette smoking
Active liver disease	Mild hypertension
Age >35 and cigarette smoker	Age >35
Porphyria	
Oestrogen dependent tumour	
Impending major surgery	
History of jaundice in pregnancy	
Major haemoglobinopathy	

Comment

The widespread use of oral contraceptives is a testament to their popularity. Serious cardiovascular complications are clearly of concern and must be explained to a woman proposing to take the pill. However, they must be explained in the perspective that risk of myocardial infarction and stroke is concentrated largely in older women who smoke and that some, at least, of the morbidity in currently available statistics can still be ascribed to the use of now obsolete high-dose oestrogen preparations.

Other uses for oestrogens

1 Replacement therapy: widely used in controlling menopausal symptoms. There is an increasing demand from postmenopausal women for adequate hormone replacement therapy. The type of preparation used will depend on whether or not the uterus is still present. If it is, then a combination of oestrogen and progesterone should be used to prevent endometrial hyperplasia/carcinoma. In the absence of a uterus, oestrogen alone is of use. Occasionally, short courses of oestrogen are required in conditions like atrophic vaginitis/vulvitis and cystitis. A long-term benefit of replacement therapy may be the prevention of osteoporosis.

2 Dysmenorrhoea.

3 Dysfunctional uterine bleeding.

4 Prostatic carcinoma: these tumours are androgen dependent and administration of oestrogen will decrease androgen production. Remission occurs in 60% of patients with advanced disease. Dose: stilboestrol, 1 mg 8 hourly. Adverse effects: nausea, vomiting, fluid retention, heart failure, feminization.

5 Breast carcinoma: in women who are more than 5 years postmenopausal, oestrogens produce a remission in approximately one-third of patients with metastatic disease. The chance of success is higher (as many as two-thirds) if the tumour possesses oestrogen receptors. Dose: stilboestrol, 5–15 mg 8 hourly.

Anti-oestrogen therapy

Tamoxifen competes with oestrogen at binding sites on oestrogen dependent breast tumours in premenopausal women. Remission occurs in about 40% of patients (Chapter 13, Section 13.1). Dose: 10 mg twice daily. Tamoxifen can cause hot flushes and uterine bleeding.

15.2 BROMOCRIPTINE

Mechanism

Bromocriptine is a dopamine receptor agonist that prevents the release of prolactin by stimulating dopamine receptors in the pituitary. It increases growth hormone (GM) release in normal subjects but suppresses GM release in acromegaly.

Pharmacokinetics

Bromocriptine is effective orally and eliminated by liver metabolism followed by biliary excretion.

Adverse effects

Nausea and vomiting may limit dose increases. Postural hypotension can occur. Constipation is common. High doses (> 20 mg/day) can produce a wide range of neuropsychiatric effects, including confusion, psychosis, dyskinesias and bizarre choreiform movements.

Clinical use and dose

Hyperprolactinaemia: up to 7.5 mg twice a day.
Postpartum suppression of lactation: 2.5 mg twice a day for 2 weeks.
Acromegaly: 5 mg 6 hourly.
Parkinsonism: high doses up to 100 mg daily (Chapter 20, Section 20.2).

15.3 DANAZOL

Mechanism

Danazol inhibits pituitary gonadotrophin release, thereby reducing ovarian function and producing atrophy of the endometrium. It also blocks oestrogen and progesterone receptors and has some androgenic activity.

Adverse effects

Avoid danazol during pregnancy: virilization of female fetus has been reported.

Danazol is not an effective contraceptive and non-hormonal methods should be used during treatment. Acne, hirsutism and voice changes occasionally occur.

Drug interactions

Danazol potentiates the action of carbamazepine and anticoagulants.

Clinical use

Endometriosis.
Menorrhagia.
Premenstrual syndrome.
Hereditary angioedema.

15.4 CLOMIPHENE

Mechanism

Clomiphene is an oestrogen receptor antagonist that prevents negative feedback of oestrogen at the hypothalamus, leading to increased secretion of FSH and LH.

Clinical use and dose

Female subfertility: 50 mg/day for 5 days.
Oligospermia: 12.5 mg/daily (monitor treatment by regular sperm counts).

15.5 TESTOSTERONE

Mechanism

Testosterone is the major male sex hormone and is responsible for secondary sexual characteristics.

Pharmacokinetics

Testosterone has an extensive first-pass metabolism: it is given either sublingually or by intramuscular injection.

Adverse effects

Testosterone causes virilization when given to women and patients with liver tumours when used in high dose. Methyltestosterone causes cholestatic jaundice.

Drug interactions

Oral anticoagulant requirements are decreased by testosterone.

Clinical use

Testosterone is used for replacement therapy and oestrogen-dependent metastases from breast cancer in premenopausal women.

15.6 DRUGS ADVERSELY AFFECTING SEXUAL FUNCTION

Several drugs can adversely influence sexual function and the more frequently used are listed in Table 15.2. Remember that patients might not volunteer information about an adverse effect which they consider embarrassing, and which they might not relate to their drug treatment.

Table 15.2. Drugs which can adversely influence sexual function

Drug	Comment
Methyldopa	Impotence; failure of ejaculation; loss of sexual drive
Clonidine	Impotence Difficulty in achieving orgasm (women)
Tricyclic antidepressants	Delayed ejaculation
Phenothiazines	Difficulties in erection and ejaculation
Phenelzine	Delayed ejaculation
Cimetidine	Impaired spermatogenesis (reversible) Impotence
Isoniazid	Menstrual disturbance
Diuretics	Impotence and reduced libido: mechanism unknown
Guanethidine	Impotence, retrograde ejaculation
Sulphasalazine	Impaired spermatogenesis (reversible)

Chapter 16
Drugs and Gastrointestinal Disease

16.1 PEPTIC ULCER

Aims

1 To relieve pain.
2 To heal the ulcer.
3 To prevent ulcer relapse or complications.

Relevant pathophysiology

The cause or causes of peptic ulceration are unknown. Peptic ulcers in the stomach or duodenum probably result from an imbalance between 'aggressive' forces of acid and pepsin and the 'defensive' factors of gastric mucus and bicarbonate secretion, gastric mucosal blood flow and the innate resistance of the gastric and duodenal mucosa. Gastric acid is a prerequisite for the development of a peptic ulcer. ('No acid, no ulcer'.) Also, the vast majority of patients with peptic ulcer have the bacterium *Helicobacter pylori* present on their gastric mucosa. The precise role of this bacterium in the production of peptic ulcers is unknown but its presence is associated with ulcer relapse.

It is important to realize that both gastric and duodenal ulceration are chronic, relapsing conditions. It is relatively simple to heal ulcers with drug therapy but more difficult to keep them healed. There is now some evidence to suggest that ulcers stay healed for longer if *Helicobacter pylori* infection is eradicated, although this is difficult to achieve in clinical practice.

Drugs used in the treatment of peptic ulcer

1 Antacids.
2 Drugs which inhibit acid secretion:
   (a) H_2-receptor antagonists.
   (b) Proton pump inhibitors: omeprazole.
   (c) Anticholinergics: pirenzepine.
   (d) Synthetic prostaglandins: misoprostol.
3 Drugs which do not inhibit acid secretion:
   (a) Chelated salts of bismuth.
   (b) Sucralfate.
   (c) Carbenoxolone.

Antacids

Mechanism

These drugs are weak alkalis so they partly neutralize free acid in the stomach. They may also stimulate mucosal repair mechanisms around ulcers, possibly by stimulating local prostaglandin release.

Pharmacokinetics

Most antacids (principally salts of magnesium or aluminium) are not absorbed from the alimentary tract to any appreciable extent. Some, such as sodium bicarbonate, are absorbed.

Adverse effects

Antacids which contain aluminium tend to cause constipation. Those containing magnesium have the opposite effect. Sodium bicarbonate in large quantities may alter acid—base status causing a metabolic alkalosis and may promote the formation of phosphate-containing renal calculi. Absorbable antacids should not be administered in the long term. Antacids with a high sodium content should be avoided in patients with impaired cardiac function or chronic liver disease.

Drug interactions

Antacids may reduce the absorption of a number of different drugs from the gut. These include digoxin, phenothiazines and tetracyclines.

Clinical use and dosage

Antacids are mainly used for symptomatic relief in patients with peptic ulcer, gastro-oesophageal reflux disease or non-ulcer dyspepsia ('indigestion'). They can accelerate the healing of peptic ulcers but must be given frequently and in high doses.

Suitable antacids are:
Aluminium hydroxide, 5–15 ml 6 hourly.
Magnesium trisilicate, 10–20 ml as required.

Drugs which inhibit acid secretion

H_2-receptor antagonists

Currently, there are four such agents available (cimetidine, ranitidine, nizatidine and famotidine). They are all competitive antagonists for histamine at the H_2-receptor found mainly on parietal cells.

Mechanism

By competing with histamine at the H_2-receptor, these drugs reduce acid secretion by the parietal cell, especially at night and in the fasting state. They are less effective in reducing food-stimulated acid secretion.

Pharmacokinetics

They are well absorbed following oral administration. They have relatively short half-lives and are largely excreted unchanged by the kidneys.

Adverse effects

These are rare and usually of a minor nature. Cimetidine is weakly antiandrogenic in man. It may rarely cause impotence or gynaecomastia. Either cimetidine or ranitidine may cause reversible mental confusion, particularly in sick elderly patients. Some potentially serious cardiac dysrhythmias have occurred following intravenous injections of H_2-receptor antagonists.

Drug interactions

Cimetidine inhibits oxidative drug metabolism by the liver. It interacts with many drugs but only three are of clinical importance. These are phenytoin, theophylline and warfarin. These three drugs are metabolized in the liver and have narrow therapeutic indices; cimetidine will slow their metabolism and may induce toxicity.

To date, no clinically relevant drug interactions have been reported with the other H_2-receptor antagonists.

Clinical use and dosage

H_2-receptor antagonists are of proven value in the treatment of duodenal ulcer, benign gastric ulcer and gastro-oesophageal reflux disease. Patients being treated for gastric ulcer should have repeated endoscopic examinations with gastric biopsy to exclude the possibility of malignancy.

Recommended doses of H_2-receptor antagonists are:

Cimetidine, 400 mg twice daily or 800 mg at night.

Ranitidine, 150 mg twice daily or 300 mg at night.

Nizatidine, 300 mg at night.

Famotidine, 40 mg at night.

These drugs can heal 75–80% of duodenal ulcers within 4 weeks and 90–95% within 8 weeks. Gastric ulcers may take longer to heal but 80–90% will heal within 8 weeks.

Although H_2-receptor antagonists are of no proven value in the management of bleeding peptic ulcer, they are used in the prophylaxis of gastric mucosal stress related haemorrhage in critically ill patients, such as those with fulminant hepatic failure.

In high doses, H_2-receptor antagonists may be successful in controlling the excessive secretion of gastric acid seen in the rare Zollinger–Ellison syndrome.

H_2-receptor antagonists are a useful adjunct to treatment in patients with chronic pancreatic exocrine insufficiency. Since they inhibit gastric acid secretion, they reduce the likelihood of exogenous pancreatic enzymes being denatured in the stomach.

Comment

The H_2-receptor antagonists are firmly established in the treatment of peptic ulceration. They give prompt symptomatic relief and can heal almost all ulcers if given for long enough. Their specific indications are as listed above. They are of no proven value in non-ulcer dyspepsia and should not be given indiscriminately for undiagnosed abdominal pains.

Some patients, such as those with frequent relapses or those with a history of an ulcer complication, should be given maintenance treatment after their ulcer has healed successfully. A reduced maintenance dose at night (e.g. 400 mg cimetidine, 150 mg ranitidine, 150 mg nizatidine, 20 mg famotidine) will reduce the spontaneous ulcer relapse rate. However, by no means all patients require maintenance treatment. In the long-term treatment of patients with peptic ulcer, successfully stopping smoking is a much more important factor.

Proton pump inhibitors: omeprazole

Mechanism

This drug is an irreversible inhibitor of the proton pump of the parietal cell. The pump is an enzyme which actively secretes hydrogen ions into the gastric lumen. Omeprazole is an extremely powerful inhibitor of gastric acid secretion.

Pharmacokinetics

Absorption is limited when initially given by mouth but this increases with repeated administration. The plasma half-life is short but there is a prolonged pharmacological effect. Omeprazole is converted to inactive metabolites in the liver.

Adverse effects

No significant adverse effects have been reported to date.

Drug interactions

Omeprazole inhibits hepatic oxidative drug metabolism. It prolongs the elimination of diazepam and phenytoin. There may also be a weak interaction with warfarin.

Clinical use and dosage

Omeprazole is indicated for the treatment of gastric or duodenal ulcers which have not healed on conventional medication, including those in patients taking non-steroidal anti-inflammatory drugs (NSAIDs). The standard dose is 20 mg once daily but this can be increased to 40 mg once daily in the rare, resistant patients.

Omeprazole is the drug of choice for the management of Zollinger–Ellison syndrome. Doses of up to 120 mg daily have been used.

Anticholinergics: pirenzepine

Mechanism

This is a relatively specific competitive antagonist of acetylcholine at the muscarinic receptor on the parietal cell. It is a weak inhibitor of gastric acid secretion.

Pharmacokinetics

Absorption is limited; most is excreted unchanged.

Adverse effects

Since selectivity of action for the stomach is only relative, pirenzepine does produce dose related anticholinergic side effects, including dry mouth, difficulty in visual accommodation, hesitancy of micturition and constipation.

Drug interactions

No important interactions are known.

Clinical use and dose

Pirenzepine is approved for the treatment of duodenal ulcer and benign gastric ulcer but healing rates are inferior to those obtained with H_2-receptor antagonists. Side effects are also more common but are limited if the total daily dose does not exceed 150 mg.

Synthetic prostaglandins: misoprostol

Mechanism

Prostaglandins suppress gastric acid secretion through an incompletely understood mechanism. They can also protect the gastric mucosa from injurious agents through a mechanism unrelated to suppression of acid secretion ('cytoprotection').

Pharmacokinetics

Misoprostol has a short plasma half-life. It may act on the stomach both locally and systemically.

Adverse effects

There is diarrhoea in up to 40% of patients, but this is usually mild and self-limiting. Misoprostol and other prostaglandins are potentially abortifacient and so should not be given to women of child-bearing age.

Clinical use and dose

The main indication is to prevent gastric mucosal damage and gastric ulcers in patients on NSAIDs. Dose is 200 μg twice to four times daily.

Comment

Misoprostol should be considered for those patients who genuinely require to take NSAIDs and who have a past history of peptic ulcer or upper gastrointestinal bleeding.

For patients already on NSAIDs who are found to have a peptic ulcer, the NSAID should be stopped if possible. However, even if the NSAID has to be continued (in a patient with rheumatoid arthritis, for example), the ulcer can be healed with any type of anti-ulcer drug. There is no specific indication for misoprostol in this situation.

Drugs which do not inhibit acid secretion

Chelated salts of bismuth: tripotassium dicitrato bismuthate

Mechanism

The means whereby bismuth salts heal ulcers are not fully understood. They do not inhibit acid secretion by the stomach. They may form an insoluble protective layer over the ulcer base, preventing further damage by acid and pepsin. They may stimulate local prostaglandin production. Bismuth is toxic to *Helicobacter pylori* but must be given with antibiotics to eradicate successfully the infection.

Pharmacokinetics

A small quantity of bismuth is absorbed following oral administration. Urinary excretion of bismuth continues for over 2 weeks after stopping a course of treatment.

Adverse effects

The liquid preparation should be avoided because of an unpleasant smell and taste and the fact that it discolours the tongue. The liquid or tablet preparation may colour the faeces black. The long-term consequences of bismuth absorption are unknown, so this drug is not recommended for continuous or repeated administration.

Comment

There is now good evidence that ulcer relapse rates are lower after healing with bismuth than after healing with H_2-receptor antagonists. This may be related to suppression of *Helicobacter pylori*.

Sucralfate (sucrose aluminium octasulphate)

Mechanism

The exact mechanism of ulcer healing by sucralfate is unknown. It may act by coating ulcer bases or by stimulating local prostaglandin release. It does not affect acid secretion.

Pharmacokinetics

Sucralfate acts locally; only small amounts of aluminium are absorbed.

Adverse effects

Constipation.

Drug interactions

Sucralfate can reduce the absorption of a number of different drugs, including phenytoin and tetracyclines.

Clinical use and dosage

Sucralfate is indicated for the treatment of duodenal ulcer and benign gastric ulcer. The usual dose is 1 g four times daily or 2 g twice daily. Healing rates are comparable to those obtained with H_2-receptor antagonists. Sucralfate should not be used in patients with chronic renal failure because of the risk of aluminium absorption and toxicity.

Carbenoxolone

Mechanism

Carbenoxolone may stimulate gastric mucus secretion but does not affect acid secretion.

Adverse effects

Carbenoxolone acts like aldosterone, so causes salt and water retention and hypokalaemia.

Drug interactions

Spironolactone counteracts the aldosterone-like effect of carbenoxolone but also reduces its therapeutic effect. Thiazide diuretics worsen the hypokalaemia.

Clinical use and dosage

Carbenoxolone has been used in the past for the treatment of benign gastric ulcer in a dose of 100 mg three times daily.

Comment

Carbenoxolone is only included here for the sake of completeness. Its use is not recommended since other drugs are available which are more efficacious and less toxic.

16.2 GASTRO-OESOPHAGEAL REFLUX DISEASE

Aims

1 To relieve symptoms.
2 To heal lesions of oesophagitis.
3 To prevent complications.

Relevant pathophysiology

In most patients, the lower oesophageal sphincter is functionally incompetent and relaxes inappropriately to allow reflux of gastric contents, containing acid and pepsin, into the oesophagus. Secretion of gastric acid is normal in most patients. Some patients have impaired clearance of refluxed material from the oesophagus.

Drugs used in the treatment of gastro-oesophageal reflux disease

1 Antacids and antacid–alginate combinations.
2 Drugs which inhibit acid secretion:
   (a) H_2-receptor antagonists.

   (b) Proton pump inhibitors: omeprazole.
3 Drugs which affect oesophageal and/or gastric motility:
   (a) Metoclopramide, domperidone.
   (b) Cisapride.

Antacids and antacid/alginate preparations

Antacids are discussed above. In combination with an alginate, they are thought to provide a protective coating to the lower oesophagus, preventing some contact with refluxed gastric contents.

Drugs which inhibit acid secretion

H_2-receptor antagonists

These are discussed above. They have generally been less successful in the management of gastro-oesophageal reflux disease than in peptic ulcer. To be effective in the treatment of gastro-oesophageal reflux disease, they may have to be given in much higher doses than in peptic ulcer (e.g. ranitidine, 300 mg 6 hourly).

Proton pump inhibitors: omeprazole

This is discussed above. To date, severe gastro-oesophageal reflux disease is the main indication for the use of omeprazole. It is superior to the H_2-receptor antagonists in treating the symptoms of this condition and in healing the oesophagitis. Unfortunately, relapse is common after stopping treatment and omeprazole has not been approved for long-term use.

Drugs which affect oesophageal and/or gastric motility

Metoclopramide, domperidone

These drugs are discussed in more detail in Section 16.4. In gastro-oesophageal reflux disease, they accelerate gastric emptying through the pylorus, increase lower oesophageal sphincter tone and may promote the clearance from the oesophagus of refluxed gastric contents.

They are seldom effective alone but can be combined with an H_2-receptor antagonist.

Cisapride

Mechanism

This drug probably promotes motility in the upper gastrointestinal tract by causing release of acetylcholine from nerve endings in the myenteric plexus. It speeds up gastric emptying and oesophageal clearance and may increase lower oesophageal sphincter tone.

Pharmacokinetics

Cisapride is extensively protein bound and is metabolized extensively in the liver.

Adverse effects

No significant adverse effects have been reported to date.

Drug interactions

No clinically important interactions are known.

Clinical use and dose

Cisapride is indicated in the treatment of gastro-oesophageal reflux disease (and in certain conditions associated with delayed gastric emptying). The usual dose is 10 mg three or four times daily. In gastro-oesophageal reflux disease, it can be combined with an H_2-receptor antagonist.

16.3 DIARRHOEA AND CONSTIPATION

Aims

1 To identify and eliminate a cause where possible.
2 If the cause is unclear, to give symptomatic relief.

Drugs used in specific conditions

Irritable bowel syndrome

This common condition is the most frequent cause of chronic, recurrent abdominal pain. It may also cause upset of bowel habit, with diarrhoea, constipation or both. The pathophysiology is poorly understood. There are abnormal motility patterns in the bowel and patients may be unduly sensitive to distension or contraction of visceral smooth muscle. Some patients' diets are deficient in fibre. There is a relationship between psychological stress and symptoms in some patients.

Mebeverine is an antispasmodic agent which does not have significant anticholinergic effects. It is useful in relieving symptoms in some patients in a dose of 135 mg three times daily.

Enteric coated capsules of **peppermint oil** are useful in relieving gut spasm in some patients. The capsules may cause heartburn if bitten into.

Pancreatic insufficiency

A preparation of exogenous pancreatic enzymes containing trypsin, lipase and amylase is given for patients with chronic pancreatic exocrine insufficiency, as in chronic pancreatitis or cystic fibrosis. H_2-receptor antagonists are frequently also given, as described above.

Drugs used in non-specific diarrhoea

Codeine phosphate

This is a useful agent for symptomatic control of diarrhoea. It raises intracolonic pressure and sphincter tone. It should not be given to patients with colonic diverticular disease and should be used only cautiously in patients with inflammatory bowel disease, and only under careful supervision.

Morphine

Kaolin and morphine mixture British Pharmaceutical Codex (BPC) is a time-honoured remedy containing only small quantities of morphine. It is unpalatable so is taken as a liquid.

Diphenoxylate

This is an opiate derivative. It is combined with atropine in the preparation 'Lomotil'. It is more expensive than codeine phosphate and probably no better.

Loperamide

Loperamide is a synthetic opiate with some anticholinergic activity. It may cause dizziness or dryness of the mouth. The usual dose is 2 mg three or four times daily.

Comment

A cause for diarrhoea must always be sought by history (including a thorough drug history) and physical examination, supplemented as appropriate by stool samples for microbiology and possibly other investigations, including sigmoidoscopy, barium enema, rectal biopsy or colonoscopy. Occasionally, the cause lies in the upper alimentary tract (e.g. malabsorption or giardiasis).

Antibiotics should not be used indiscriminately for patients with undiagnosed diarrhoea.

Drugs used in non-specific constipation

Drugs which increase faecal bulk

These consist of non-absorbable polysaccharides, as in bran, ispaghula or sterculia. They are generally effective in simple constipation, particularly where the intake of dietary fibre is poor. They are the agents of choice where treatment is likely to be prolonged.

Stimulant laxatives

These agents stimulate intestinal motility, probably through an effect on the myenteric nerve plexus. Examples are senna and bisacodyl. Prolonged use leads to hypotonicity of the bowel and thereby eventually exacerbates chronic constipation.

Stool softeners

The best known agent in this group is liquid paraffin. It acts by lubricating the faeces, which aids passage along the bowel. It may cause slight perianal irritation. Long-term use can lead to malabsorption of fat-soluble vitamins. It is not indicated for infants, as inhalation of the liquid may produce a lipoid pneumonia.

Osmotic laxatives

These agents retain water in the bowel. They increase faecal bulk and moisten faeces. Examples are lactulose and salts of magnesium.

Comment

The commonest cause of constipation is lack of dietary fibre and most cases will respond to a high-fibre diet. Both the constipation and diarrhoea associated with diverticular disease may improve with a high-fibre diet.

16.4 NAUSEA AND VOMITING

Aims

1 To establish an underlying cause and give specific treatment if possible.
2 To give symptomatic treatment.

Relevant pathophysiology

Vomiting is controlled by two separate brainstem centres: the vomiting centre and the chemoreceptor trigger zone. The trigger zone may be activated endogenously or exogenously by toxins or by drugs such as opiates. Activation of the trigger zone stimulates the vomiting centre. The act of vomiting is controlled by the vomiting centre, mainly through vagal action. The vomiting centre has afferent input from the gut, higher cortical centres and the vestibular apparatus. Muscarinic receptors and histamine H_1-receptors are highly concentrated around the area of the vomiting centre.

Drugs used in treatment of vomiting

Anticholinergic drugs: hyoscine

Mechanism

They compete with acetylcholine at muscarinic receptors in the gut and CNS and have antispasmodic action in the gut wall. They may be successful in motion sickness because of their central action.

Adverse effects

Adverse effects are drowsiness plus typical anticholinergic effects of dry mouth, blurred vision and difficulty in micturition.

Clinical use and dose

A 0.3–0.6 mg dose of hyoscine is usually adequate prophylaxis for motion sickness.

Antihistamines: promethazine

Mechanism

Antihistamines are competitive antagonists of histamine at H_1-receptors, acting mainly on the vomiting centre rather than on the chemoreceptor trigger zone. They have weak anticholinergic effects.

Adverse effects

Adverse effects are drowsiness, occasional insomnia and euphoria. Central effects are accentuated by alcohol.

Clinical use and dose

Antihistamines are used in motion sickness or in vestibular disorders. They are also widely used in the treatment of allergic rhinitis and other allergic reactions (Chapter 13, Section 13.1).

Promethazine is given at a dose of 25 mg 8 hourly.

Dopamine antagonists

Phenothiazines: chlorpromazine, prochlorperazine

Mechanism

The general clinical pharmacology of phenothiazines is described in Chapter 19. These drugs act mainly on the chemoreceptor trigger zone. They have dopamine receptor antagonist properties as well as anticholinergic and other actions.

Adverse effects

Prolonged use may produce Parkinsonian type tremor or other dyskinesias.

Clinical use and dose

Phenothiazines are effective in a variety of situations, including the vomiting of chronic renal failure and neoplastic disease, and drug induced vomiting.

Recommended doses are:

Chlorpromazine, 25–50 mg 8 hourly.

Prochlorperazine, 5–25 mg orally or 12.5 mg i.m.

Metoclopramide

Mechanism

Metoclopramide is a central dopamine receptor antagonist, effective at blocking stimuli to the chemoreceptor trigger zone. It also has effects on upper gastrointestinal tract motility, as described above.

Adverse effects

Metoclopramide may cause acute extrapyramidal reactions, such as opisthotonus, oculogyric crisis or other dystonias. These can be treated with an intravenous anticholinergic agent, such as benztropine (Chapter 19).

Metoclopramide raises serum prolactin levels and may cause gynaecomastia by virtue of its antidopaminergic effects.

Drug interactions

Metoclopramide potentiates the extrapyramidal side effects of phenothiazines.

Clinical use and dose

Metoclopramide is effective in most causes of vomiting, apart from motion sickness. The usual dose is 10 mg 8 hourly, orally or parenterally.

Domperidone

Mechanism

Domperidone is a dopamine antagonist, effective at the chemoreceptor trigger zone.

Adverse effects

Domperidone is less likely to cause extrapyramidal reactions than metoclopramide. It raises prolactin levels and may produce cardiac dysrythmias following rapid intravenous injection.

Clinical use and dose

Domperidone is effective in most situations, especially nausea and vomiting related to cytotoxic drug therapy. The usual dose is 10–20 mg 4–8 hourly, orally or parenterally.

Cannabinoids: nabilone

Mechanism

Tetrahydrocannabinol is the active constituent of marijuana. Nabilone is a synthetic cannabinoid used in the treatment of nausea and vomiting during cytotoxic therapy. Its mode of action is unclear.

Adverse effects

Nabilone causes drowsiness, dizziness and dryness of the mouth. Euphoria and hallucinations are rare.

Clinical use and dose

Nabilone at a dose of 1–2 mg twice daily is of value in treating patients receiving cytotoxic agents. Prolonged use may produce toxic effects on the CNS.

Serotonin antagonists: ondansetron

Mechanism

Ondansetron is a selective antagonist of serotonin at 5-HT_3-receptors. Its exact mode of action in controlling nausea and vomiting is unclear but it has both CNS and peripheral actions.

Adverse effects

Ondansetron causes constipation and headache; flushing may occur.

Clinical use and dose

Ondansetron is indicated for the treatment of nausea and vomiting associated with cytotoxic therapy or radiotherapy. The dose and rate of administration depends on the severity of the problem and on the chemotherapy used.

16.5 INFLAMMATORY BOWEL DISEASE

Aims

1 To obtain remission in periods of relapse.
2 To prolong periods of remission.

Relevant pathophysiology

Ulcerative colitis and Crohn's disease are chronic inflammatory conditions of unknown aetiology. Both are characterized by episodes of remission and relapse. Drug treatment is aimed at controlling inflammation and bringing about remission. Treatment of these conditions is not only pharmacological but also depends on psychological support, correction of nutritional deficiencies and possibly surgery.

Drugs used in the treatment of inflammatory bowel disease

Corticosteroids

These agents are discussed in detail in Chapter 14.

Steroids are of proven value in the treatment of acute relapses of ulcerative colitis and Crohn's disease. They may be given rectally, orally or intravenously depending on the extent and severity of the condition.

Rectal steroids (e.g. hydrocortisone hemisuccinate, 100 mg in 100 ml fluid twice daily) are given in mild to moderate attacks of ulcerative colitis limited to the left side of the colon. In more severe or extensive cases, 40–60 mg oral prednisolone daily should be given. The dose of prednisolone should be reduced as symptoms improve, and ultimately stopped. High doses of intravenous hydrocortisone are given as part of the management of acute fulminating ulcerative colitis.

Steroids are of no value for ulcerative colitis in remission and should be withdrawn once clinical remission is achieved. There is no good evidence that Crohn's disease is helped by long-term steroids.

Sulphasalazine

Mechanism

This has two components, sulphapyridine and 5-aminosalicylic acid (5-ASA). It is thought that 5-ASA is the active component exerting some local anti-inflammatory effect.

Pharmacokinetics

When taken orally, only a small proportion of the dose is absorbed; most reaches the colon intact. Once in the colon, bacteria split the drug into its two components.

Sulphapyridine is absorbed into the circulation and is metabolized by the liver. The rate of its removal from the body depends on the acetylator status of the patients. Almost all the 5-ASA remains within the colon.

Adverse effects

These are mainly due to sulphapyridine. Nausea, vomiting, headache and skin rashes are quite common. Blood dyscrasias, methaemoglobinaemia and acute pancreatitis have been reported. Reversible male infertility is common with this drug. Some side effects are more troublesome in slow acetylators.

Clinical use and dose

In relapses of ulcerative colitis or colonic Crohn's disease, sulphasalazine is given in doses of up to 4 g daily with steroids. During remission of ulcerative colitis, sulphasalazine is given in a dose of around 2 g daily and can be continued indefinitely unless side effects are a problem.

Mesalazine

Mechanism

This is a controlled-release preparation of 5-ASA.

Pharmacokinetics

5-ASA is released in the terminal ileum and colon. Only small quantities are absorbed.

Adverse effects

Since there is no sulphapyridine in this preparation, it lacks most of the side effects of sulphasalazine.

Clinical use and dose

Mesalazine is indicated for maintenance of remission of ulcerative colitis. The usual dose is 400 mg three times daily. It is also now indicated as part of the management of mild to moderate attacks of ulcerative colitis in doses of up to 800 mg three times daily.

Olsalazine

Mechanism

This drug (sodium azodisalicylate) consists of two molecules of 5-ASA linked by an azo bond. Colonic bacteria split the azo bond to release 5-ASA within the colon.

Pharmacokinetics

5-ASA is released in the colon and only small amounts are absorbed.

Adverse effects

As for mesalazine.

Clinical use and dose

Olsalazine is used for the maintenance of remission of ulcerative colitis. The usual dose is 500 mg twice daily.

16.6 DRUGS ADVERSELY AFFECTING GASTROINTESTINAL FUNCTION

Virtually any drug may cause nausea, vomiting or diarrhoea and a detailed drug history is essential in patients with such complaints. Some specific drug induced gastrointestinal problems are listed in Table 16.1.

Diarrhoea is common in patients receiving antibiotics. This is usually attributed to an alteration in the intracolonic bacterial flora. In some patients a colitis may result from antibiotic therapy—antibiotic associated colitis or pseudomembranous colitis. This is due to the proliferation of *Clostridium difficile* in the bowel and the secretion of an endotoxin. Treatment of this condition depends on the prescription of an antibiotic which is poorly absorbed when given orally. Two suitable agents are vancomycin and metronidazole.

Table 16.1. Some drugs with adverse effects on the gut

Drug	Comment
Antacids containing aluminium; sucralfate	Constipation
Antacids containing magnesium	Diarrhoea
Oral iron salts	Nausea; constipation or diarrhoea (only nausea is dose related); darkens stools (as does bismuth)
Antibiotics	Oral and/or oesophageal candidiasis; diarrhoea
Aspirin/non-steroidal anti-inflammatory drugs (NSAIDs)	Dyspepsia; gastric erosions (with or without significant bleeding); may increase formation of gastric ulcers; increased risk of perforation or bleeding of existing gastric or duodenal ulcer; NSAIDs may cause ulceration, stricture or perforation of small intestine; NSAIDs may promote relapse of inflammatory bowel disease
Oral potassium supplements	Ulceration or perforation at sites of stasis (e.g. oesophageal or intestinal stricture)

Chapter 17
Drugs and the Blood

17.1 ANAEMIA AND HAEMATINIC DEFICIENCIES

Aims

1 To relieve symptoms.
2 To correct the underlying disorder.
3 To replace any deficiencies: iron, vitamin B_{12}, folic acid.

Relevant pathophysiology

The cellular constituents of the blood—the red cells, white cells and platelets—exist as a result of the balance between production and destruction. Anaemia occurs when the concentration of haemoglobin in the blood falls below the normal for the age and sex of the patient. The lower limits of normal are:

1 For adult males: 13.0 g/dl.
2 For adult females: 11.5 g/dl.

The balance between production and destruction may be disturbed by:

1 Blood loss.
2 Impaired red cell formation: haematinic deficiency or bone marrow depression.
3 Increased red cell destruction: haemolysis.

Iron, vitamin B_{12} and folic acid are essential for normal marrow function. Deficiency of any or all of these results in defective red cell synthesis and eventual anaemia. As each of the agents plays a different part in cellular production in the marrow, individual deficiencies are manifested in different ways. Accurate diagnosis is therefore essential before any specific agent is given. Lack of iron causes a hypochromic, microcytic anaemia with low serum ferritin. Lack of vitamin B_{12} or folic acid causes a macrocytic anaemia with a megaloblastic bone marrow. If the marrow is deprived of either or both vitamin B_{12} and folic acid the blood picture and the marrow look the same, but it is essential to determine which substance is missing. If folic acid is given to a patient who has vitamin B_{12} deficiency neurological damage, subacute combined degeneration of the cord may be provoked or aggravated.

Iron deficiency anaemia

Iron

As iron is usually absorbed from the gut, a satisfactory response is achieved in most patients when iron salts are given orally. Several ferrous salts are available. There is little to choose between them although they vary greatly in cost. The cheaper salts such as ferrous sulphate should be used unless gastrointestinal adverse effects are severe. Slow-release preparations should be avoided because of unreliable absorption. The duration of treatment, and its success, depends on the underlying cause of the anaemia. Haemoglobin should rise by approximately 0.1–0.2 g/dl (100–200 mg/100 ml) per day or 1 g/week. The achievement of normal haemoglobin levels should then be followed by a further 6 months' treatment in an attempt to replenish iron stores throughout the body.

Adverse effects

Some people cannot tolerate oral iron preparations. The main complaints are nausea, epigastric discomfort, constipation and diarrhoea. A change in the ferrous salt form may help but improvement may be related to a lower content of iron in the alternative preparation.

Dose

Ferrous sulphate is given at a dose of 200 mg three times daily until anaemia is corrected and iron stores are replenished.

Parenteral iron

Oral iron therapy occasionally fails to achieve its objective because of lack of patient cooperation, severe adverse effects or gastrointestinal malabsorption. Two parenteral routes are then available:

1 Deep intramuscular injection.

2 Intravenous infusion.

The total dose of parenteral iron required is calculated for each patient on the basis of body weight and haemoglobin level.

Dose

Iron dextran is given by deep intramuscular injection, 1 ml (50 mg) on the first day, 2 ml (100 mg) daily or at longer intervals, depending on the response, or by slow intravenous infusion over a period of 6–8 h. The infusion rate should be increased slowly and the patient observed carefully for signs of a type I hypersensitivity response (Chapter 13, Section 13.2).

Iron sorbitol is given by deep intramuscular injection only; initially 1.5 mg iron/kg to a maximum of 100 mg per injection.

Megaloblastic anaemia

Vitamin B_{12}

Vitamin B_{12} deficiency demands that vitamin B_{12} should be injected in adequate doses for life. Usually the underlying disease, such as pernicious anaemia, cannot be corrected and the vitamin therefore must be supplied by a route which bypasses the defective absorption mechanism in the gut. Treatment should correct the anaemia and then maintain a normal blood picture. It should arrest, reverse or prevent lesions of the nervous system and replenish depleted stores.

Preparations available are hydroxocobalamin and cyanocobalamin. Both are suitable for intramuscular injection and are equally effective, but hydroxocobalamin is now widely used because of its slower elimination from the body.

A dramatic response often follows within 2–3 days of the start of vitamin B_{12} therapy. Symptoms improve and the haemoglobin concentration rises progressively to normal. An early index of success is a rise in the reticulocyte count, which reaches a peak after about 1 week and then gradually declines to normal in the next 2 weeks.

Marrow changes reverse rapidly.

Adverse effects

These are rare and probably related to contamination or impurities in the injected solution.

Dose

Hydroxocobalamin is given at a dose of 1 mg daily by intramuscular injection for 1 week, then at 2 monthly intervals for life.

Folic acid

Folic acid deficiency in Western countries is frequently the result of low dietary intake. Less commonly it is the consequence of malabsorption. Pregnancy makes such demands on iron and folic acid stores in the mother that it has been routine for iron and folic acid to be prescribed throughout pregnancy.

Dose

An oral dose of 5–15 mg daily is given initially, then 5 mg daily for 3–4 months, depending on the cause. When combined with iron for prophylactic use in pregnancy, 200–500 μg are given daily.

Erythropoietin

Erythropoietin is a glycoprotein secreted by the kidney under conditions of hypoxia. It stimulates the proliferation of erythrocyte progenitor cells. Recombinant human erythropoietins are used in the treatment of anaemia associated with chronic renal failure in patients on dialysis. Side effects include hypertension, thrombosis at vascular access sites, flu-like symptoms and seizures.

Comment

Whatever the type of anaemia, a cause must always be sought. Anaemia is an observation, not a diagnosis, and there could be an important underlying cause requiring treatment.

17.2 DRUG INDUCED ANAEMIA

Drug induced blood loss

Drugs used to relieve pain and inflammation in rheumatoid and osteoarthritis are often associated with chronic, occult blood loss from the gastrointestinal tract.

Aspirin ingestion is a well recognized cause of this type of anaemia and all other non-steroidal anti-inflammatory drugs, e.g. indomethacin, ibuprofen, etc., carry the same risk (Chapter 12, Section 12.2).

Drug induced megaloblastic anaemia

Two important mechanisms result in drug induced megaloblastic anaemia:

1 Interference with cellular DNA synthesis by cytotoxic drugs such as cytosine arabinoside, 5-fluorouracil or 6-mercaptopurine.

2 Interference with folate absorption or use of anticonvulsants such as phenytoin and phenobarbitone or the cytotoxic drug methotrexate which inhibits dihydrofolate reductase.

Drug induced marrow depression: aplastic anaemia

This occurs when cellular activity in the bone marrow is suppressed and is usually associated with the suppression of white cell and platelet formation (pancytopenia).

Drugs causing aplastic anaemia usually incorporate a benzene ring with closely attached amino groups. The outcome depends on the dose and the length of exposure, and to less well defined factors such as the degree of susceptibility, idiosyncracy or hypersensitivity exhibited by an individual.

Certain drugs have a high risk of causing aplastic anemia. These include cytotoxic drugs and gold salts. In other cases this is a rare idiosyncratic adverse effect, e.g. with antimicrobials such as chloramphenicol and the sulphonylureas.

Some drugs have a tendency to suppress white cells, e.g. phenylbutazone, meprobamate and chlorpromazine, while others inhibit platelet production, e.g. gold salts.

Unless the risk is acceptable, as in the treatment of some forms of malignant disease, aplastic anaemia should be prevented at all costs. The risks can be minimized by avoiding known marrow depressants, especially in patients with a history of allergy or idiosyncracy. If the risk is accepted, then every effort should be made to detect early signs and symptoms of bone marrow depression. The patient should be advised that sore throat, fever malaise and bruising may be an indication. Regular peripheral blood examination is of limited value but should nevertheless be performed. In many circumstances, where the degree of exposure to the causative agent has not been excessive, withdrawal of the agent leads to recovery within 2–3 weeks. Otherwise, intensive therapy is required, including comprehensive antibiotics, transfusion of blood products, administration of androgens and corticosteroids and, in extreme cases, bone marrow transplantation.

Drug induced haemolytic anaemia

A haemolytic anaemia occurs when the rate of red cell destruction is increased and red cells survive for a shorter time than the normal 100–200 days. Many drugs can reduce red cell survival:

1 Those that inevitably cause haemolytic anaemia (direct toxins).

2 Those that cause haemolysis because of hereditary defects in red cell metabolism.

3 Drugs that cause haemolysis because of the development of abnormal immune mechanisms.

Direct toxins

Drugs and chemicals that have powerful oxidant properties are likely to cause haemolysis. Damage by these agents results in fragmentation and irregular contraction of red cells, spherocytosis, basophilic stippling, Heinz bodies, methaemoglobinaemia and sulphaemoglobinaemia. In addition to many domestic and industrial agents, haemolytic anaemia may follow:

1 Phenacetin-containing analgesics, which were popular but have now been withdrawn because they were associated with chronic haemolytic anaemia and renal interstitial damage and papillary necrosis.

2 Sulphones, used in the treatment of leprosy and sulphonamides, including sulphasalazine and dapsone.

Interaction with hereditary defects in red cells

Glucose-6-phosphate dehydrogenase deficiency in Negroes and Mediterranean races may give some protection against falciparum malaria, but the red cells in these individuals are abnormally sensitive to oxidizing agents, resulting in haemolysis.

A large number of compounds may cause this haemolytic reaction, notably:

1 Antimalarial drugs, e.g. primaquine and pamaquin.

2 The sulphones used in leprosy, e.g. dapsone, and other antibiotics.

Immune mechanisms

Drugs can be associated with two immune haemolytic mechanisms.

Immune haemolytic anaemia

Antibodies may be formed against the drug or its metabolites. Antibodies can only be demonstrated *in vitro* in the presence of the drug. They may be stimulated by the drug binding directly to red cells forming a drug–red cell complex (the hapten cell mechanism, e.g. penicillin and cephalothin) or by the drug itself with subsequent adsorption on to the red cell surface. Activation of complement then causes lysis (immune complex mechanism, e.g. quinidine, *p*-aminosalicylic acid and rifampicin).

Autoimmune haemolytic anaemia

Antibodies are formed against the red cells. They can be demonstrated *in vitro* in the absence of the drug. This not uncommon form of haemolytic anaemia has been associated most often with the antihypertensive drug methyldopa. While at least 15% of patients on methyldopa develop a positive direct antiglobulin test, less than 0.1% develop overt haemolytic anaemia. If the drug is withdrawn, the haemoglobin level recovers but it may take many months for the antiglobulin test to become negative. Other drugs occasionally causing this kind of haemolytic anaemia are levodopa and mefenamic acid.

17.3 DRUG INDUCED NEUTROPENIA

The most common adverse effect of drugs on the white cell system is a reduction in the number of neutrophils below the lower limit of normal (neutropenia).

Drugs causing this do so either as part of aplastic anaemia (pancytopenia) or as a selective neutropenia which does not involve the red cells or platelets. Drugs causing pancytopenia have been discussed in relation to aplastic anaemia.

Several drugs occasionally cause selective neutropenia, e.g. carbimazole, sulphonamides, chloroquine.

Treatment of an established case of neutropenia calls for:

1 Immediate withdrawal of the offending agent.

2 The prevention or control of infection in protective isolation if the neutropenia is severe.

17.4 DRUG INDUCED THROMBOCYTOPENIA

Platelets may be reduced in number (thrombocytopenia) or function by drugs and chemicals. This may be part of aplastic anaemia or selective thrombocytopenia. The latter is a rare effect of various drugs, including thiazides, sulphonamides and sulphonylureas, and sodium valproate.

Treatment of an established case includes:

1 Immediate withdrawal of the offending agent.

2 Administration of corticosteroids.

3 Transfusion of platelet concentrate.

Comment

Whenever a disorder of blood cell formation is observed and an adverse drug effect suspected, take a careful drug history and consult reference books describing adverse effects.

Chapter 18
Anaesthesia and the Relief of Pain

18.1 RELEVANT PATHOPHYSIOLOGY

Sensory receptors for pain are found in all tissues of the body. A variety of noxious stimuli (thermal, chemical, mechanical or electrical) cause them to respond and lead to the subjective experience of pain.

1 The first-order afferent neurones transmitting pain impulses are of two types:

(a) The rapidly conducting (12–30 m/s) small diameter myelinated fibres of the A group (delta).

(b) The slow (0.5–2 m/s) non-myelinated C fibres.

Both rapid and slow conducting fibres enter the substantia gelatinosa of the spinal cord in the dorsal roots.

2 Second-order neurones carry the pain stimuli to the thalamus in the lateral spinothalamic tracts. Branches from both A and C fibres form synapses with cells in the substantia gelatinosa. The A fibres excite while the C fibres inhibit the substantia gelatinosa cell. The sensitivity of the substantia gelatinosa cells to impulses of the A and C fibres is controlled by descending fibres from higher centres.

3 From the thalamus, third-order neurones convey pain impulses to the post-central gyri of the cerebral cortex. The thalamus is the main region responsible for the integration of pain input but the cortical area is concerned with the exact and meaningful subjective interpretation of pain.

The transducing qualities of free nerve endings are affected by chemical changes in the immediate vicinity, e.g. changes in the concentrations of potassium or calcium ions, acetylcholine, noradrenaline, 5-hydroxytryptamine, histamine, bradykinin and prostaglandins. Bradykinin and related peptides are formed in extracellular fluid whenever there is tissue damage and account for the vascular and exudative changes of inflammation. Bradykinin sensitizes and stimulates nerve endings and causes pain. The analgesic effects of aspirin and other non-steroidal anti-inflammatory drugs result from the impaired release of mediator by mechanisms including inhibition of prostaglandin synthesis (Chapter 12, Section 12.2).

Within the CNS, opiate receptors are localized in the substantia gelatinosa and in the limbic areas of the brain. It appears that endogenous opiates released as neurotransmitters from specific opiate-containing neurones act on these sites to modify pain sensation. Leucine and methionine enkephalins are pentapeptides which are equipotent with morphine. β-Endorphin is a 31 amino acid polypeptide formed from β-lipotropin, a pituitary hormone. It has 48 times the analgesic activity of morphine. The discovery of endogenous opiates provides a rational basis for the use and actions of morphine-like drugs. Substance P, an 11 amino acid peptide, may be another transmitter in the pain pathway. It is present in the spinal cord in the central terminals of the A and C fibres and may be released as the neurotransmitter for the first-order neurones.

Principles of drug treatment

From a practical point of view, there are two types of pain:

1 Visceral pain is a dull, poorly localized pain, e.g. peritoneal pain.
2 Somatic pain is sharply defined, e.g. pain of a fractured femur.

Pain is a valuable symptom of underlying pathology and may be vital in the diagnosis of disease, e.g. in management of the acute abdomen. Unquestioning prescription of an analgesic drug is to be avoided but so also is inadequate administration of relief to a patient in distress.

There is a pronounced placebo effect in the treatment of pain. Thirty per cent of patients in pain experience some relief from a doctor taking an interest in their pain and prescribing any drug.

18.2 OPIOID ANALGESICS

Morphine

Mechanism of action

Morphine produces a range of depressant effects by a central action on specific opiate receptors within the CNS and in peripheral tissues.

The CNS effects include analgesia, euphoria and sedation; depression of respiration; depression of the vasomotor centre resulting in hypotension; cough suppression; release of antidiuretic hormone; miosis and nausea and vomiting. Peripheral effects include smooth muscle contraction with reduced motility of the gastrointestinal tract; reduced secretion of gastrointestinal tract; biliary spasm; urinary retention; constriction of bronchi partly due to histamine release; vasodilatation and itching.

Pharmacokinetics

Morphine is unreliably absorbed after oral administration and subject to high first-pass metabolism. However, a slow-release oral preparation is now available which results in delayed but sustained therapeutic plasma morphine concentrations. The drug can be given intravenously, intramuscularly or subcutaneously. After intramuscular injection, peak brain concentrations occur between 30 and 45 min but relatively little of the administered drug crosses the blood–brain barrier.

The major route of elimination is conjugation with glucuronic acid to form morphine-3-monoglucuronide, which is excreted in the urine. Only a very small amount of free morphine appears in the urine, bile or faeces. About 90% of the administered dose is eliminated within the first 24 h.

Adverse effects

Many of the adverse effects of morphine represent an extension of its pharmacological effects as a result of relative overdosage. They include:

1 Respiratory depression, periodic breathing or apnoea.

2 Hypotension.

3 Nausea and vomiting.

4 Constipation.

5 Tremor.

6 Urticaria and itch.

7 Tolerance and addiction to the drug, which develop readily even when used in clinical practice.

Drug interactions

Morphine delays the absorption of other drugs when they are given orally. In addition, its depressant effects are potentiated by other drugs, such as phenothiazines, tricyclic antidepressants and monoamine oxidase inhibitors. Morphine will, in turn, potentiate the effect of most hypnotics, and all volatile anaesthetic agents.

Clinical use and dose

1 The relief of visceral and traumatic pain.

2 The relief of anxiety and pain after myocardial infarction of haematemesis.

3 In acute left ventricular failure (pulmonary oedema) to reduce preload by venodilation (Chapter 7).

4 Before as well as during anaesthesia, as part of a balanced anaesthetic technique.

The usual dose for relief of severe pain is 10–15 mg i.m. every 4 h as required to relieve pain.

Other opioid analgesics

Many opioid drugs are available and their properties are summarized in Table 18.1.

Papaveretum

This is a solution containing the pure alkaloids of opium. It has the same uses as morphine.

Diamorphine or heroin

This is more potent and more lipid soluble than morphine. It is metabolized to monoacetylmorphine and then morphine. It is claimed to be less sedative and less emetic than morphine but there is little evidence for this. It is used in acute myocardial infarction and is claimed to cause less marked hypotension than morphine. It is highly addictive.

Codeine or methylmorphine

The actions of codeine are similar to those of morphine but it is a less potent analgesic. It is used as a cough suppressant, and also to control diarrhoea, and in combination with aspirin or paracetamol as a mild analgesic. It is metabolized to morphine.

Table 18.1. Comparison of opioid analgesic drugs

	Dose (mg)	Route	Duration of action (h)	Notes
Natural opiates				
Morphine	10–15	i.m., s.c.	4	
	10–30	Oral as sustained release	8	Slow onset needs regular dosage to be useful
Papaveretum	20	i.m., s.c.	4	
Semi-synthetic				
Diamorphine	5	i.m., s.c.	4	
Oxycodone	10	i.m.	4–6	Used in chronic pain
	30	Rectal	4–8	
Dihydrocodeine	50	i.m., s.c.	4	
	30–60	Oral.	4	
Synthetic				
Pethidine	100–150	i.m., s.c.	2–3	
Pentazocine	20–40	i.m., s.c.	4	Agonist antagonist
Buprenorphine	0.3	i.m., s.c.	8	Partial agonist
	0.3	Sublingual	8	Slow onset
Butorphanol	1–4	i.m.	4	Agonist antagonist
Dextromoramide	5–8	i.m.	2–3	
	10	Oral	3	Used in chronic pain
Levorphanol	1.5–4.5	Oral/i.m.	4–6	Chronic pain
Dipipanone	10	Oral	5–6	Chronic pain
Methadone	5–10	Oral/i.m.	5–6	Chronic pain

Pethidine

This is a widely used synthetic narcotic analgesic, which may cause more severe nausea and hypotension than morphine. It is more sedative and has a more rapid onset with a shorter duration of action. Smooth muscle contraction is less prominent and, therefore, it is used in biliary and ureteric colic. Constipation and miosis do not occur to the same extent. Its major metabolite, norpethidine, is active and may accumulate and cause convulsions in patients with renal impairment. The risk of toxicity may be increased in patients taking other drugs which induce hepatic enzymes.

Fentanyl and alfentanil

These are opioids used intravenously during anaesthesia. They have a very short duration of action (20–30 min for fentanyl). Fentanyl is lipophilic and can be absorbed transdermally and by inhalation.

Partial agonists and opiate antagonists

Buprenorphine

This is a partial agonist and antagonist at opiate receptors. It is a potent long-lasting analgesic drug which can be absorbed sublingually. Dependence or addiction potential is claimed to be low. Respiratory depression is not reversed by the opiate antagonist naloxone except in very high dose (15 mg or more). Hallucinations can occur. Note that it is not advisable to give buprenorphine to augment inadequate analgesia from morphine and more potent agents.

Pentazocine

This is another drug with agonist–antagonist properties. It produces respiratory depression, hallucinations, less nausea than morphine and is claimed to result in less dependence or addiction. As it increases workload on the heart it is not recommended in patients with myocardial infarction.

It is not advisable to give pentazocine to augment inadequate analgesia from morphine and more potent agents.

Nalbuphine and meptazinol

These are synthetic opioids used parenterally in the treatment of surgical and chronic pain.

Naloxone

This is a specific opioid antagonist without agonist activity. It is used to antagonize all of the actions of opioid analgesic drugs. It precipitates withdrawal symptoms if given to addicts or the neonate born to a mother addicted to narcotics. Naloxone may be given intravenously or intramuscularly in a dose of 0.4–1.2 mg. When given intravenously, the onset of action occurs within 1–2 min and it lasts 20–30 min. Thus, if it is used to reverse an opioid that has a longer duration of action it should be given repeatedly, by intravenous infusion or intramuscularly.

18.3 LOCAL (REGIONAL) ANAESTHESIA

Transmission of impulses in peripheral nerves is associated with depolarization of the nerve cell membrane, which is the result of an increased membrane permeability to sodium ions. Local anaesthetic agents produce a localized, reversible block to nerve conduction by reducing the permeability of the membrane to sodium. Most of the clinically useful local anaesthetic agents act by displacing calcium from the receptor site on the internal surface of the cell membrane, resulting in blockade of the membrane sodium channel. These agents may exist in the charged and uncharged form in solution. The uncharged form diffuses more readily through the neural sheath while the charged form attaches to the receptor. The relative proportion of the charged and uncharged form depends upon the pK_a of the drug, the pH of the solution and the pH at the injection site. The smaller the nerve fibre, the more sensitive it is to local anaesthetic block. Thus it is possible, though practically difficult, to block pain and autonomic fibres and leave proprioception, i.e. touch and movement.

Local anaesthetics are administered locally and do not rely on the circulation to take them to their site of action. However, uptake into the systemic circulation terminates their effects. The rate of systemic absorption is determined by:

1 Pharmacokinetic properties of the drug.
2 Vascularity of the injection site.

3 Concentration of the solution used.

4 Rate of injection.

A vasoconstrictor, such as adrenaline, may be used in solution with the local anaesthetic to delay systemic absorption, prolong the local block and limit toxicity.

Local anaesthetics are weak bases with pK_a values between 7.5 (mepivacaine) and 8.9 (procaine). Marked changes in the ratio of ionized to non-ionized drug occur with changes in acid–base balance. They are extensively bound to plasma proteins. Differences in binding between agents may influence the intensity and duration of effect and placental transfer.

Local anaesthetic drugs are of two types:

1 *Esters*, e.g. procaine, which are metabolized in the plasma by esterases.

2 *Amides*, e.g. lignocaine, which are extensively metabolized in the liver, the clearance being dependent on liver blood flow. With the exception of prilocaine, which is a secondary amine, all the amides in clinical use are tertiary amines. In the liver, *N*-dealkylation of the tertiary amine produces a more soluble secondary amine which may be active and is in turn dealkylated. Very little of an injected dose of local anaesthetic is excreted unchanged in the urine.

The physicochemical and pharmacokinetic properties of several local anaesthetics are shown in Table 18.2.

Table 18.2. Comparison of opioid analgesic drugs

Agent	Relative dosage	pK_a	$t_{1/2}$ (h)	Onset	Duration
Amides					
Lignocaine	1.0	7.9	1.6	Rapid	Medium
Bupivacaine	0.25	8.1	2.7	Slow	Long
Prilocaine	1.0	7.9		Slow	Medium
Cinchocaine	0.25			Rapid	Long
Mepivacaine	1.0	7.6	1.9	Rapid	Medium
Etidocaine	0.5	7.7	2.7	Rapid	Long
Esters					
Cocaine	1.0		*	Slow	Medium
Procaine	2.0	8.9	*	Slow	Short
Amethocaine	0.25	8.5	*	Slow	Long
Chloroprocaine	3.0	8.7	*		

* $t_{1/2}$ is very short owing to hydrolysis in plasma.

Lignocaine

Lignocaine has both local and systemic effects. Local effects include loss of pain and other sensations, vasodilatation and loss of motor power. Systemic effects occur following absorption from the site of local administration or following systemic administration and result from generalized membrane stabilization. Myocardial excitability is depressed. Adverse effects are due to overdosage and include anxiety and excitement progressing to sedation, disorientation, lingular and circumoral anaesthesia, restlessness, twitching, tremors, convulsions and unconsciousness. Coma may be accompanied by apnoea and cardiovascular collapse.

A 1 or 2% solution of lignocaine is used for local infiltration regional intravenous and or extradural analgesia. The maximum safe dose for a 70 kg man is 200 mg without adrenaline and 400 mg with adrenaline. The first effects are noted 5–10 min after administration, and the duration of action is of the order of 2–3 h. Lignocaine is also used in the treatment of ventricular tachyarrhythmias (Chapter 6, Section 6.2) as it possesses Class I antiarrhythmic activity.

Other local anaesthetics

Prilocaine

This is equipotent with lignocaine and can be used for all types of local analgesia. It is less toxic than lignocaine because of its greater degree of tissue uptake. Large doses may produce methaemoglobinaemia, which is caused by a metabolite, *O*-toluidine. It is available in 0.5 and 1% solutions. The maximum dose is 300–400 mg. The drug is widely used for intravenous regional anaesthesia.

Bupivacaine

This is an amide which is four times as potent as lignocaine and considerably longer lasting. It is available as a 0.25, 0.5 or 0.75% solution and the maximum dose is 100–150 mg. This agent must not be used for intravenous regional anaesthesia as it is toxic in high doses.

Cocaine

This is an ester and is unique in that as well as local anaesthetic properties it is a CNS stimulant. It is used clinically for topical analgesia and for its central euphoriant effects in the management of terminal malignant disease, often together with opiate analgesics.

Procaine

This is an ester that has a short duration of action and extremely poor penetration because of its vasodilator properties and its high pK_a values which makes it ionized at physiological pH.

18.4 GENERAL ANAESTHESIA

Modern anaesthesia is characterized by the so-called balanced technique in which drugs are used specifically to produce analgesia, sleep, muscle relaxation and abolition of reflexes. Nowadays, a single drug is very rarely used to produce all the components of surgical anaesthesia.

Intravenous anaesthetic agents

These drugs are used to produce a rapid and pleasant induction of sleep. In almost all cases anaesthesia will be maintained by other agents and thus it is rapidity of onset and not brevity of action that is the most desirable property. The mechanism of action of these agents is not known but it is thought that they act in the reticular activating system of the brain. They are all highly lipid-soluble agents and cross the blood–brain barrier rapidly. Their rapid onset of action is due to this rapid transfer into the brain and high cerebral blood flow. Action is terminated by distribution of the drugs to less well perfused tissues.

Barbiturates

Thiopentone

Thiopentone, the sulphur analogue of pentobarbitone, is the most widely used intravenous anaesthetic. After administration of 4 mg/kg, sleep occurs in one arm–brain circulation time (15–20 s) but this may be delayed in patients with cardiac disease or shock. Loss of consciousness is pleasant and lasts for 3–5 min. After administration, the initial decay of plasma concentration is very rapid and the half-life of the initial distribution phase is 2.5 min. Elimination is by hepatic metabolism and the terminal half-life is 6.2 h (Table 18.3). Thus the drug is not suitable to be given as repeat injections to maintain anaesthesia because accumulation occurs with a very prolonged duration of action.

Table 18.3. Comparison of opioid analgesic drugs

Drug	Distribution volume (l/kg)	Clearance (ml/min)	Plasma half-life $t_{1/2}$ (h)
Thiopentone	1.6	144	6.2
Methohexitone	1.1	825	1.6
Ketamine	3.3	1296	3.4
Etomidate	4.5	740	4.6

The adverse effects of thiopentone include respiratory depression, myocardial depression and vasodilatation, resulting in a lowered arterial pressure. Laryngeal reflexes are not depressed until deep narcosis results and stimulation of the larynx may result in laryngeal spasm. The drug has no analgesic properties.

In the event of an extravascular injection, necrosis and ulceration of the tissues may result because of the alkalinity of the solution. The anaesthetist must take great care that thiopentone is not injected into an artery since this results in precipitation of crystals of the drug, with thrombosis of the artery and gangrene of the limb. This complication is less severe when a 2.5% solution of thiopentone is used instead of the 5% solution. Thiopentone, like all barbiturates, may exacerbate porphyria.

Methohexitone

This is an oxybarbiturate which is three times as potent as thiopentone. The initial decline in plasma concentrations because of distribution is similar to that seen after thiopentone but the elimination phase is more rapid. Adverse effects include respiratory depression, muscle twitching and involuntary movements. It is used to induce anaesthesia in outpatients.

Non-barbiturate anaesthetics

Ketamine

This is a derivative of phencyclidine. It may be administered intravenously or intramuscularly and has both analgesic and anaesthetic properties. It is extensively used in underdeveloped countries and has been safe in relatively inexperienced hands. It produces full surgical anaesthesia but the form of this anaesthesia is different from other agents like barbiturates. Distribution of the drug throughout the body is very rapid and the metabolic half-life is of the order of 2.5 h. When given in large doses, dreams and hallucinations may occur on awakening. This has limited its usefulness. These psychic sequelae may be abolished by benzodiazepines. Other adverse effects include hypertension.

Etomidate

This is an imidazole derivative with a very short duration of action owing to rapid distribution. It has minimal effect on myocardial contractility and is preferred in very sick patients. It is metabolized in the liver and has a half-life of 4.6 h. Injection may be painful and causes muscle twitching with involuntary movements. Nausea and vomiting are common. A high dose, especially by infusion, may impair adrenal steroid responses to stress, as the drug blocks 11-β-hydroxylation in the adrenal cortex and may interfere with synthesis of cortisol.

Inhalation anaesthetic agents

These agents, usually with others, such as intravenous analgesics, are used to maintain a state of general anaesthesia after induction. The depth of anaesthesia produced by these drugs is related to the tension or the partial pressure of the agent in the arterial blood. Since the alveolar epithelium of the lung presents virtually no barrier to their diffusion, the alveolar concentration or partial pressure of the drug in the alveoli determines the depth of anaesthesia. This alveolar concentration is influenced by:

1 The concentration of the drug in the inspired gas.
2 Alveolar ventilation.
3 Cardiac output.
4 The solubility of the drug in the blood.

As a general rule, drugs with a low blood–gas solubility, such as nitrous oxide, cyclopropane and halothane, act rapidly and drugs with a high blood–gas solubility, such as ether, act slowly.

The potency of these agents is related to, but is not dependent on, fat solubility. The minimum alveolar concentration (MAC) is the alveolar concentration which produces a state of surgical anaesthesia in 50% of patients. Put another way, it is the dose that abolishes movement in response to incision in 50% of patients.

In practice, clinical signs are used to monitor anaesthetic administration. MAC is a population median which varies with age and other factors.

Nitrous oxide

This is a gas at room temperature. It cannot produce surgical anaesthesia when administered alone as its MAC is over 100%. It is used in a concentration of 50–80% to produce analgesia. Prolonged exposure to nitrous oxide may result in bone marrow depression.

Halothane

This is a potent, non-irritant, non-inflammable halogenated hydrocarbon, which is a liquid at room temperature and must be vaporized before use. Eighty per cent of an administered dose is excreted by the lungs and the remainder is metabolized by the liver. Hepatic damage very rarely occurs 7–10 days after halothane anaesthesia and may be due to production of a toxic metabolite. Multiple exposures over a short period of time increase the frequency of liver damage. In fact, concern over liver damage and associated legal complications are now reducing the use of halothane.

Halothane depresses respiration and the myocardium. Bradycardia and arrhythmias may occur if carbon dioxide retention is present. Vasodilatation and hypotension are also seen.

The MAC is 0.75% and halothane is normally given as a 1–2% concentration in a mixture of oxygen and nitrous oxide.

Enflurane

This is a halogenated ether. Its properties are remarkably similar to those of halothane, but it has more respiratory depression and may produce changes in the electroencephalograph that are similar to epilepsy for a few days after anaesthesia. It is less soluble in blood than halothane and so is more rapidly acting. Its MAC is 1.7% and as the liver metabolizes much less enflurane than halothane the risk of hepatitis may be reduced.

Isoflurane

This is an isomer of enflurane. The MAC is 1.2%. Its onset of action is more rapid than that of halothane or enflurane. It has less respiratory depressant and arrhythmogenic actions and over 99% is eliminated unchanged via the lungs.

Comment

Halothane, enflurane and isoflurane can be given in a closed circuit with a carbon dioxide absorber. This approach economizes on gas and reduces environmental pollution.

18.5 NEUROMUSCULAR BLOCKING DRUGS

When an electrical impulse in a motor nerve reaches the nerve ending it releases acetylcholine at the neuromuscular junction. Acetylcholine acts on nicotinic cholinergic receptors on the muscle membrane, resulting in a wave of depolarization. The acetylcholine is then destroyed rapidly by a specific cholinesterase.

Neuromuscular blocking drugs may interfere with neurotransmission in one of two ways:

1 Prolongation of the normal depolarization, e.g. suxamethonium.

2 Competitive inhibition of acetylcholine at the receptors, e.g. tubocurarine, pancuronium.

These drugs are used during anaesthesia to:

1 Produce muscle paralysis for any operation which will be assisted by neuromuscular blockade, but particularly for abdominal surgery.

2 Facilitate tracheal intubation.

3 Ventilate the lungs in cardiothoracic surgery or in intensive therapy.

4 Prevent fractures during electroconvulsive therapy.

After administration, the anaesthetist must always ventilate the patient's lungs since paralysis includes all voluntary muscle, notably the respiratory muscles. The use of these drugs is an integral part of a balanced anaesthetic technique, but great care must be taken to ensure that the patient is unconscious and anaesthetized and not just paralysed.

Factors that influence the action of neuromuscular blocking drugs are:

1 Muscle blood flow (the most important factor). Muscles with high blood flow have the earliest onset and shortest duration of action.

2 Changes in temperature.

3 pH.

4 Potassium concentrations influence the degree of paralysis.

5 Aminoglycoside antibiotics prolong competitive blockade by reducing acetylcholine release.

6 Drugs that produce central muscle relaxation, e.g. benzodiazepines or halothane, prolong the muscle paralysis.

7 Renal disease, since most competitive blockers are excreted unchanged in the kidney to a greater or lesser extent. Atracurium, is, however, metabolized in the blood.

8 Hereditary atypical cholinesterase markedly prolongs the effect of suxamethonium.

Suxamethonium

This is a very short-acting depolarizing neuromuscular blocking drug. A dose of 1 mg/kg produces muscle fasciculations within 1 min followed by complete paralysis for 5–10 min.

Respiration must be maintained artificially. The drug is broken down very rapidly by plasma cholinesterase. In patients with the genetically determined abnormality and atypical enzyme, paralysis is prolonged for 6–24 h and artificial ventilation of the lungs must be continued throughout this period. Adverse effects of suxamethonium include bradycardia, muscle pains and raised intraocular pressure.

Tubocurarine

This is a monoquaternary alkaloid which produces competitive neuromuscular paralysis. After 15–30 mg intravenously, the paralysis is maximal at 4 min and 50% recovery occurs at 50–60 min. The kidneys are the principal route of elimination, with the biliary system an alternative that becomes more important in renal failure. Neuromuscular blockade may be reversed at the end of surgery by administering an anticholinesterase such as neostigmine. This drug is always given with atropine, which prevents the muscarinic effects of acetylcholine and allows the nicotinic effects to be manifest. The adverse effects of tubocurarine include hypotension, which is due to histamine release. This adverse effect has now markedly reduced its use and atracurium and vecuronium have largely replaced it.

Vecuronium

This is a monoquaternary ammonium analogue of pancuronium. It causes less tachycardia and is shorter acting. It is a drug designed to fit the receptors and because it has few side effects is particularly favoured in patients with cardiac disease.

Atracurium

This, likewise, has few cardiovascular side effects. It has a very short duration of action because of rapid non-enzymatic degradation in plasma. It is particularly favoured in patients with renal or hepatic disease.

Comment

Atracurium and vecuronium are being increasingly used in place of tubocurarine in anaesthetic practice. Both new drugs are more selective for the nicotinic receptor.

Chapter 19
Drugs and Psychiatric Disease

The last 30 years have seen major changes in psychiatric practice and treatment, with the advent of the now familiar range of psychotropic drugs and the trend away from custodial care and towards restoring individual patients to a place in the community. The introduction of the phenothiazines in the 1950s transformed the lives of many schizophrenics by abolishing troublesome symptoms and permitting a return to more normal behaviour. Next came the antidepressants, a welcome adjunct to the effective but cumbersome and, to some, distasteful electroconvulsive treatment. Since the 1960s lithium has been used effectively in acute mania and prophylactically in bipolar affective illness. Last, but by no means least, those most widely prescribed of all drugs—the proliferating array of benzodiazepines—are used for their anxiolytic and sedative effects alone or as adjuncts to other forms of treatment in the whole range of psychiatric illness.

Psychiatric diagnostic categories have a disconcerting tendency to merge. Attempts to clarify by reclassification have led to a proliferation of overlapping terminology. In general, where a particular illness does not fall clearly into a diagnostic category, treatment is directed at relief of the predominating symptoms. Table 19.1 presents a working outline of the major categories in which drug treatment is likely to be required.

Table 19.1. Classification of psychiatric diseases

Psychoses	*Neuroses*
Functional:	Anxiety
Manic (unipolar)	Phobic states
Manic–depressive (bipolar)	Obsessive, compulsive
Depressive (unipolar)	Depressive (reactive depression)
Schizophrenia	Hysterical
Paranoid psychoses	
	Less commonly, behavioural aspects of drug dependence, alcoholism and personality disorders may require drug treatment
Organic:	
Acute and chronic brain syndromes	
Drug induced	

Comment
The classification of psychiatric diseases is controversial and complex, with frequent overlap. It is important to try to characterize the principal underlying abnormality, as specific drug treatment is available for most of these categories. Misdiagnosis may exacerbate psychiatric symptoms; for example, sedative benzodiazepines given to a depressed patient may lead to further obtundation of function and even increased liability to suicide. Tricyclic antidepressants may precipitate or aggravate psychotic symptoms in a schizophrenic patient.

19.1 ANXIOLYTICS

Aim

The aim is to control symptoms of anxiety without interfering with normal physical or mental function.

Relevant pathophysiology

The experience of anxiety is a universal phenomenon. Excessive anxiety or its physical manifestations, or a perception of excessive anxiety is very common, and it accounts in part for the wide and excessive use of anxiolytic drugs or minor tranquillizers (15–20% of the population at any time). In Britain, as in the USA, the anxiolytic benzodiazepines are the most widely prescribed group of drugs. Medical practitioners, conditioned to 'treat', find it extremely difficult to acknowledge that a patient's problem lies outside the scope of medical treatment.

The principal groups of drugs used in the management of anxiety are the benzodiazepines, the β-receptor blockers and recently developed agents affecting 5HT systems.

Comment
Anxiety in appropriate circumstances is a normal response. If anxiety symptoms are frequent or persist in a severe form, they may interfere with normal function. Such pathological anxiety is an indication for assessment and possibly short-term drug treatment.

Benzodiazepines

Mechanism

Benzodiazepines have a relatively selective action on the limbic system, cerebral cortex and the ascending amine systems that govern arousal. There is no good evidence that they act directly by modifying endogenous brain catecholamine or serotonin mechanisms, but benzodiazepines do potentiate gamma-aminobutyric acid (GABA) transmission. Recently, the identification of specific binding sites for benzodiazepines has led to speculation that these 'receptors' are normally present to be activated by an, as yet, unidentified 'endogenous benzodiazepine', which is lacking in anxiety states.

Benzodiazepines do not have analgesic properties. However, an amnesic action is useful in addition to sedation and is utilized as premedication for minor investigation procedures like gastroscopy and bronchoscopy. Several studies of anxiety have confirmed the anxiolytic efficacy of benzodiazepines and their superiority to barbiturates.

The benzodiazepines currently available range from very short-acting drugs such as flurazepam or temazepam, which are used as hypnotics, to longer-acting agents such as diazepam, chlordiazepoxide and oxazepam, which are most useful as anxiolytics. Variations in pharmacokinetics and metabolism are responsible for these differences.

Pharmacokinetics

Diazepam is rapidly absorbed from the gastrointestinal tract and extensively metabolized by oxidation in the liver. It forms several active metabolites, including oxazepam, which is used therapeutically in its own right. The plasma half-life is long (24 h) and its duration of effect even longer, as the active metabolites have half-lives of several days. The half-life may be increased in the elderly, who may also be more sensitive to the drug.

Oxazepam is an active metabolite of diazepam. It is cleared by conjugation in the liver and has a half-life of 10–20 h.

Medazepam is also metabolized in the liver to diazepam. These agents have few clear advantages over diazepam.

Chlordiazepoxide was one of the earlier benzodiazepines. It is still used as an anxiolytic, and is the drug of choice in serious alcohol withdrawal states.

Adverse effects

Benzodiazepines are drugs of dependence. The risk of physical dependence is apparently greater with short-acting agents. It is important that prescriptions should be limited to short-term use (no longer than 6 weeks) and in the case of anxiety only if the condition is severely disabling.

Other adverse effects include:

1 Drowsiness, agitation, ataxia and lightheadedness, especially in the elderly.

2 Incontinence, nightmares and confusion.

3 Excessive salivation.

4 Changes in libido

5 Respiratory depression, hypotension.

6 Impaired alertness with motor and intellectual dysfunction, e.g. driving, operating machinery.

7 Paradoxical stimulant effects in some violent patients.

8 Disinhibition can lead to suicidal behaviour.

9 Withdrawal can be associated with rebound increased agitation, hallucinations and epileptic seizures.

10 Thrombophlebitis may follow intravenous diazepam.

11 Psychological adjustment to bereavement may be inhibited by benzodiazepines.

Drug interactions

Benzodiazepines have additive or synergistic effects with other centrally acting drugs—antihistamines, alcohol, barbiturates. This may increase the impairment of motor or intellectual function or worsen respiratory depression.

Diazepam and chlordiazepoxide do not interfere with the metabolism of other drugs and do not interact with warfarin.

Clinical use and dose

Benzodiazepines are appropriate in the short-term management (2–4 weeks) of severe disabling anxiety. Chlordiazepoxide is the treatment of choice in delirium tremens.

Diazepam: orally, 4–30 mg daily in divided doses titrated to control symptoms and continued only as long as is necessary; intramuscularly or slow intravenous injection, 10 mg repeated after 4–6 h if required. Diazepam is used as a sedative in acutely agitated hospitalized patients or as premedication before minor procedures.

Doses of other anxiolytics are shown in Table 19.2.

Table 19.2. Anxiolytic drugs and dose range used

Drug	Group	Daily dose (mg)
Chlordiazepoxide	Benzodiazepines	75–100
Diazepam	Benzodiazepines	4–30
Lorazepam	Benzodiazepines	1–10
Medazepam	Benzodiazepines	10–30
Oxazepam	Benzodiazepines	30–120
Meprobamate	Glycerol derivative	1.2–2.4
Propranolol	Beta-blocker	40–160

Comment

Use the lowest possible dose.

The use of benzodiazepines to treat mild anxiety is unjustifiable. Long-term use is to be avoided. If a patient has taken a benzodiazepine for a long time, the drug should be withdrawn slowly, at a rate determined by the severity of the withdrawal syndrome.

Other drug treatment of anxiety

β-Receptor blockers

β-Receptor blockers reduce cardiovascular and other β-receptor mediated effects of increased sympathetic activity. Most experience has been acquired with propranolol, the non-selective beta-blocker. The clinical pharmacology and adverse effects of beta-blockers are discussed in Chapter 8, Section 8.1. Beta-blockers should be used with caution in patients with a past history of asthma, peripheral vascular disease, cardiac failure or bradyarrhythmias.

Dose

Propranolol: 40–160 mg daily in divided doses.

Serotonergic agents

Buspirone is a $5HT_{1A}$ receptor agonist for which reasonable evidence of clinical efficacy exists. It does not appear to interact with the same receptors as the benzodiazepines, but early claims of freedom from physical dependence should be treated with caution. The $5HT_3$ receptor antagonists represent another class of potentially dependence-free anxiolytics which are currently being developed.

Barbiturates

There is now no place for phenobarbitone or other long-acting barbiturates in the management of anxiety. Benzodiazepines are more effective anxiolytics with less serious consequences of accidental or suicidal overdose. The dependence potential and withdrawal problems with barbiturates are also more serious than with benzodiazepines.

Chlormethiazole

Chlormethiazole has few advantages over benzodiazepines, prolonged use may lead to dependence and severe respiratory depression can occur.

Comment

Anxiety symptoms should only be treated with drugs if they are severe and interfere with the patient's lifestyle or if alternative social or psychotherapy is not possible or appropriate. Treatment should be regularly revised and stopped as soon as possible. Benzodiazepines are effective but beta-blockers may be an alternative, with less dependence problems and abuse potential.

19.2 HYPNOTIC DRUGS AND THE TREATMENT OF INSOMNIA

Aim

By short-term use the aim is to restore normal restful sleep without a residual hangover the next day and to aid a return to normal sleep without drugs.

Relevant pathophysiology

Insomnia is an interference with the quality or quantity of sleep and is a very common complaint. Insomnia is a subjective symptom and reflects what the patient considers to be the 'normal' length and quality of sleep. Individuals vary in their expectation of sleep. Requirements for sleep may vary and diminish with advancing age. A reduced duration of total sleep is common in the elderly and may not be pathological.

The treatment of sleep disorders requires:

1 An assessment of the type of sleep disorder.

2 Assessment of accompanying symptoms of anxiety or depression and their treatment.

3 Diagnosis and treatment of other physical symptoms interfering with sleep, e.g. pain, nocturnal dyspnoea or urinary frequency.
4 Consideration of non-pharmacological strategies, including changes in lifestyle. Simple measures like bathing, exercising, enriched milk drinks or modest alcohol intake at bedtime may help.

Drug treatment should only be offered when the alternatives above have been excluded, and where there is evidence of frequent and marked sleep impairment. Hypnotics should ideally be used for short periods of days or weeks when required, and not given for regular long-term use.

Comment
A successful hypnotic should act rapidly, allow the subject to wake if necessary without severe sedation and be free from residual hangover effects in the morning. Unfortunately, few of the available agents meet these criteria.

Benzodiazepines

Mechanism

Benzodiazepines exert hypnotic effects by similar mechanisms to their anxiolytic actions but at higher doses. At the peak of drug action, in addition to the anxiolytic effect, the drugs affect brain arousal systems by potentiating the inhibitory effects of GABA.

Nitrazepam, flurazepam and temazepam are widely used. They induce sleep within 20–40 min of dosing and produce sleep with a reduction in deep sleep (stage 4) and a reduction in rapid eye movement (REM) sleep.

Residual hangover effects with cumulative adverse reactions in chronic dosing may occur with nitrazepam and flurazepam, which have a long half-life and an active metabolite, respectively.

Benzodiazepines can lead to dependence and should only be used for severe disabling insomnia for periods of less than 6 weeks.

Pharmacokinetics

These drugs are rapidly absorbed and are highly non-ionized at plasma pH 7.4. This, together with their lipid solubility, favours fast penetration of the blood–brain barrier. They are metabolized by the liver and the elimination half-life differs (Table 19.3). Temazepam appears to have the advantage of a short half-life and no active metabolites. Residual impairment is less with temazepam than with other benzodiazepines.

Table 19.3. Benzodiazepine hypnotic drugs

Drug	Plasma half-life (h)	Active metabolite
Nitrazepam	20 +	None
Fiurazepam	2–4	Yes, with long half-life
Temazepam	5–6	None

Adverse effects

Benzodiazepines are drugs of dependence. Other unwanted effects include:

1 Over-sedation, especially in the elderly and those taking alcohol or other sedative agents during the day.

2 Respiratory depression, particularly in chronic lung disease.

3 'Hangover' or residual effects are more common with barbiturates and long-acting benzodiazepines.

4 Rebound insomnia and vivid dreams may occur after stopping hypnotics and be associated with withdrawals features, including fits.

5 Behavioural activation and paradoxical agitation have been observed with benzodiazepines, as with sedative antihistamines, in children and young adults.

Clinical use and dose

Benzodiazepines are indicated in the short-term management of severe, disabling insomnia.

Temazepam: 10–30 mg
Nitrazepam: 5–10 mg
Flurazepam: 15–30 mg
} 30 min before bedtime.

Comment

Hypnotic drugs should only be used for short periods of time. They should certainly not be prescribed without very careful thought. Other physical, psychiatric and social factors may well require attention.

19.3 ANTIDEPRESSANTS

Aims

The main aims are to relieve symptoms of depression, restore normal social behaviour and to prevent further episodes.

Relevant pathophysiology

Depression is common in all populations. Pathological feelings of sadness and despair may be associated with physical and emotional withdrawal. Depressive illnesses are a common factor in suicide.

Psychotic depression is characterized by despair with physical symptoms, e.g. anorexia, sleep disturbance, weight loss. Hallucinations and delusions of unworthiness are common. Episodes may be recurrent (unipolar depression) or alternate with mania (bipolar or manic depressive psychosis).

Drug induced depression may be caused by a range of drugs, including sedatives, steroids, opiates and the antihypertensive methyldopa. The causative drug should be withdrawn if possible.

The neurochemical basis of depression may involve functional underactivity of limbic and forebrain neurones in which noradrenaline or serotonin act as transmitters. The amine hypothesis is supported by biochemical measurement of transmitters and metabolites *in vivo* in cerebrospinal fluid and in brain tissue at postmortem. There is further support from the therapeutic actions of drugs that modify amine turnover.

Monoamine oxidase inhibitors block the breakdown of intraneuronal noradrenaline and serotonin and may increase transmitter overflow.

Tricyclic antidepressants block neuronal reuptake (uptake 1) of noradrenaline into noradrenergic neurones, or re-uptake of serotonin into serotonin neurones. They may alter transmitter levels in the synaptic cleft. The long-term therapeutic effects of the tricyclics and tetracyclics probably depend on chronic changes in pre- and postsynaptic receptor sensitivity.

Fluvoxamine and L-tryptophan increase (in different ways) serotonin levels.

Comment

The diagnosis of depression is complicated by frequent non-specific somatic symptoms of anorexia, malaise, weight loss and constipation. Conversely, depression often accompanies non-psychiatric physical illness. Suicide by self-poisoning or other means is a serious complication of depression.

Tricyclic antidepressants

Mechanism

This group of drugs includes the closely related agents amitriptyline, nortriptyline, imipramine and desipramine. They competitively block neuronal uptake of noradrenaline and serotonin into nerve endings and in the short term increase transmitter levels in the synaptic cleft. In the long term these agents lead to down-regulation of pre- and postsynaptic α-adrenoceptors and serotonin receptors in the brain.

All tricyclics have a range of other pharmacological properties that may contribute to their therapeutic actions and adverse effects:

1 α-Receptor blockade.
2 Anticholinergic effects.
3 Non-specific sedative actions.

The therapeutic response to tricyclics develops over 2–3 weeks. Suicide by overdose of antidepressant is not uncommon during this lag period during treatment.

Recent reports suggest that long-term tricyclic treatment is superior to placebo in reducing the frequency of recurrent depressive symptoms. Amitriptyline, which has more sedative properties, may be useful in agitated depression or where insomnia is troublesome. Imipramine, with less sedative properties, is indicated in those who have marked motor retardation.

Pharmacokinetics

Tricyclics are extensively metabolized by the liver. The half-life of amitriptyline is > 24 h and the formation of metabolites with antidepressant activity further extends the duration of drug activity. Once-daily dosing, ideally at night, is indicated for most tricyclics.

Hepatic metabolism of tricyclics is determined by genetic and environmental factors. There are wide differences in plasma level when the same dose is given to

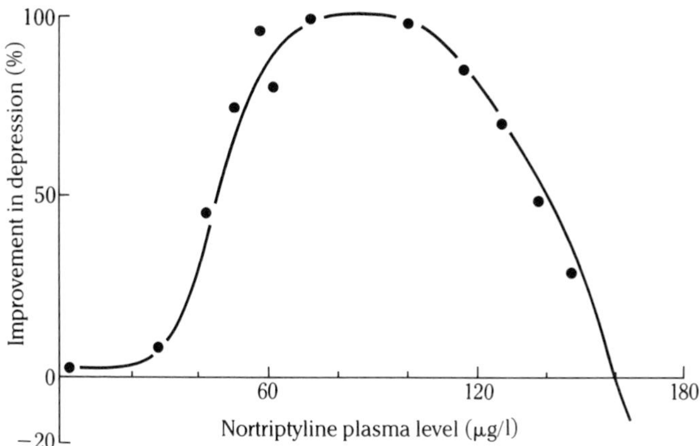

Fig. 19.1. Relationship between drug plasma level and effect with nortriptyline.

a group of individuals. Thus the dose of tricyclic should be titrated individually, with therapeutic response or adverse effects as end points.

Studies with nortriptyline have shown an unusual relationship between drug plasma level and effect (Fig. 19.1). At low drug levels and also at high drug levels there is little effect, while optimal effect is seen within a very narrow concentration range (50–150 μg/l) or therapeutic window. This has led some to propose routine drug level monitoring as a guide to antidepressant therapy.

Adverse effects

1 Sedation and confusional states, especially with amitriptyline.

2 Anticholinergic effects, e.g. dry mouth, constipation, urinary symptoms and precipitation of glaucoma.

3 Postural hypotension, especially in the very young and old.

4 Cardiac tachyarrhythmias (seen in overdose) and conduction defects that are quinidine/procainamide-like. May occur more frequently in patients treated with long-term tricyclics.

5 Self-poisoning by tricyclic overdose is common and its management is discussed further in Chapter 21, Section 21.2.

6 Fits may occur on withdrawal of tricyclics.

Clinical use and dose

Imipramine: 25–75 mg orally, titrated to 100–200 mg daily.

Amitriptyline: as a single dose.

They may also be useful in nocturnal enuresis and hyperactivity syndrome in childhood.

Other related antidepressants

Monocyclic, bicyclic and tetracyclic drugs have been developed with similar properties to the tricyclics.

Serotonin-selective antidepressants

The newest generation of antidepressants is typified by the bicyclic agent fluoxetine. It exerts its effects through a highly specific blockade of serotonin re-uptake. Efficacy in depressive illness is well established. Adverse reactions are qualitatively different from, and tend to be less severe than, the traditional tricyclics. The most commonly occurring side effects are nausea and agitation (occurring in about one-sixth of patients) but one distinct advantage is remarkable safety in overdose. Claims, mainly from North America, of increased suicide and a tendency to aggressive disinhibition in patients taking fluoxetine have so far not been substantiated. A dangerous 'hyperserotonin' syndrome has been described when used in combination with monoamine oxidase inhibitors or lithium. Fluoxetine has a long elimination half-life (3 days) which allows the drug to be taken once a day, usually at a dose of 20 mg.

Mianserin

This is a tetracyclic compound which is useful in depression but is not a potent uptake blocker. Therapeutic activity is similar to the tricyclics, as is the lag in response.

Anticholinergic side effects and cardiovascular reactions appear to be less common with mianserin. However, serious blood dyscrasias can occur in patients treated with this drug, and this is particularly likely in the elderly.

A 30–60 mg daily dose is given at bedtime, increasing if necessary and if tolerated to 200 mg daily.

There is no indication that combinations of tricyclic drugs with related compounds are of any benefit over one drug used in optimal dose.

Comment

Tricyclic antidepressants are widely used in the treatment of acute depression and may reduce the frequency of recurrent episodes. There is a delay of 14–21 days before the therapeutic effect can be seen. The dose should be determined individually. Plasma level monitoring may help in optimizing the response in poor responders.

Monoamine oxidase inhibitors

Mechanism

Phenelzine, tranylcypromine and iproniazid are non-competitive irreversible antagonists of monoamine oxidase (MAO). They block MAO type A, in contrast to selegiline which is described in Chapter 20. The enzyme is blocked not only in brain monoamine neurones but also in peripheral neurones, enterocytes in the gut wall and platelets. Inhibition of MAO leads to increases in serotonin, noradrenaline and dopamine in the brain.

The problems with MAO inhibitors result from widespread enzyme inhibition. These drugs are rarely used now. Indications are therapeutic failure with tricyclic or tetracyclic drugs, hypochondriasis, phobic states and atypical depression.

When used, the response may be delayed for 2–3 weeks. Recovery of MAO is slow (2–3 weeks) after the drug is stopped as it requires synthesis of a new MAO enzyme.

Adverse effect

1 Postural hypotension.
2 Headache.
3 Anticholinergic side effects.
4 Drug induced liver damage (phenelzine and isocarboxazid).
5 Hypertensive crisis.

The most important adverse effect is hypertensive crisis following amine-containing foods, beverages or drugs. Inhibition in the gut wall of MAO allows absorption of tyramine and other sympathomimetic substances in food or drink. These are usually metabolized to inactive products by MAO during absorption. The amines are taken up from the circulation by peripheral sympathetic nerve endings. They displace endogenous noradrenaline from storage sites (indirect sympathomimetic action) and this leads to hypertension, tachycardia and headache.

Severe paroxysmal hypertension may cause a cerebrovascular accident. Foods rich in tyramine, particularly cheese, meat, yeast extract and red wine, should be avoided.

Comment

The dangers of hypertension, the limitations on food intake and the availability of alternatives have greatly reduced the role of monoamine oxidase inhibitors in depression.

19.4 NEUROLEPTIC DRUGS (ANTIPSYCHOTICS, MAJOR TRANQUILLIZERS)

Aims

The main aims are to reverse cognitive, affective and motor disturbances and to restore the patient to as near normal a life in society as possible.

Relevant pathophysiology

The neuroleptics are used in acute schizophrenia to diminish disturbance due to delusional thinking, hallucinations, inappropriate behaviour and anxiety. In chronic schizophrenia these drugs are thought to diminish relapse in a proportion of patients if given in adequate dose. However, they are less useful than at first hoped in this chronic group. In affective disorders the neuroleptics are used to control manic symptoms and behaviour. Occasionally they are used in depression where anxiety, agitation or delusions are prominent. They are also used in drug induced psychoses.

The pathophysiology of mental illness is still unclear and the mechanisms by which drugs exert their effect are still largely hypothetical. The 'dopamine hypothesis' which proposed an over-activity of the brain–dopamine system in schizophrenia is the most favoured explanation for the antipsychotic effects of neuroleptics. The finding of increased dopamine concentrations in the brains of both treated and untreated schizophrenics, together with the dopamine receptor antagonistic effects of neuroleptics, are in keeping with this hypothesis. More recently it has been proposed that there is a deficiency of the excitatory amino acid L-glutamate in certain brain areas which, through polysynaptic connections, leads to disinhibition of dopamine neurones. While this clearly suggests therapeutic possibilities, research is at an early stage.

Phenothiazines

Mechanism

Neuroleptic antipsychotics all act as competitive antagonists of dopamine receptors in the central nervous system and compete for dopamine binding sites *in vitro*.

This series of drugs shows a range of other pharmacological properties which may be of importance in determining the profile of adverse effects for an individual drug.

1 Anticholinergic activity is considerable with thioridazine and much less with fluphenazine.

2 α-Receptor blockade is prominent with chlorpromazine and thioridazine and less with fluphenazine.

3 Sedation occurs with chlorpromazine and thioridazine.

Chlorpromazine, thioridazine and trifluoperazine are among the agents used for long-term oral therapy. Fluphenazine in depot preparations may be given by intramuscular injection.

Extrapyramidal (Parkinsonian) adverse effects often occur and may require to be controlled by temporary co-administration of anticholinergic drugs such as procylidine, benzhexol, orphenadrine and benztropine (Chapter 20, Section 20.2).

Pharmacokinetics

Chlorpromazine is absorbed orally and metabolized by the liver to many active and inactive metabolites. It has a plasma half-life of over 16 h which, together with the long-lived active metabolites, makes once-daily dosing practical. No clear-cut therapeutic range can be defined because of the presence of unquantitated active metabolites and a wide range of interindividual responses in patients. Plasma or urine drug levels are only of help in assessing compliance. First-pass metabolism is immense—of the order of 80%.

Adverse reactions

Dose related adverse reactions from known pharmacological properties:

1 Dopamine receptor blockade, e.g. extrapyramidal dystonia in the young, Parkinsonism in the elderly.

2 Increased prolactin, e.g. galactorrhoea, infertility and impotence.

3 Anticholinergic effects, e.g. blurred vision, constipation, urinary hesitancy, dry mouth, tachycardia or arrhythmias.

4 α-Receptor blockade, e.g. postural hypotension.

5 Tardive dyskinesia; these involuntary choreoathetoid movements, unlike acute dystonia, may persist even after withdrawal of the neuroleptic drug. They may be aggravated by anticholinergic drugs and treatment is generally unsatisfactory. Benzodiazepines, diazepam and clonazepam may be helpful.

6 Neuroleptic malignant syndrome (potentially fatal hyperthermia, muscle rigidity and autonomic dysfunction).

7 Hyperthermia in the elderly.

8 Other adverse effects include sedation, confusion, nightmares and insomnia.

Hypersensitivity reactions not related to dose are:

1 Cholestatic jaundice with portal infiltration occurs in 2–4% of patients, usually early in treatment. It presents the biochemical features of cholestasis and resolves slowly on drug withdrawal.

2 Agranulocytosis occurs rarely.

3 Skin rashes, including photosensitivity dermatitis and urticaria, may be seen.

Clinical use and dose

Chlorpromazine: orally 100 mg daily, increasing up to 1 g gradually if required.
Chlorpromazine: intramuscular injection, 25–50 mg 6–8 hourly as required to control acute symptoms.

Neuroleptics administered in lower doses are used in nausea and vomiting (Chapter 16, Section 16.3), hiccough, vertigo and labyrinthine disturbances, and during drug withdrawal reactions.

In acute attacks of mania, phenothiazines in high doses are used. They are widely used as premedication in anaesthesia (Chapter 18, Section 18.4).

Fluphenazine

This is another phenothiazine derivative. As the decanoate or enanthate ester it can be given as a depot by intramuscular injection at intervals of 14–40 days. Outpatient treatment of schizophrenia is aided by the use of these depot formulations and the ensuing improvement in compliance. Patients with psychoses are notoriously 'poor compliers' with medical instructions if not under close supervision.

Adverse effects of fluphenazine are similar to those of chlorpromazine but sedation and anticholinergic adverse effects are less common. Extrapyramidal adverse effects are correspondingly more common, particularly dystonia and akathisia or restlessness. Liver and bone marrow toxicity and skin rashes have been reported, as with most other phenothiazines.

Dose

Fluphenazine decanoate: 25 mg by injection into the gluteal muscles every 15–40 days. A test dose (12.5 mg) should be given when treatment is begun, to assess possible extrapyramidal reactions.

Non-phenothiazine neuroleptics

Newer antipsychotic agents have been introduced which are not phenothiazine derivatives but share the property of dopamine receptor blockade:

1 Haloperidol, which is a butyrophenone.
2 Pimozide, which is a diphenylbutylperidine.
3 Flupenthixol, which is a thioxanthene.
4 Sulpiride, which is a substituted benzamide.

These agents are less sedating than chlorpromazine and thus useful in withdrawn psychotic patients. Extrapyramidal reactions occur with all of these, but are particularly troublesome with flupenthixol and haloperidol. Pimozide is said to cause fewer dystonic reactions, especially at low doses, but may precipitate a dangerous cardiac conduction defect. Flupenthixol as the decanoate can be given by intermittent (2–4 weeks) intramuscular injection. Clozapine (a dibenzazepine) is effective in approximately one-third of otherwise treatment-resistant cases. It may cause agranulocytosis and prescription is permitted only for hospital in-patients who have weekly blood monitoring.

Comment

Neuroleptic antipsychotic drugs have a major place in the management of functional psychoses. The dose should be determined individually from response and adverse effects. Depot intramuscular preparations may be useful for long-term out-patients' management. Adverse effects are common and may be disabling or even dangerous. Patients on long-term antipsychotic medication should be under close medical supervision.

Neuroleptics should not be used in the management of simple anxiety as an alternative to anxiolytics or minor tranquillizers.

19.5 LITHIUM

Relevant pathophysiology

Mania and hypomania are characterized by a pathologically elevated mood and disinhibited behaviour. It may present on its own or may be part of a manic depressive (bipolar affective disorder) syndrome. Mania is characterized by cheerfulness with motor over-activity, non-stop talk, flight of ideas, grandiosity and a progressive lack of contact with reality.

Treatment of an acute manic episode includes sedation with haloperidol or other major tranquillizers, together with general supportive measures. Specific therapy with lithium salts is used both in the acute attack and for prophylaxis between attacks. Lithium is also now recognized to have a place in the prophylaxis against recurring depressive psychosis.

Lithium carbonate

Mechanism

The monovalent lithium cation, given as the carbonate salt, modifies the affect in mania. The mechanism of action of lithium is not clear. It appears to substitute for the sodium and potassium cations in cellular transport processes. It has effects on the release of monoamine neurotransmitters and alters intracellular and extracellular ion concentrations, fluxes across excitable membranes and the concentrations of 'second messengers' such as inositol phosphate. Lithium may take several days to achieve its effect.

Pharmacokinetics

Lithium is rapidly and completely absorbed after oral dosing. It is not metabolized and is excreted unchanged by the kidney with a half-life of 12 h. Lithium is distributed in total body water, slowly enters cells and reaches steady state levels after dosing for 5 days. There is a very narrow therapeutic range for lithium (0.6–1.2 mmol/l), with severe adverse effects occurring at higher levels. Monitoring of drug levels in plasma is essential for optimal control of therapy (Chapter 2). Change in renal function is the most important factor modifying elimination and thus plasma levels. Lithium clearance is 0.2 times the creatinine clearance, and the dose must be modified in the presence of renal impairment and in the elderly. The sodium and potassium status of the patient also influences lithium levels and response. Thus dehydration, salt depletion or diuretic therapy all tend to increase the plasma drug concentration.

Adverse effects

These are more common and severe when the plasma lithium level exceeds 1.2 mmol/l or in the presence of salt depletion or diuretic therapy:

1 Nausea and vomiting.
2 Drowsiness, confusion and fits.
3 Ataxia, nystagmus and dysarthria.
4 Hypothyroidism by interference with iodination; rarely hyperthyroidism.
5 Oedema and weight gain.
6 Nephrogenic diabetes insipidus.

Drug interactions

Lithium levels rise following the introduction of diuretics. Other drugs altering sodium balance (e.g. steroids, ACE inhibitors) may have the same effect. Lithium potentiates the neurotoxicity of haloperidol and flupenthixol. Owing to the wide range of further possible interactions, always check carefully before administering another drug with lithium.

Dose

Lithium carbonate: 0.4–2.0 g daily in divided doses, depending on renal function and drug plasma levels achieved.

Other drugs used in mania

Haloperidol and other antipsychotic major tranquillizers have long been used in the management of acute mania. Symptoms are controlled, but it is not clear whether the duration of the manic episode is reduced. These drugs are useful in the treatment of acute attacks.

Haloperidol or chlorpromazine have been used successfully and may be used either alone or in combination with lithium carbonate so long as the dose of haloperidol does not exceed 15 mg/day and the plasma lithium concentration does not exceed 0.8 mM.

Adverse effects are those of the dopamine receptor blocking and anticholinergic properties of these drugs, particularly drug induced Parkinsonian or dystonic reactions (Chapter 19, Section 19.4).

Comment

Lithium carbonate is used for long-term prophylaxis in bipolar affective disorder and recurring depressive illness, and it is used together with phenothiazines for control of symptoms in acute attacks. The daily dose of lithium depends on renal function and should be determined individually. Monitoring of lithium plasma levels is essential for optimal treatment without unacceptable adverse effects.

19.6 DRUG INDUCED PSYCHIATRIC DISEASE

Central nervous system adverse effects of drugs are common, especially in the case of lipid-soluble drugs with specific effects on:

1 Receptors.
2 Transmitter synthesis.
3 Degradation of transmitters.
4 Electrophysiological effects on excitable membranes.

A careful history of recent drug ingestion is an essential feature of the evaluation of a patient with psychiatric illness and, where possible, the first step in the management of drug induced psychiatric symptoms should be withdrawal of the offending drug.

There are many well documented examples of drugs causing behavioural adverse effects, and these are summarized in Table 19.4.

19.7 ABUSE OF PSYCHOACTIVE DRUGS

Abuse of drugs and related agents has been noted with increased frequency in young people in urban communities. Therapeutic drug use may also lead to dependence, e.g. benzodiazepines used for anxiety or insomnia, or opiate analgesic abuse in patients first treated for chronic severe pain. However, the concept of drug misuse or abuse must be judged in a cultural and historical context. Attitudes to the non-therapeutic use of cannabis and even opiates differ greatly throughout the world.

The problems of drug abuse are:

1 The direct specific toxic effects, e.g. respiratory depression with opiates.
2 Generalized actions on mood, disinhibition of social behaviour and impaired level of consciousness.
3 Short-term consequences of drug withdrawal, e.g. psychological and physical symptoms of dependence.
4 Long-term medical complications of the contemporary drug ‘subculture’, e.g. hepatitis, septicaemia, AIDS and bacterial endocarditis.

Table 19.4. Drug induced psychiatric disease

Depression	
Antihypertensives	Steroids
Methyldopa	Corticosteroids
Clonidine	Oral contraceptive pill
Reserpine	Analgesics
Propranolol	Opiates
Guanethidine	Non-steroidal anti-inflammatory drugs
Sedatives	*Others*
Barbiturates	Levodopa
Ethanol	Tetrabenzine
Benzodiazepines	Methysergide
Neuroleptics	
Phenothiazines and other antipsychotics	
Organic psychoses	
Sympathomimetics (amphetamine) and the amphetamine-derived 'designer' drug 'ecstasy'	
Anticholinergic drugs (atropine, benzhexol)	
Levodopa and dopamine agonists (bromocriptine, apomorphine)	
Steroids (prednisolone, dexamethasone)	
Phencyclidine (PCP: 'angel dust')	
Cannabis	
Anxiety and anxiety symptoms	
Sympathomimetics (amphetamine, ephedrine, phenylpropanolamine, etc.)	
β_2-Adrenoceptor agonists (isoprenaline, salbutamol, terbutaline)	
Drug withdrawal states	
Benzodiazepines, clonidine, barbiturates, opiates and alcohol	

Psychoactive drugs, like analgesics or sedatives, have a high potential for abuse because of:

1 *Central effects.* They modify mood or behaviour, leading to either pleasurable experiences or depersonalization or intoxication and unconsciousness.

2 *Tolerance.* If there is tolerance to the effect with regular use and thus a need to increase the dose to get the same effect, then not only is the drug-taking habit reinforced but there is a greater risk of chemical toxicity or adverse effects at the higher doses.

3 *Withdrawal symptoms.* Symptoms on withdrawal of the abused drug further reinforce the need for continued drug use (or abuse). While these withdrawal symptoms may often be psychological, in the case of benzodiazepines, opiates and barbiturates, physical symptoms on withdrawal create further dependence or 'addiction'.

Drugs with a high abuse potential can be divided into:

1 Therapeutic agents:
  (a) Benzodiazepines.
  (b) Barbiturates.
  (c) Other hypnotics and sedatives.
  (d) Opiate analgesics and analogues, including dextropropoxyphene.

2 Non-therapeutic agents ('street' drugs):
(a) Cannabis.
(b) Cocaine.
(c) Opiates.
(d) Amphetamines; their therapeutic use now is very limited.
(e) LSD, psylocybin, phencyclidine and other hallucinogens.
(f) Solvents.
(g) Alcohol.

Comment

The management of drug abuse is not easy and involves:

1 Management of acute pharmacological toxicity.

2 Treatment of any acute medical complications, e.g. septicaemia, endocarditis.

3 Psychiatric assessment and treatment of any underlying psychopathology.

4 Controlled planned withdrawal of the drug, if necessary, with temporary substitution, e.g. methadone for heroin.

5 Long-term measures such as family or community support (Alcoholics Anonymous), psychotherapy or drug therapy (disulfiram for alcoholics).

Chapter 20
Drugs and Neurological Disease

20.1 EPILEPSY

Aim

Anti-epileptic drug treatment should prevent generalized or focal seizures without impairing cognition or coordination.

Pathophysiology

Epilepsy is a paroxysmal disorder of cerebral function involving aberrant bursts of electrical activity. Epilepsy may be:

1 Generalized. Generalized seizures are those in which epileptic discharges arise deep in the brain and involve both cerebral hemispheres widely and simultaneously from the outset. Consciousness is always lost. They are further subdivided into tonic–clonic (previously 'grand mal'), absence (previously 'petit mal'), myoclonic, tonic or clonic. The epileptic activity of partial seizures (simple or complex) may spread to become generalized, in which case the seizure is said to be secondarily generalized.

2 Partial. Partial seizures are those in which epileptic activity emanates from a focal area of the brain. These may be simple partial when consciousness is retained or complex partial when the patient is unaware of the event. Symptoms and signs depend on the site of onset and can be motor, sensory, autonomic or psychic. Seizures arising from the temporal lobe are the most common. Partial seizures may be a consequence of cerebral damage (at birth or following trauma), infection, tumour or infarction.

Epileptic fits must be distinguished from other causes of loss of consciousness as treatment is different. The diagnosis is based on the history of repeated, short, stereotyped events. An 'aura' or warning can be helpful for indicating a focal onset to the episode. As the patient is often unconscious during the seizure, a witness is always useful and sometimes essential. Following an attack, the patient may be confused, complain of a throbbing headache and feel very tired. He or she may ache all over, have bitten his or her tongue or mouth and have been incontinent of urine. Often a period of sleep is necessary for full recovery, which may take several hours or even days.

A seizure is a symptom, not a pathological diagnosis. It is important to determine whether epilepsy is primary (no underlying lesion and often a family history) or secondary (to cerebral damage, tumour or other neurological disorders) by appropriate investigations.

Principles of drug treatment

Treatment should be begun with a single anti-epileptic drug. Small doses are used initially to allow titration to the optimal dose with the avoidance of cognitive and psychomotor side effects. If one first-line drug does not abolish the seizures, a second should be substituted. Up to 80% of patients can be controlled fully on a single anticonvulsant drug, although not necessarily the first one to be tried. Some patients appear resistant to all currently available drugs and here the end point must be to reduce the number of seizures to as few as possible without producing unacceptable sedation. A seizure diary is an essential aid to assessing control.

The choice of anticonvulsant depends on the type of seizures:

1 Tonic–clonic:
   (a) Sodium valproate }
   (b) Carbamazepine } first line.
   (c) Phenytoin, second line.

2 Absence:
   (a) Sodium valproate, first line.
   (b) Ethosuximide, second line.

3 Myoclonic:
   (a) Sodium valproate, first line.
   (b) Clonazepam, second line.

4 Partial:
   (a) Carbamazepine }
   (b) Phenytoin } first line.
   (c) Sodium valproate, second line.
   (d) Vigabatrin, adjunctive therapy.

Therapeutic drug monitoring

Monitoring plasma concentrations of anticonvulsant drugs may help to optimize the dose. A drug level, however, can only be regarded as a guide around which to alter the dosage according to the patient's clinical condition. Therapeutic drug monitoring is particularly useful to ensure compliance and to help manage combinations of anticonvulsant drugs which invariably interact. The target range is best defined for phenytoin and least useful for sodium valproate.

Anti-epileptic drugs

A summary of indications, dosage, clinical use and target ranges is shown in Table 20.1.

Carbamazepine

Carbamazepine, a tricyclic derivative, is particularly effective for the treatment of partial and tonic–clonic fits. It is also the drug of choice in trigeminal neuralgia and is also used in other painful conditions.

Table 20.1. Indications, dosages and target ranges of commonly used anticonvulsant drugs

Drug	Indications	Starting dose	Maintenance daily range	Dosage interval	Target range
Carbamazepine	Partial and generalized tonic–clonic seizures	100–200 mg	400–2000 mg	b.d.*	4–10 mg/l (17–42 μmol/l)
Clobazam	Adjunctive therapy in refractory epilepsy	10 mg *nocte*	10–40 mg	o.d.–b.d.	None
Clonazepam	Myoclonic and generalized tonic–clonic seizures	0.5–1 mg	2–8 mg	o.d.–b.d.	None
Ethosuximide	Absence seizures	500 mg	500–2000 mg	o.d.–b.d.	40–100 mg/l† (283–708 μmol/l)
Phenobarbitone	Partial and generalized tonic–clonic, clonic and tonic seizures	30–60 mg	60–240 mg	o.d.–b.d.	10–40 mg/l† (40–172 μmol/l)
Phenytoin	Partial and generalized tonic–clonic seizures; status epilepticus	100–200 mg	100–700 mg	o.d.–b.d.	10–20 mg/l (40–80 μmol/l)
Primidone	Partial and generalized tonic–clonic seizures	125–250 mg	250–1500 mg	o.d.–b.d.	5–12 mg/l† (23–55 μmol/l)
Sodium valproate	Primary generalized epilepsies; partial seizures	200–400 mg	400–3000 mg	b.d.	50–100 mg/l† (347–693 μmol/l)
Vigabatrin	Adjunctive therapy in refractory partial epilepsy	0.5 g	2–3 g	b.d.	None

* b.d. possible in all patients with controlled-release formulation.
† Target range less helpful.

Pharmacokinetics

Extensively metabolized in the liver, carbamazepine is a powerful enzyme inducer. It can induce its own metabolism so that the elimination half-life falls from an initial 24–48 h following a single dose to as low as 8 h on chronic dosing. The target range of 4–10 mg/l (17–42 μmol/l) is less well established than for phenytoin, possibly because of the formation of an active metabolite.

Adverse effects

1 Concentration dependent:
(a) Diplopia.
(b) Dizziness.
(c) Headache.
(d) Nausea.
(e) Unsteadiness.
(f) Hyponatraemia.

2 Idiosyncratic:
(a) Morbilliform rash in 5–15% of patients.
(b) Hepatotoxicity }
(c) Leucopenia } rare.
(d) Stevens–Johnson syndrome }

Drug interactions

Pharmacokinetic interactions with carbamazepine are common. The drug accelerates the breakdown of hormones, so most women on oral contraceptives require a daily oestrogen dose of 50–100 μg. Carbamazepine also induces the metabolism of corticosteroids, theophylline, haloperidol and warfarin. Inhibition of its metabolism with resultant neurotoxicity can occur with cimetidine, danazol, dextropropoxyphene (in compound preparation with paracetamol), diltiazem, isoniazid, verapamil and viloxazine.

Dose

Carbamazepine must be introduced in a low dose (100–200 mg once or twice daily) to offset the development of neurotoxicity; the dose can then be increased every 4–6 weeks to a maintenance amount that controls the fits. Tolerance to the central nervous side effects usually occurs but these symptoms often provide a ceiling to dosage in patients with refractory epilepsy. The controlled-release formulation may be helpful in such cases.

Sodium valproate

Sodium valproate is effective for all types of generalized epilepsy, particularly tonic–clonic, absence and myoclonic seizures. It can be used also for partial fits. It is relatively free of sedative side effects.

Pharmacokinetics

Sodium valproate is well absorbed, degraded in the liver to a number of metabolites, some of which are active, and extensively protein bound. The half-life is short

(7–17 h). There is no relationship between concentration and effect and so the target range of 50–100 mg/l (347–693 μmol/l) is not clinically useful in management.

Adverse effects

1 Concentration dependent:
- (a) Anorexia, nausea and vomiting.
- (b) Tremor.
- (c) Hair loss or curling.
- (d) Peripheral oedema.
- (e) Weight gain.

2 Idiosyncratic:
- (a) Hepatotoxicity, (b) Pancreatitis, (c) Thrombocytopenia } rare.
- (d) Spina bifida in babies exposed *in utero* (1%).

Drug interactions

Sodium valproate is a minor inhibitor of drug metabolism. It can increase the concentrations of other anti-epileptic drugs.

Dose

The starting dose should be low (200–400 mg twice daily) and increased according to seizure control and reported side effects. Sodium valproate can be prescribed twice daily in all patients. Its full pharmacological action may not occur for some weeks after steady state concentrations have been achieved.

Phenytoin

Phenytoin is effective for the prophylaxis of partial and generalized tonic–clonic seizures. Because of its saturation kinetics and impressive side effect profile, there is a move away from using phenytoin as a drug of first choice.

Pharmacokinetics

Phenytoin is variably absorbed and its metabolism by the liver is capacity limited and binding sensitive. Its metabolism is saturable at therapeutic concentrations and so a small increment in dose can produce an unexpectedly large increase in serum level. Conversely, the concentration can fall precipitously when the dose is modestly reduced. The target range of 10–20 mg/l (40–80 μmol/l) is useful in helping to decide the size of an increment in dose.

Adverse effects

Symptoms of neurotoxicity become increasingly likely as plasma levels exceed 20 mg/l (80 μmol/l). However, the diagnosis of toxicity should be made on clinical grounds. Patients will complain of mental slowing and unsteadiness of gait. Examination will reveal nystagmus and ataxia (heel–toe walking is especially sensitive). This is an important diagnosis to make, as persistent toxicity can result in permanent cerebellar damage.

1 Concentration dependent:
 (a) Anorexia, nausea and vomiting.
 (b) Gum hyperplasia, acne, hirsutism and facial coarsening.
 (c) Aggression, sedation, impaired memory and depression.
 (d) Nystagmus and ataxia.
 (e) Vitamin D and folic acid deficiencies.

2 Idiosyncratic:
 (a) Blood dyscrasias.
 (b) Rash and Stevens–Johnson syndrome.
 (c) Teratogenicity in exposed babies.
 (d) Drug induced systemic lupus erythematosus.
 (e) Reduced serum IgA.
 (f) Dupytren's contracture.
 (g) Lymphadenopathy.
 (h) Peripheral neuropathy.

Drug interactions

Phenytoin is commonly implicated in drug interactions. It is an enzyme inducer, capable of reducing the concentration and so the efficacy of other lipid-soluble drugs, such as anticoagulants, corticosteroids, cyclosporin, oral contraceptives and theophylline. Because its metabolism is saturable, it provides a target for enzyme inhibitors, such as allopurinol, amiodarone, cimetidine, imipramine, metronidazole and some phenothiazines and sulphonamides.

Dose

The unusual kinetic profile makes phenytoin difficult to use without the help of concentration monitoring. The starting dose should be 200–300 mg daily in adults. If seizures persist, the dose is best adjusted with reference to a measured concentration. If the level is less than 8 mg/l (20 μmol/l), an increment of 100 mg is appropriate; patients with concentrations between 8 and 12 mg/l (20–60 μmol/l) can have an extra 50 mg; at about 12 mg/l, the dose should be increased by a maximum of 25 mg on each occasion.

Phenobarbitone

Phenobarbitone has been in clinical use since 1912. It is as good as carbamazepine and phenytoin in abolishing partial and tonic–clonic seizures. The main drawback lies in its adverse effects on cognition and behaviour. Sedation and drowsiness overlap with its anticonvulsant properties at therapeutic doses. For this reason it has been relegated to a second-line agent.

Pharmacokinetics

Phenobarbitone is largely metabolized in the liver but a substantial proportion of the drug is excreted unchanged by the kidneys. It has a long elimination half-life (72–144 h), which permits once daily dosing for some patients, usually in the evening. Tolerance makes the target range of 10–40 mg/l (40–172 μmol/l) unhelpful and the toxic threshold imprecise.

Adverse effects

Phenobarbitone can produce fatigue, listlessness and tiredness in adults and insomnia, hyperkinesia and aggression in children (and confusion in the elderly) Subtle impairment of mood, memory and learning capacity occur at all ages. Others problems include:

1 Decreased libido.
2 Hypocalcaemia.
3 Folate deficiency.
4 Rash.
5 Hepatotoxicity.
6 Dupuytren's contracture.

Interactions

Phenobarbitone is the prototype enzyme inducer. It will accelerate the breakdown of most lipid-soluble drugs, including warfarin, oral contraceptives, sulphonylureas and other anticonvulsants.

Dose

Phenobarbitone should be started at a low evening dose to allow tolerance to the sedative effects to take place (30–60 mg in adults, 4 mg/kg in children). Unfortunately, tolerance can also develop to its anticonvulsant properties and rapid withdrawal of the drug can lead to an increase in seizure frequency.

Other anticonvulsants

Ethosuximide

Ethosuximide is still widely used to treat generalized absences in children and adolescents. In children over 6 years, 500 mg/day is a reasonable starting dose, with 250 mg/day added as required at weekly intervals. Toxicity is dose related and usually involves the gastrointestinal tract (nausea, vomiting, abdominal pain, hiccough) and central nervous system (lethargy, dizziness, ataxia, psychosis). Routine concentration monitoring is unnecessary in most children.

Primidone

Primidone is largely metabolized to phenobarbitone. Efficacy is similar to its metabolite but it produces more side effects. There is little reason to recommend primidone over phenobarbitone for those few patients in whom treatment with a barbiturate is contemplated.

Clonazepam

Clonazepam is a 1,4-benzodiazepine which is effective against myoclonic and tonic–clonic seizures. Sedation and tolerance are particular problems. Exacerbation of seizures can occur when the drug is withdrawn.

Clobazam

Clobazam is a 1,5-benzodiazepine which is less sedative than clonazepam. It is useful as an adjuvant anticonvulsant in refractory partial epilepsy, particularly in patients with an anatomical basis for their seizure disorder, e.g. an inoperable tumour. Because of the high likelihood of tolerance, it is often prescribed intermittently for premenstrual exacerbations or as 'cover' for special events, such as holidays, weddings and surgery.

Vigabatrin

Vigabatrin is the first drug to be specifically designed as an anticonvulsant. It is an irreversible inhibitor of the enzyme GABA transaminase, which catalyses the breakdown of the natural anticonvulsant and inhibitory neurotransmitter GABA. Vigabatrin is particularly useful as adjunctive therapy in patients with refractory partial epilepsy. Sedation and behavioural side effects are major drawbacks. Because of a propensity to produce psychosis, it should not be given to patients with a background of mental illness. Like all other anticonvulsants, treatment should be begun with 500 mg daily and can be increased at monthly intervals to the standard dose of 1 g twice daily.

Status epilepticus

Status epilepticus can be defined as a seizure lasting more than 30 min or several distinct episodes without restoration of consciousness. Generalized tonic–clonic status is a life-threatening disorder that requires prompt treatment. The longer the fitting continues, the more difficult it is to control and the higher the morbidity and mortality. Management is as follows:

Immediate

1 Remove false teeth and turn the patient on to his or her side.
2 Give diazepam intravenously (10 mg over a few seconds).
3 If fits continue, give another 10 mg over 30 s.
4 Adminster 10 litres oxygen/min via a high-flow mask.
5 Take blood for urea and electrolytes, glucose and anticonvulsant levels.

Subsequent

1 Infuse 15–18 mg/kg phenytoin in 0.9% saline at 50 mg/min.
2 Monitor cardiac rhythm.
3 If known to have tumour, give high-dose dexamethasone.
4 If alcoholic, administer intravenous thiamine (100 mg).

This regimen will abolish seizures in more than 90% of patients.

Refractory

For resistant cases, other options are available:

1 Chlormethizole infusion.
2 Intravenous phenobarbitone.
3 Paraldehyde infusion.
4 Intravenous lignocaine.

Rarely, a patient will need to be anaesthetized with thiopentone, paralysed and ventilated in the Intensive Care Unit. Status epilepticus still has a significant mortality of 5–10%.

Maintenance regimen

When seizures have been abolished, an appropriate oral regimen should be instituted immediately. If poor compliance has been the precipitating factor in a patient known to have epilepsy, a loading dose of the previous anticonvulsant should be provided. In an untreated patient, oral phenytoin would be an appropriate initial choice. The dose can be determined by monitoring serum phenytoin concentrations.

Comment

Complete abolition of seizures with anticonvulsant monotherapy can be expected in more than 80% of patients. There is little evidence that more than 10% of patients with refractory epilepsy benefit from treatment with two drugs and much more that polypharmacy produces cognitive impairment and complex drug interactions. There is even less support for combinations of more than two anticonvulsants.

In patients with refractory epilepsy once all reasonable monotherapy options have been exhausted, it is time to add a second first-line drug or perhaps clobazam or vigabatrin if the problem is complex partial seizures. In some patients, the law of diminishing returns will require doctor and patient to accept that some seizures will still occur. In this situation, the aim is to balance maximum seizure control with optimum quality of life. Combinations of high doses of sedative anticonvulsants will produce intolerable sedation and sometimes simplification of the drug regimen actually will be beneficial. A few simple rules should be followed:

1 Choose the correct drug for the seizure type.

2 Start at a low dose and titrate slowly to avoid toxicity and allow tolerance to any central nervous side effects.

3 Monitor drug levels if seizure control is not readily attained.

4 Keep regimen simple, with once or twice daily dosing.

5 Counsel to provide the patient with an understanding of the prophylactic nature of the treatment, which will improve compliance.

6 Avoid polypharmacy whenever possible.

20.2 EXTRAPYRAMIDAL DISEASES

Aim

The aim is to correct imbalance between dopamine and acetylcholine in the striatum and restore motor function while minimizing neurological, psychiatric and cardiovascular adverse effects of treatment.

Relevant pathophysiology

Parkinsonism is most common in older age groups (> 55 years) and is characterized by:

1 Tremor at rest (pill rolling type).
2 Rigidity (lead pipe or cog wheel type).
3 Hypokinesia (paucity of spontaneous movement).

These are associated with a loss of a dopamine-containing neuronal pathway from the substantia nigra to the corpus striatum and low dopamine levels in the striatum.

A Parkinsonian syndrome may result from:

1 Idiopathic nigrostriatal degeneration (Parkinson's disease)—common.
2 Postencephalitic—after viral infection.
3 Drug induced
   (a) Phenothiazines and other antipsychotic drugs are dopamine receptor blockers.
   (b) Other drugs—methyldopa, reserpine, tetrabenazine—deplete striatal dopamine.
4 Other rarer causes include:
   (a) Manganese poisoning.
   (b) Carbon monoxide poisoning.
   (c) Cerebrovascular disease.
   (d) Wilson's disease.

Principles of drug treatment

Parkinsonism results neurochemically from:

1 Absolute loss of dopamine in the striatum.
2 Relative increase in the actions of acetylcholine in the basal ganglia.

Rational drug treatment thus consists of restoring the dopaminergic–cholinergic balance in the striatum by:

1 Increasing dopamine effects, with levodopa or bromocriptine.
2 Blocking acetylcholine actions, with anticholinergics.

Although those with mild disease may start on anticholinergic drugs, the major disability of Parkinsonian patients is hypokinesia with difficulty walking, dressing and eating. When this appears, levodopa is given, often in addition to anticholinergics.

Physiotherapy, occupational therapy and social support are important adjuncts to treatment but stereotactic surgery has very little place nowadays.

Levodopa

Mechanism

As the immediate precursor of dopamine in catecholamine synthesis, levodopa is decarboxylated in the brain to replenish striatal dopamine. Dopamine itself cannot be given as it is not absorbed orally and does not cross the blood–brain barrier. Adverse effects of levodopa result from the effects of dopamine and other active amines formed in the brain and periphery. Levodopa is now used together with a peripheral, or extracerebral, decarboxylase inhibitor, carbidopa or benserazide. Peripheral decarboxylase inhibitors block dopamine formation from levodopa outside the brain, but they are polar drugs which themselves do not cross the blood–brain barrier and thus do not influence brain decarboxylation.

Peripheral decarboxylation inhibitors:

1 Prevent extracerebral adverse effects due to formation of catecholamines:
(a) Arrhythmias.
(b) Hypertension.
(c) Nausea and vomiting.

2 Reduce the daily dose of levodopa required.

Pharmacokinetics

Levodopa is absorbed from the jejunum and may compete with dietary aromatic amino acids. It has a short plasma half-life (1–2 h), but in many patients it can be given two or three times daily. However, long-term treatment may lead to dramatic changes in performance which are improved by smaller, more frequent doses.

Adverse effects

These result from the pharmacological effects of dopamine, noradrenaline and metabolites. They are usually dose related. Psychiatric adverse effects may require drug withdrawal.

1 Dyskinesia, new involuntary movements, commonly dose limiting.

2 Fluctuations in motor performance occur frequently with long-term (> 5 years) treatment ('on–off' effects). They may be helped by careful dose titration or drug-free periods.

3 Psychiatric effects, psychosis, depression or mania. Confusion is common in elderly patients.

4 Postural hypotension.

5 Nausea and vomiting, early in treatment, worse on levodopa alone.

6 Cardiac arrhythmias, especially with levodopa alone.

7 Open angle glaucoma.

Clinical use and dose

Levodopa and carbidopa (Sinemet), and levodopa and benserazide (Madopar) are taken two or three (or more) times daily in an individually titrated dose: starting at 200–300 mg of levodopa and increasing up to 1 g daily of levodopa.

Comment

Levodopa dose must be titrated individually to obtain the maximum improvement in motor function while minimizing adverse effects. The efficacy of levodopa falls off with long-term treatment, indicating that the underlying neurological disease progresses and is not reversed by levodopa treatment.

Anticholinergic drugs

Mechanism

These are synthetic atropine-like drugs that competitively block the muscarinic cholinergic receptor. Several are available, including:

Benzhexol.
Benztropine.
Orphenadrine.

There is a modest therapeutic effect in Parkinsonism, with improvement in tremor and rigidity. The dose is increased to the maximum tolerated without adverse effects. Anticholinergic drugs are usually used together with levodopa preparations or alone in mild early disease. There are few differences between anticholinergics and no justification for using more than one drug from this group at any time.

Adverse effects

Adverse effects are those of blockade of muscarinic cholinergic receptors.

1 Central nervous system, e.g. confusion, disorientation, sedation and rarely psychosis.
2 Cardiovascular, e.g. tachycardia, arrhythmias.
3 Gastrointestinal, e.g. dry mouth, constipation.
4 Urinary, e.g. hesitancy, frequency.
5 Paralysis of visual accommodation and glaucoma.

Doses

Benzhexol: 2–15 mg.
Orphenadrine: 100–400 mg.
Benztropine: 0.5–4 mg.

These are given daily in two or more divided doses, starting at low levels and increasing if tolerated. Benztropine and orphenadrine can be given intravenously or intramuscularly in the treatment of phenothiazine induced dystonia.

Other anti-Parkinsonian drugs

Amantadine

This has modest anti-Parkinsonian effects. It is relatively free of adverse effects but may cause confusion if given at night. It can be tried in patients who cannot tolerate levodopa. It also has antiviral activity (Chapter 10, Section 10.5). The beneficial effect of long-term amantadine is disputed.

Bromocriptine

This is a direct dopamine receptor agonist, which has a similar range of actions and at least as severe adverse effects as levodopa. It has no clear advantage over levodopa in the majority of patients. The clinical pharmacology of bromocriptine is described in Chapter 15, Section 15.2. New dopamine receptor agonists like lisuride and pergolide appear to be promising.

Selegiline

This is a selective type B MAO inhibitor which may be used together with levodopa. It may improve the response in some patients with 'on–off' fluctuations in performance. Type A MAO inhibition (Chapter 19, Section 19.3) has no place in the treatment of Parkinsonism.

Apomorphine

This potent dopamine receptor agonist, which is given subcutaneously, may be helpful at late stages in the disease.

Drug induced extrapyramidal symptoms

These are most commonly seen following phenothiazines in the treatment of schizophrenia and other psychoses, and also after anti-emetics with dopamine receptor blocking properties, e.g. prochlorperazine, metoclopramide.

The symptoms depend on the age of the patient:

1 Parkinsonian syndrome in older patients.

2 Acute dystonic reactions with rigidity, muscle spasm and opisthotonus in younger patients. These may progress to tardive dyskinesia.

3 Tardive dyskinesia (Chapter 19, Section 19.4).

Levodopa should not be given for drug induced Parkinsonism.

Treatment is by reduction in dose (or cessation of the drug if possible). Alternatively, long-term anticholinergic drugs (benztropine or benzhexol) may be given. Acute dystonic reactions respond rapidly to intravenous benztropine or orphenadrine.

Chorea

Chorea, either Huntingdon's (the familial form) or secondary to cerebrovascular damage in the basal ganglia, is characterized by repetitive semi-purposive movements which resemble levodopa induced dyskinesia.

The neurochemistry of chorea is not established, but functionally may include overactivity of dopamine systems in the basal ganglia due to deficiency of the inhibitory transmitter GABA.

Chorea has been treated with:

1 Tetrabenazine, which depletes dopamine from nerve endings. Adverse side effects are sedation, depression and Parkinsonism.

2 Haloperidol (a butyrophenone) or phenothiazines, which act as dopamine receptor blockers and cause Parkinsonism or dystonic reactions as common adverse effects.

3 Sodium valproate, which elevates brain levels of GABA.

In many patients with chorea, the adverse effects limit the use of these agents.

Dystonia

Slowly sustained abnormal movements affecting the eyes (blepharospasm) or neck (torticollis) respond to intramuscular botulinum toxin. This treatment is expensive but effective.

Comment

Treatment of extrapyramidal diseases involves the adjustment of the level of cholinergic and dopaminergic activity in the basal ganglia. This requires increasing dopamine effects in Parkinsonism and reducing dopamine effects in chorea.

Adverse effects result both from overcorrection of the local transmitter function and more distant consequences on both brain and peripheral receptors or modification of neurotransmitter function.

20.3 MIGRAINE

Headache is a frequent symptom which, rarely, is caused by underlying neurological disease and is most often ascribed to 'tension'. Treatment is usually symptomatic, often by self-medication with 'over-the-counter' preparations.

Relevant pathophysiology

Migraine is a specific, common, often familial, form of vascular headache. Onset in older patients (40 years) may suggest an underlying cerebral lesion (tumour or vascular malformation). If symptoms begin at a younger age no underlying cause is usually found.

Characteristically, an attack of migraine consists of:

1 A premonitory period of listlessness, often with visual disturbance and flashing lights or focal neurological features lasting up to 30 min.

2 A unilateral headache spreading from behind the eye. The headache is constant and throbbing, and may be accompanied by photophobia, nausea and vomiting. It may last 6–12 h or rarely for several days.

The initial aura and warning symptoms or focal neurological features are believed to be caused by vasoconstriction of intracranial blood vessels, although neural mechanisms are also likely to be implicated. The later headache is the result of vasodilatation of extracerebral and intracerebral vessels. Migraine may be provoked by humoral agents, vasoactive amines, prostaglandins or peptides in a proportion of patients. Tyramine or tyramine-containing foods may precipitate headaches in some patients with migraine. The therapeutic efficacy of serotonin antagonists suggests that serotonin (5-hydroxytryptamine or 5-HT) may also contribute.

In addition, there is evidence that selective serotonin agonists (5-HT_{ID}) can improve symptoms and prevent migraine attacks in a high proportion of patients without unacceptable side effects. These drugs are currently under intensive investigation.

Principles of drug treatment

Management of migraine consists of:

1 Avoidance of precipitating factors, e.g. cheese, chocolate, meat extract or alcohol.

2 Symptomatic treatment of the acute attack with simple analgesics. Ergotamine preparations, bed rest and anti-emetics are required in more severe cases.

3 Prophylactic treatment, if the frequency of attacks justifies it, with serotonin antagonists (pizotifen) or β-receptor blockers (propranolol).

Prophylaxis is indicated if a patient has more than 2–3 attacks per month or finds that migraine interferes with their life.

Ergotamine

Ergotamine is still widely used for the management of the more severe attacks. Ergot alkaloids are α-receptor blockers and also have direct vascular effects causing vasoconstriction. Thus they can modify the constriction and dilatation believed to underlie the symptoms. Ergotamine may also block serotonin receptors.

Ergotamine may be given in several ways during the prodromal phase of the migraine attack: sublingually, rectally by suppository, subcutaneously, intramuscularly, or by inhalation.

Gastrointestinal irritation together with migraine induced nausea and vomiting and gastric stasis make oral dosing of little use.

Ergotamine may be given together with an anti-emetic.

Adverse effects

1 Nausea and vomiting.
2 Abdominal pain and cramps.
3 Withdrawal headache.
4 Peripheral vasoconstriction with Raynaud's phenomenon in patients with coexisting peripheral vascular disease.

Ergotamine is contraindicated in pregnancy and in patients with cerebrovascular or peripheral vascular disease.

Dose

Ergotamine tartrate: sublingually, 1–2 mg to a total dose of 6–8 mg per attack or 12 mg/week; rectally, 2 mg repeated after 1 h to the same total dose as above; by aerosol, 360 μg inhalation repeated up to six inhalations daily or 15 per week.

Metoclopramide may be used in the management of an acute attack of migraine both to prevent nausea and vomiting (Chapter 16, Section 16.3) and to speed gastric emptying and facilitate absorption of orally administered analgesics.

Comment

Ergotamine is used for treatment of the acute attack and never prophylactically. Proprietary preparations often contain caffeine, analgesics or anti-emetics. 5-HT_{ID} agonists such as sumatriptan may offer high efficacy with fewer side effects, not only in control of the acute attack but also in prophylaxis.

Prophylaxis of migraine

Pizotifen

This serotonin-receptor antagonist also has anticholinergic properties.

Adverse effects include drowsiness, weight gain and dizziness. It is given orally as 0.5 mg two or three times daily in the long term to reduce the frequency of acute migraine attacks.

Propranolol

Propranolol is a non-selective β-receptor blocker that has been found to reduce the frequency of migraine attacks in many patients. It is given orally in daily doses of 40–80 mg. Adverse effects are discussed in Chapter 10.

Diazepam

This and other benzodiazepines may be useful if anxiety appears to be a precipitating factor.

Clonidine

This α_2-receptor agonist, used in low doses (50–100 μg), was claimed to reduce the frequency of attacks. It is less widely used now.

Methysergide

This is a serotonin-receptor blocker, which although effective may lead to retroperitoneal fibrosis with long-term use and should only be considered in severe cases resistant to other agents. It is very effective in 'cluster headaches'.

Comment

Migraine prophylaxis depends on the avoidance of identified precipitating factors and, if required, long-term treatment with pizotifen or propranolol as prophylaxis to reduce the frequency of acute attacks.

Acute attacks are controlled by simple analgesics, supplemented if required by ergotamine and anti-emetics, or more recently, by the 5-HT_{10} agonist, sumatriptan.

Chapter 21
Drugs and Endocrine Disease

21.1 DIABETES MELLITUS

Pathophysiology

Diabetes mellitus comprises two separate disorders:

1 Non-insulin dependent diabetes mellitus (NIDDM) is a disorder of middle-aged and elderly patients and has a very strong genetic basis. The early stages are characterized by resistance to the action of insulin and hyperinsulinaemia. With time, insulin secretion declines and pancreatic failure occurs as a late event. The underlying cause of the disorder remains obscure: there are strong associations with essential hypertension and obesity, and subjects have a very high risk of arterial disease.

Weight reduction improves the metabolic abnormalities, including the insulin resistance; drugs to increase insulin secretion from the pancreas or the peripheral action of insulin are given, but in later stages of the disease when insulin deficiency occurs insulin therapy may become necessary.

2 Insulin dependent diabetes mellitus (IDDM) is due to autoimmune destruction of pancreatic islet cells, possibly occurring as a late consequence of occult viral pancreatitis. The disease is characterized by absolute insulin deficiency and subjects require insulin therapy from the outset. There is a tendency to develop ketoacidosis owing to unrestrained lipolysis, fatty acid degradation and formation of ketone bodies.

Insulin deficiency (either absolute or relative) results in profound metabolic abnormalities, including altered carbohydrate, fat and protein metabolism. Both types of diabetes mellitus are associated with the long-term complications of nephropathy, retinopathy and neuropathy. In addition, both are associated with a high risk of atherosclerosis.

Aims of treatment

The purpose of treatment is to restore metabolism, including glucose homeostasis, to normal. There is some evidence to suggest that this might delay or prevent the development of the long-term consequences of diabetes mellitus.

Insulin

Insulin is synthesized as a prohormone in the pancreatic beta cells and secreted into the circulation as a mature dimer composed of two peptides linked by disulphide bridges. The main actions of insulin are:

1 Glucose transport into muscle and fat cells.
2 Increased glycogen synthesis.
3 Inhibition of gluconeogenesis.
4. Inhibition of lipolysis and increased formation of triglycerides.
5 Stimulation of membrane bound energy-dependent ion transporters (e.g. sodium/potassium ATPase).
6 Stimulation of cell growth.

Pharmacokinetics

Insulin in destroyed in the gut and must be given parenterally. It is degraded in the liver and kidney and has a half-life (either endogenous or exogenous) of approximately 9 min. It should be recognized that insulin is normally secreted into the portal circulation and there is a high level of extraction by the liver. Insulin administration (either subcutaneous or intravenous) will always result in an unphysiological relationship between the amount of insulin systemically and the amount of insulin in the portal circulation.

Adverse effects

1 Local effects following subcutaneous injection of insulin can lead to either loss of fat (lipo-atrophy) or hypertrophy of fat (lipo-hypertrophy). These reactions are unusual since the advent of human or highly purified animal insulins.
2 Antibodies may develop to insulin (this is not seen with human insulin) and binding of insulin to antibody may result in prolongation and attenuation of the action of insulin.
3 Hypoglycaemia is the most frequent and potentially most serious adverse effect. This is normally due to decreased carbohydrate intake, unaccustomed exercise, administration of too much insulin or ingestion of alcohol. Symptoms and signs are those of adrenergic activation (sweating, tachycardia, systolic hypertension and hunger) and of neuroglycopenia (visual disturbance, drowsiness, seizures and coma).

Insulin formulation

The majority of patients starting insulin treatment are now given human insulin, which is genetically engineered or chemically modified from insulin made from porcine pancreas. Insulin was previously made from bovine or porcine pancreas, and patients started on these preparations may continue to use them. Current porcine insulins are highly purified. There is some evidence to suggest that human insulin may be associated with more rapid onset of hypoglycaemia and altered awareness of hypoglycaemia, and this can cause problems for patients who convert from more traditional insulin preparations.

In order to prolong its biological action, insulin is given by subcutaneous injection, thereby slowing its rate of delivery to the circulation. Absorption can be slowed further by combining the insulin with protamine (a basic protein) or zinc or both, the resulting preparation having a slower onset but longer duration of action. A further modification in the rate of absorption depends on whether the insulin preparation is amorphous or crystalline, the latter dissolving more slowly. Broadly

Table 21.1. Insulin formation

Duration of action	Examples	Peak effect (h)	Duration of action (h)
Short	Insulin injection (soluble insulin)	2–4	6–12
Intermediate	Isophane insulin	5–12	12–24
	Insulin zine suspension (amorphous)	3–6	12–16
Long	Protamine zinc	5–14	24–30
Mixed	Biphasic (short + intermediate)	2–10	18–20
	Insulin zinc suspension (intermediate + long)	3–8	16–24

speaking, insulin preparations can be divided into four categories—short, intermediate, long and mixed—depending on their onset and duration of action following subcutaneous administration (Table 21.1).

Dose

Insulin is available in the uniform strength of 100 units/ml. The dose, frequency of administration and combination of insulin formulations depend on numerous factors which vary greatly between individuals. The majority of patients need a long-acting insulin given either once or twice daily to provide basal blood sugar homeostasis, as well as more frequent injections of a short-acting insulin to mimic the physiological increase of insulin secretion associated with meals. A typical regimen would be soluble and isophane insulin twice daily, although newly diagnosed patients may now be given more frequent injections of soluble insulin by means of convenient, commercially available pen injector devices. Most patients now monitor glycaemic control by measuring capillary blood glucose levels using glucose oxidase impregnated sticks. In this way patients can adjust their own dose of insulin to maintain blood sugar levels as near normal as possible during the day.

Oral hypoglycaemic drugs

Sulphonylureas

Mechanism

Sulphonylureas act primarily by stimulating pancreatic β cells to produce more insulin. Functioning pancreatic tissue is, therefore, necessary for their action. In addition they inhibit both gluconeogenesis and insulin degradation in the liver and possibly increase insulin receptor density. An unrelated action of chlorpropamide is to increase the release and effect of antidiuretic hormone.

Adverse effects

All sulphonylureas can cause symptomatic hypoglycaemia, which is the most frequent adverse reaction. Chlorpropamide can cause prolonged hypoglycaemia, particularly when renal function is reduced, e.g. in old age. Much less frequently the sulphonylureas are associated with allergic reactions (mainly rashes) gastro-intestinal symptoms, bone marrow suppression and cholestatic jaundice, which can be either allergic or dose related.

There are two problems peculiar to chlorpropamide. First, the effect on antidiuretic hormone may result in hyponatraemia. Second, a proportion of patients (up to one-third) experience flushing when they take alcohol. This is an autosomal dominant trait and may involve endogenous opiods since it is reversed by naloxone.

Glymidine is a sulphapyramidine that does not cross-react with sulphonylureas if skin sensitivity occurs.

Drug interactions

The interactions described for insulin apply also to sulphonylureas. It is important to warn patients that alcohol may potentiate the hypoglycaemic effect. It addition, sulphonamides (including co-trimoxazole) can enhance the hypoglycaemic effect of sulphonylureas.

High-dose aspirin can decrease the renal excretion and therefore enhance the hypoglycaemic action of chlorpropamide.

Clinical use and dose (Table 21.2)

The majority of patients are now started on a drug with a short half-life (e.g. gliquidone, glipizide or glibenclamide). The risks of hypoglycaemia with chlorpropamide make it unsuitable in the elderly and in patients with renal or cardiac failure.

Table 21.2. Sulphonylureas currently in clinical use

	Half-life (h)	Clearance route	Dose (mg)	Frequency of daily dose
Acetohexamide	2–5	M (A)	250	2–3
Chlorpropamide*	36	K	100–500	1
Glibenclamide	6	M	5	1–3
Glibornuride	8	M	12.5–75	1
Gliclazide	12	M	40–320	1
Glipizide	2–4	M	2.5–7.5	2–3
Gliquidone	$1\frac{1}{2}$	M	15–45	2–3
Glymidine	5–8	M (A)	500	1–3
Tolazamide	8	M (A)	100–500	1–2
Tolbutamide	5–8	M	500	2–4

M, metabolized by liver; K, excreted unchanged by kidney; A, active metabolites.
* A small proportion of chlorpropamide is metabolized to active products but renal elimination is the major route of clearance.

Biguandies (metformin)

Mechanisms

The mechanisms are uncertain, but the following effects are likely to contribute:

1 Decreased glucose absorption from the gut.
2 Increase glucose entry to cells.
3 Anorectic effects.

Pharmacokinetics

Metformin is excreted unchanged by the kidney.

Adverse effects

Lactic acidosis is the most serious, though uncommon, problem. It carries a high mortality and is more common in patients with renal, hepatic or cardiac dysfunction. The more frequent adverse effects affect the gastrointestinal tract: nausea, vomiting and diarrhoea.

Dose

Metformin: 0.5–1 g 8 hourly.

Clinical use, benefits and risks of insulin and oral hypoglycaemic drugs

Changes in insulin formulation (e.g. human insulin), the technology of insulin delivery (availability of infusion pumps and pen injector devices) and technology for home monitoring of blood glucose allow much stricter control of glucose homeostasis in insulin-taking patients. There is increasing interest in measures which might prevent the development of long-term complications of diabetes. In this context, there is evidence that strict control of high blood pressure may retard the development of diabetic nephropathy. There is also interest in drugs which may delay the development or progression of diabetic neuropathy: drugs which inhibit the reduction of aldose within nerve cells may prevent the accumulation of sorbitol, which is implicated in the pathogenesis of neuropathy. Long-term evidence that these drugs are of benefit is still awaited.

Increasing understanding of the links between NIDDM, essential hypertension, obesity and atherosclerosis and identification of hyperinsulinaemia as a potential risk factor for atherosclerosis may account for the failure of hypoglycaemic therapy to reduce the high cardiovascular mortality in patients with NIDDM. The absolute importance of weight reduction as a means of improving insulin sensitivity and reducing hyperinsulinaemia in these patients should be emphasized.

Diabetic emergencies

Hypoglcyaemic coma

Causes

Coma is usually precipitated by missing a meal, unaccustomed exercise or taking too much insulin or sulphonylurea.

Clinical features

Coma can present with a wide range of neurological signs. Every medical emergency arriving with mental impairment, coma or other neurological signs must have a capillary glucose checked on arrival.

Treatment

A 50 ml dose of 50% dextrose is given intravenously and repeated as necessary. Alternatively, 1 mg glucagon is given intravenously or intramuscularly which is useful if the patient is difficult to restrain. Glucagon may be given to patients to retain at home for administration by relatives as emergency treatment for hypoglycaemia.

Ketoacidosis

Causes

Infections are the most common identifiable cause. Myocardial infarction, trauma and inadequate insulin dosage are other causes.

Clinical features

Typically these patients are dehydrated, hyperventilating and may have impaired consciousness. Blood glucose is usually markedly elevated and arterial hydrogen ion concentration is low. Body potassium content is decreased although the plasma potassium concentration is high, reflecting the need for insulin to transport potassium across cell membranes.

Treatment

This is based on four measures:

1 Fluid to replace dehydration.
2 Insulin to control hyperglycaemia.
3 Potassium to counter hypokalaemia.
4 Bicarbonate to counter acidosis.

Typical deficiencies would be: water, 6 litres; sodium, 600 mmol (mEq); potassium, 400 mmol (mEq).

Fluid

1000 ml isotonic saline in 30 min.
1000 ml isotonic saline in 1 h.
1000 ml isotonic saline in 2 h.
1000 ml isotonic saline in 4 h.
500 ml isotonic saline 4 hourly.

Note

Use a central venous pressure line in the elderly or those with cardiac disease. If serum sodium rises above 155 mmol/l (mEq/l), use half normal saline.

Insulin

Soluble insulin, 6 units/h, is given by infusion pump. A double rate is given if the glucose level is not falling at 2 h.

When blood glucose is <15 mmol/l (270 mg/100 ml), change to 5% glucose infusion at the rate of 500 ml 4 hourly (add 13 mmol/l potassium chloride) and give 3 units/h insulin. Continue until the patient is eating.

Potassium

Giving insulin and correcting acidosis lowers plasma potassium. Hypokalaemia is a major cause of morbidity in treating ketoacidosis. Give 20 mmol/h from the beginning, adjusting as shown in Table 21.3 for plasma potassium. Continuous monitoring of the electrocardiogram should be undertaken; changes in T-waves give an early indication of important changes in plasma potassium.

Table 21.3. Potassium regimen in patients with diabetic acidosis

mmol (mEq)/h	Plasma K^+ mmol (mEq)/l
39	< 3
26	3–4
20	4–5
13	5–6
0	> 6

Bicarbonate

The above treatment is normally sufficient to restore normal acid–base balance, correct dehydration and normalize blood sugar concentrations. Severely acidotic patients can be given bicarbonate, although this has been associated with serious fluid disequilibrium and development of cerebral oedema. For this reason the use of bicarbonate is not routinely recommended.

Comment

Successful treatment of ketoacidosis depends on frequent monitoring of, and rapid response to, biochemical and haemodynamic indices.

Remember that there is often an underlying cause. If you suspect infection, treat with antibiotics after relevant culture specimens have been obtained.

Hyperosmolar, non-ketotic hyperglycaemic coma

Cause

The cause is obscure. It usually occurs in the elderly or non-insulin dependent diabetics.

Features

Typical laboratory findings are very high blood glucose, raised urea, raised sodium and a high plasma osmolality.

Treatment

Isotonic saline is given or half normal if plasma sodium is >150 mmol (mEq)/l. Adjust the rate of infusion with a central venous pressure line. Give insulin as for ketoacidosis and possibly heparin, as these patients are prone to thrombosis.

21.2 THYROID DISEASE

Hyperthyroidism

Pathophysiology

The majority of patients with hyperthyroidism have Graves' disease, which is an autoimmune disorder characterized by antibodies directed against and stimulatory for the thyroid stimulating hormone (TSH) receptor. The peak incidence is in middle-aged females. The disorder can be chronic, but in a substantial proportion of patients a single episode of hyperthyroidism may enter remission either spontaneously or following treatment with antithyroid drugs. Remission is more likely in patients who have mild disease with minimal enlargement of the thyroid gland.

Toxic multinodular goitre and solitary toxic thyroid adenoma can also cause hyperthyroidism. Patients with these disorders will not enter remission following a course of treatment with antithyroid drugs and are best managed by destructive therapy (either surgery or radioactive iodine)

General principles of treatment

1 Symptomatic therapy: some of the peripheral manifestations of thyroid hormone excess, such as tachycardia and tremor, will respond to β-adrenoreceptor blockade. Non-selective beta-blockers (such as propranolol) are of value, as the tremor of thyrotoxicosis responds to β_2- but not β_1-antagonists.

2 Radioactive iodine (^{131}I) causes a radiation thyroiditis and so reduces hormone reduction by the gland.

3 Thyroid hormone synthesis can be interrupted by drugs such as carbimazole.

Less commonly, drugs can be used which block iodine uptake by the thyroid (potassium perchlorate) or block thyroid hormone release (potassium iodide).

Thiourylene antithyroid drugs

These drugs (carbimazole, methimazole, propylthiouracil) all share a similar chemical structure. Methimazole is a product of carbimazole metabolism and is the active compound. Methimazole is widely used in the USA and Europe while carbimazole is available in the UK.

These drugs act to inhibit thyroid hormone synthesis by:

1 Inhibition of iodide oxidation.

2 Inhibition of iodination of tyrosine.

3 Inhibition of coupling of iodotyrosines.

Propylthiouracil also inhibits the conversion of T_4 to T_3; as T_3 is the active hormone, this may have some additional therapeutic benefit. Carbimazole/methimazole may also inhibit some of the immunological aspects of Graves' disease, and this may be a factor in increasing the likelihood of development of remission in some patients.

As antithyroid drugs do not alter the secretion of preformed thyroid hormone, the effects on circulating thyroid hormone levels and on the symptoms of thyrotoxicosis are not apparent for some time (2–4 weeks).

Pharmacokinetics

Carbimazole is hydrolysed in plasma to methimazole. Methimazole is accumulated in thyroid tissue, and as the intrathyroidal duration of action is at least 12 h the drugs need only be given twice daily. Carbimazole/methimazole and propylthiouracil cross the placenta and can therefore result in fetal hypothyroidism and goitre development. Pregnant patients given antithyroid drugs need to be given the lowest dose possible for this reason. The drugs are secreted in breast milk (propylthiouracil to a lesser extent than carbimazole/methimazole), and this can result in neonatal hypothyroidism.

Adverse effects

1 All of the drugs will cause hypothyroidism and goitre enlargement when given chronically. This can be prevented by reducing the dose of the drug or by giving the patient thyroid hormone (see below).

2 The most common side effect is urticarial rash. A substantial proportion of patients who develop a rash when on carbimazole will also do so on propylthiouracil.

3 The most serious side effect is granulocytopenia, which may progress to agranulocytosis. Patients should be given a written warning at the start of treatment about this possible side effect (which is rare) and should be instructed to report any sore throat or fever immediately.

4 Arthralgia, hepatitis and serum sickness type reactions are all rarely seen with these drugs.

Clinical use and dose

Carbimazole: 30–60 mg daily is normally used. Most patients will respond to 20 mg twice daily. To prevent hypothyroidism, the dose can be reduced thereafter to around 5–10 mg per day. A more efficient procedure is to continue with the initial dose and to add thyroid hormone (thyroxine, 0.1–0.15 mg per day) once the patient has become euthyroid. There is now good evidence that this approach results in a higher remission rate in patients with Graves' disease.

Methimazole: this drug is not available in the UK. A dose of 10–15 mg twice daily will control the majority of patients with thyrotoxicosis.

Propylthiouracil: an initial dose of 100 mg three times per day will control the majority of patients.

Patients with Graves' disease who may enter remission are often given antithyroid drugs for up to one year. If remission seems likely at that point, drugs may be withdrawn and the patients followed to detect subsequent relapse. This approach is not appropriate for patients who do not have disease which will enter remission (e.g. multinodular goitre), for patients in whom relapse of thyrotoxicosis would be harmful (e.g patients with cardiac disease) or in patients in whom remission is very unlikely (patients with very large goitres or where the immune markers of Graves' disease are very high). Antithyroid drugs may also be used to prepare patients before destructive therapy in the form of either thyroid surgery or radioactive iodine.

Radioactive iodine

Radioactive iodine is well absorbed orally and causes a radiation thyroiditis. There is little radiation dose to other tissues. The advantages of radioactive iodine are its simplicity (normally a single dose), low cost and safety. The major disadvantage is the occurrence of hypothyroidism. Early hypothyroidism (within a few months) is a dose related phenomenon. Where large doses are given, up to 90% of patients may become hypothyroid after the first dose. With lower doses, between 10 and 20% of patients will be hypothyroid. Thereafter, late hypothyroidism will affect between 2 and 4% of patients per year. This is an inexorable phenomenon and the majority of patients given radioactive iodine will eventually become hypothyroid. For this reason some centres prefer to give a large ablative dose at the outset. There is no evidence of any carcinogenic risk following radioactive iodine treatment. There have been concerns about genetic hazard, and for this reason patients with reproductive capacity have not routinely been given radioactive iodine. There are no data to suggest that there is a hazard to such patients, and in the USA radioactive iodine is the treatment of choice in the majority of patients with thyrotoxicosis. In the UK there is still some reluctance to treat women of child-bearing years with ^{131}I.

Potassium iodide

Iodide has multiple actions on the thyroid. The most important is an immediate reduction in thyroid hormone release and for this reason potassium iodide is used in thyroid crisis. The drug will also inhibit thyroid hormone formation and iodide trapping.

Potassium perchlorate

This drug prevents thyroid iodide uptake. It has been associated with the development of aplastic anaemia and is now not used in routine clinical practice.

β-Adrenoreceptor blockade

This has been discussed above. Propranolol reduces peripheral conversion of T_4 to T_3, and also provides some symptomatic relief. It should be emphasized that beta-blockers have no effect on the underlying process of Graves' disease or on thyroid hormone secretion (Chapter 8, Section 8.1).

Thyroid crisis

This condition has a high mortality and is characterized by fever, tachycardia, dehydration and confusion. Potassium iodide along with carbimazole are used: patients also require general supportive measures, including rehydration, intravenous beta-blocker therapy and steroids.

Hypothyroidism

This can result as a consequence of previous treatment of thyrotoxicosis, congenital dysfunction or as a consequence of autoimmune thyroiditis. Lithium (used in the treatment of bipolar affective disorders) inhibits thyroid hormone release and can result in hypothyroidism requiring treatment.

Thyroid replacement therapy

Treatment is directed at replacing thyroid hormone levels in the circulation: pituitary secretion of TSH can be used as a guide to the adequacy of therapy. Two preparations are available: thyroxine (T_4) and triiodothyronine (T_3), although the latter is rarely used.

Mechanism

T_3 binds to nuclear receptors and regulates gene transcription. This leads to multiple metabolic actions. T_4 is converted to T_3 in cells by a deiodinase enzyme. In some tissue (e.g. the pituitary) there is an obligatory requirement for a high percentage of T_3 to be derived from intracellular T_4 conversion. For this reason T_4 is a more effective hormone in suppression of TSH than T_3 and is therefore the preferred thyroid hormone for replacement.

Pharmacokinetics

Both T_4 and T_3 are adequately absorbed following oral administration. T_4 has a half-life of about a week and T_3 about 2 days. Both undergo conjugation in the liver and enterohepatic circulation.

Adverse effects

These are related to the physiological and pharmacological actions of thyroid hormone. Elderly patients, or those known to have ischaemic heart disease, must receive low initial doses with slow increments since angina or myocardial infarction can be precipitated. In patients at risk of these problems it is sensible to prescribe beta-blocker therapy when starting thyroid hormone replacement. Thyroid hormone excess produces the usual clinical features of thyrotoxicosis.

The correct dose of thyroxine is assessed by measurement of serum TSH concentrations. There is some evidence that chronic T_4 excess can result in osteoporosis.

Dose

Thyroxine: starting dose is 0.05 mg/day (0.025 mg/day if elderly or with heart disease), with dose increments every 2–3 weeks, depending on thyroid function. The average dose in patients is 0.125 mg/day. Thyroxine is also used postoperatively in thyroid carcinoma:

1 To replace endogenous thyroxine.

2 To suppress TSH, as many tumours are TSH dependent.

The dose of thyroxine used under these circumstances is higher than that given as replacement therapy, and is normally in the region of 0.2 mg/day.

21.3 CALCIUM METABOLISM

Vitamin D (calciferol)

Mechanism

Vitamin D is formed in the skin from the precursor 7-dehydrocholesterol by the action of ultraviolet light. Vitamin D is also derived from dietary sources. Calciferol is inactive, and its biological effect depends on hydroxylation to 1,25-dihydroxycholecalciferol (1,25-DHCC). Renal hydroxylation is increased by parathormone, and for this reason patients with hypoparathyroidism and patients with renal failure are resistant to treatment with calciferol.

The major effect of 1,25-DHCC is to increase the intestinal absorption of calcium. In addition, the hormone promotes calcium mobilization from bone and may also increase renal calcium and phosphate reabsorption. All of these actions will increase serum calcium.

Pharmacokinetics

Vitamin D is fat soluble and bile is necessary for absorption. There is enterohepatic circulation of vitamin D.

Adverse reactions

Hypercalcaemia and its consequences are the major problem; serum calcium should be monitored regularly during treatment.

Drug interactions

Anticonvulsants and other drugs can induce the enzymes which metabolize vitamin D and can produce deficiency states of rickets or osteomalacia.

Clinical use and dosage

Calcium and vitamin D tablets BP contain, in addition to calcium salts, 12.5 μg ergocalciferol and are used for prophylaxis and treatment of rickets and osteomalacia in the dose of 12.5–125 μg/day.

Calciferol tablets, high-strength BP, contain 250 μg cholecalciferol or ergocalciferol and are used to treat resistant rickets or hypoparathyroidism in the dose of 1.25–3.75 mg/day.

1-α-Hydroxycholecalciferol (1-α-HCC)

Mechanism

1-α-HCC is hydroxylated to 1,25-DHCC in the liver.

Adverse effects

It may cause hypercalcaemia, and regular monitoring of serum calcium is essential.

Clinical use and dose

Renal rickets: 1-hydroxylation of vitamin D can be impaired in chronic renal failure. 1-α-HCC is given at the dose of 1 μg/day in addition to phosphate binding drugs. Parathormone is necessary for renal 1-hydroxylation of vitamin D and for this reason patients with this condition should be given either 1-α-cholecalciferol or 1,25-dihydroxycholecalciferol. A dose of 3–5 μg/day of 1-α-hydroxycholecalciferol is sufficient.

Vitamin D resistant rickets: 1–3 μg/day.

1,25-Dihydroxycholecalciferol

This is available for use in renal rickets at a dose of 1–3 μg/day. Regular monitoring of serum calcium essential.

Calcitonin

Mechanism

This lowers serum calcium by decreasing osteoclastic bone resorption and increasing renal calcium excretion.

Adverse effects

Nausea and flushing of the face are quite common. Inflammation can occur at the injection site.

Clinical use and dose

Calcitonin is given by intramuscular or subcutaneous injection.

For hypercalcaemia, 4–8 units/kg daily are given. In addition, it may have a role in Paget's disease complicated by fractures or severe pain.

Diphosphonates

Diphosphonates can be used to treat Paget's disease of bone. These compounds act by altering the rate of bone turnover by binding to hydroxyapatite crystals. Etridronate disodium is orally absorbed, and may be useful in reducing bone pain in Paget's disease. The dose is 5 mg/day for up to 6 months.

Hypercalcaemia

Severe hypercalcaemia can occur in hyperparathyroidism or due to a non-metastatic consequence of malignancy, where the production of a parathormone-related peptide is responsible. Rehydration with saline, given along with a loop diuretic such as frusemide, is the initial treatment of choice. Glucocorticoids (prednisolone, 30–50 mg/day) have been used widely in the past, although the response of calcium can be slow. Diphosphonates (palmidronate, etridronate) are effective and can be given intravenously.

Anterior and posterior pituitary

Hormones

Hypopituitarism results in failure of production of thyroid, adrenal, ovarian and testicular steroids; therapy with these preparations has been considered elsewhere. Growth hormone deficiency requires growth hormone replacement treatment in childhood—genetically engineered growth hormone is available and is administered in a dose of 0.5–0.7 IU/kg/week. This treatment is given by daily subcutaneous injection.

Diabetes insipidus

This can arise as a consequence of hypothalamic or pituitary dysfunction. Patients with intact thirst sensation present with polyuria and polydipsia; those with absent thirst (sometimes seen following head injury and hypothalamic syndromes) can have marked polyuria without polydipsia, resulting in severe hypernatraemia. Treatment is with synthetic antidiuretic hormone arginine vasopressin (DDAVP), given either intramuscularly or by nasal spray.

Pharmacokinetics

DDAVP is broken down by vasopressinase, and the activity of this increases during pregnancy leading to an increase in dosage requirement.

Dosage

DDAVP: 10–20 μg/day by nasal spray; 1–4 μg by intramuscular injection.

Section 3

Chapter 22
Self Poisoning

Self poisoning by drugs or other agents is a modern epidemic; it accounts for around 10% of acute medical admissions in the UK. Except in very young children, self poisoning is usually intentional.

Cases of intentional self poisoning may be divided into two groups:

1 Those who genuinely attempt suicide; this group has a high incidence of depressive psychosis and schizophrenia.

2 Those who use self poisoning to draw attention to their plight or to manipulate their social situation. Patients in this group often have inadequate personalities and often act impulsively and afterwards regret their action. Alcohol is involved in more than one-third of such cases.

It is clearly important in due course to make the distinction between the two in planning long-term management, but it has little relevance to immediate therapy.

22.1 GENERAL MANAGEMENT OF POISONING

Patients should be admitted to hospital, even if the degree of poisoning is trivial. This avoids an immediate repetition of the attempt and allows psychiatric evaluation once the drug effects have passed.

Initial assessment

History

Unless immediate cardiorespiratory resuscitation is required, the first thing to be done when the patient presents is to try to obtain an adequate relevant history. It is often necessary to question relatives or friends. Certain questions are of special importance:

1 Has the patient actually taken an overdose? Patients have occasionally been treated on inadequate evidence, perhaps because a past history of drug abuse suggested this as the likely cause of an impaired conscious level.

2 What drug or drugs were taken? Although most drugs require similar general supportive management, in some cases particular toxic effects can be anticipated, or enhancement of drug elimination might be appropriate.

3 How much drug? This may matter less and estimates may be vague. Nevertheless, some guide to the potential seriousness of the problem is valuable in planning therapy. For example, 100 paracetamol tablets always cause serious toxicity; 10 nitrazepam tablets never do.

4 Is the patient also taking other drugs, not necessarily in overdose, and is alcohol involved? For example, phenobarbitone, a hepatic enzyme inducer, worsens the hepatotoxicity caused by paracetamol. Alcohol obviously causes greater impairment of consciousness than might be expected from the dose of drug taken, and it may provoke hypothermia by vasodilatation.

5 Is there a past history of impaired consciousness or convulsions? The patient may be in a post-ictal state.

6 How was the drug obtained? This may appear of no immediate consequence, but the information may enable something to be done to help prevent another self-poisoning episode in future.

7 How was the self poisoning recognized? Manipulative rather than suicidal attempts are often associated with a place and time when discovery is likely or are followed by self-referral to medical help.

Clinical examination

A comprehensive clinical examination may well have to be deferred but particular attention should be paid at least to the following aspects.

Level of consciousness

This should not be described vaguely as 'drowsy' or 'comatose'. Coma is conventionally divided into four grades (Table 22.1). This is the minimum documentation required to permit assessment of the subsequent clinical course.

Drug induced coma often has certain features which help in differentiation from other causes:

1 Pupil reflexes are preserved, although this might be difficult to detect if the pupil is small.

2 Reflex eye movements are absent. The two reflexes involved are doll's eyes, in which rotation of the head produces contralateral deviation of the eyes, and the caloric reflex, in which instillation of cold water into the ear produces ipsilateral eye deviation.

Cardiovascular status

Hypotension is a common problem but serious elevations of blood pressure can also occur. Arrhythmias are common and tricyclic antidepressants may cause both tachycardia and heart block.

Respiratory status

Respiration can be compromised either by depression of the respiratory centre or aspiration into the lungs.

Table 22.1. Grades of coma

Grade I:	Drowsy but responds to vocal commands
Grade II:	Unconscious but responds to minimal stimuli
Grade III:	Unconscious and responds only to maximum painful stimuli
Grade IV:	Unconscious and completely unresponsive

Temperature

Hypothermia below 35°C worsens the prognosis, especially in the elderly. If the axillary temperature is found to be low, the rectal temperature should be checked.

Evidence of other cause of impaired consciousness

Is there any evidence of head injury or are there localizing neurological signs? Severe poisoning can sometimes cause false localizing brainstem signs, but in general their presence raises the suspicion of another cause of coma.

Removal of ingested drug

An attempt should be made to prevent further drug from being absorbed, unless the risk from overdose is judged to be small.

Further absorption can be prevented in two ways:

1 By recovering drug from the stomach.
2 By adsorbing residual drug with medicinal charcoal.

Recovering drug from stomach

Unabsorbed drug can be removed from the stomach by:

1 Gastric lavage.
2 Induced emesis.

This can be worthwhile up to 6 h after ingestion or 12 h with agents such as aspirin or drugs with anticholinergic effects, including tricyclic antidepressants and antihistamines, because these cause gastric atony.

Gastric lavage

Gastric lavage involves putting a wide-bore tube into the stomach and instilling warm water (500 ml). After a minute the water is removed and any tablet recovered is retained for identification. The procedure may have to be repeated five or six times until no further drug is obtained. Care is required in the comatose patient. A suction tube should be applied to the pharynx to test for the presence of a gag reflex. If it is absent it is essential to have a cuffed endotracheal tube in place before gastric lavage is undertaken, thus avoiding aspiration. Gastric lavage can be traumatic. It must be undertaken with very great care if a corrosive poison has been taken and is contraindicated if petroleum distillate has been swallowed. The technique is impracticable in young children.

Induced emesis

Induced emesis is effective, but less predictable, and its use is restricted to the conscious patient. It should not be used for corrosives or petroleum products. The agent used is Syrup of Ipecacuanha. This is safer than any other emetic agent. Emesis is usually produced within 20 min. If it is not, the dose can be repeated. Saline should not be used to induce emesis. It is not very effective and deaths have been caused by hypernatraemia when the risk of death without any treatment at all was very small.

Adsorbing drug

Effervescent activated charcoal (Medicoal) adsorbs residual drug, but 10 g of charcoal are needed to adsorb 1 g of drug. Large doses appear to be safe and the usual initial dose of 50 or 100 g of charcoal will adsorb the equivalent of 10–20 paracetamol tablets. Since release of the drug from charcoal may eventually occur, repeated dosing (below) is often worthwhile.

Continued management

With many drugs this amounts to support of the vital functions until the toxic effects of the drug have worn off.

Central nervous system

Convulsions can usually be controlled by intravenous chlormethiazole or diazepam. Convulsions that cannot be brought quickly under control by these means should be treated by muscle paralysis and ventilation since prolonged convulsions risk further brain damage.

Cardiovascular system

Tachyarrhythmias are treated conventionally, and heart block may require temporary transvenous cardiac pacing. Hypotension can often be corrected by raising the foot of the bed and giving intravenous fluids, such as plasma or high molecular weight dextran.

The place of vasoconstrictor drugs is now controversial. Their use may compromise renal blood flow and other tissue perfusion. However, if the drug taken in overdose has caused vasodilatation, this can be reversed with metaraminol, 5 mg i.v., and this may be of value if intravenous fluids are contraindicated by cardiac failure.

Respiratory system

Modest respiratory depression can be treated with high concentrations of oxygen but more severe respiratory problems require ventilation. Measurement of arterial blood gases is the most reliable guide to the extent of respiratory depression.

Hypothermia

This should be corrected by wrapping the patient in foil to prevent further heat loss and by nursing in a warm atmosphere. If the patient is on a ventilator, warmed, humidified air is an effective method of raising the temperature.

Optimal management requires the resources of an intensive therapy unit, and provided such support is available an uncomplicated recovery can be expected in a great majority of cases of self poisoning.

Enhancing drug elimination

This can be attempted by a number of means. It can alter the time course of recovery but there is little evidence that the overall outcome is changed. Grade IV coma does, however, carry a significant mortality and in this case any attempt at hastening drug elimination is justified if only to prevent complications such as hypostatic pneumonia and thromboembolic disease.

Repeated dose activated charcoal (aspirin, digoxin, theophylline, tricyclics and most anticonvulsants)

Repeated dosing with oral activated charcoal enhances the elimination of many toxins and drugs. It is thus worthwhile in cases of severe poisoning unless a known non-adsorbable drug is responsible. The main agents for which charcoal is unhelpful are alcohol, cyanide and metals. Administration of up to 50 g 4 hourly may be continued for several days. Since charcoal is unpleasant to swallow, a nasogastric tube may be required. The only major risk is that of aspiration in an unconscious patient. The use of activated charcoal as an adjunct to other manoeuvres could not be criticized in severe poisoning.

Forced alkaline diuresis (aspirin, phenobarbitonex herbicides)

This can be employed only with drugs that are distributed mainly in the extracellular fluid and are largely excreted unchanged in the urine. The rationale is that the greater the proportion of drug in ionized form the less renal tubular reabsorption takes place, since only lipophilic non-ionized compounds readily cross cell membranes. Ionization of acid drugs is encouraged by an alkaline medium. Accordingly, by rendering the urine alkaline (pH 7.5–8.5) more acid drug is excreted.

The technique of forced alkaline diuresis involves the administration of 1 litre of 5% dextrose and 500 ml of 1.2% sodium bicarbonate in the first hour with a further 1 litre dextrose and 500 ml bicarbonate over the next 3 h. Although this can be effective in increasing drug elimination, three potential problem areas have to be monitored carefully:

1 Precipitation of water intoxication and pulmonary or cerebral oedema, especially in the elderly. In that age group, central venous pressure should be measured. In general, if less than 350 ml urine in phenobarbitone or herbicide poisoning, or less than 150 ml urine in aspirin poisoning is excreted in the first hour, 40 mg frusemide i.v. should be added. Patients with aspirin poisoning are dehydrated initially.

2 Serious alkalosis. Close monitoring of plasma pH is required. With aspirin, the pH at presentation is variable. The drug ultimately causes acidosis, but this may be preceded by a respiratory alkalosis caused by hyperventilation.

3 Hypokalaemia. The intracellular flux of potassium which accompanies this treatment causes hypokalaemia; 10–20 mmol potassium as potassium chloride may have to be added to each 500 ml of infusion fluid. Some authorities recommend doing this from the start, but it is probably best to adjust potassium supplementation in the light of continuing frequent serum electrolyte measurements.

Forced diuresis is not without hazard and should be reserved for moderate to severe toxicity. In the case of salicylates, this means a plasma concentration above 3.5 mmol/l. It has been suggested recently that rendering the urine alkaline with sodium bicarbonate without additional fluid is at least as effective in enhancing aspirin excretion as the full forced diuretic regimen. This modification at least avoids the risk of fluid overload. In the presence of severe metabolic disturbance in salicylate poisoning, haemodialysis is a safer and effective alternative.

Forced acid diuresis, substituting arginine or lysine hydrochloride (10 g for 30 min) for the bicarbonate used in forced alkaline diuresis, is rarely employed. However, it may be helpful in quinine, amphetamine or fenfluramine overdosage.

Haemodialysis (lithium, severe alcohol poisoning)

Peritoneal dialysis is not advisable because peritoneal blood flow may be compromised in severely poisoned, hypotensive patients.

Haemodialysis is reserved for lithium (> 3 mmol/l) and severe alcohol poisoning, and for salicylate poisoning with severe metabolic disturbance. When renal function is normal, it has no advantage over forced alkaline diuresis for long-acting barbiturate or herbicide poisoning.

Haemoperfusion (theophylline, barbiturates, glutethimide, meprobamate, methaqualone, salicylates, chloral hydrate)

This technique involves the passage of blood through a column containing activated charcoal or resin onto which the drug is adsorbed. It is a major procedure requiring arterial and venous access. Formerly there was a risk of charcoal embolization, thrombocytopenia and defibrination. Refinements to the columns, with the introduction of the resin amberlite XAD-4 have improved matters. Haemorrhage, air embolism, infection and loss of a peripheral artery remain significant risks. It is undertaken only if the following criteria are satisfied.

The patient must:

1 Be severely poisoned with grade IV coma, major haemodynamic problems, respiratory depression or hypothermia.
2 Be deteriorating clinically in spite of full resuscitative and supportive measures.
3 Have developed complications, such as pneumonia, septicaemia or shock lung.
4 Have a high plasma drug level.

Even in these circumstances the technique is of value only if:

1 The drug adsorbs onto charcoal or resin.
2 A significant proportion of the drug is in the plasma compartment.
3 Toxicity is related to the plasma level.

22.2 SPECIAL FEATURES OF CERTAIN DRUG OVERDOSE

Most cases of drug overdose can be managed by the conservative supportive measures discussed. A number of drugs deserve individual mention, however, because of particular clinical features or therapeutic measures warranted.

Barbiturates

It used to be thought that the formation of large skin blisters in overdosed patients was characteristic of barbiturates. It is now recognized that any coma may be responsible for their appearance in pressure areas. They are of no diagnostic value.

Medium-acting barbiturates, such as butobarbitone or amylobarbitone, are metabolized by the liver. In contrast with phenobarbitone toxicity, forced alkaline diuresis is of no value in treating overdose with these agents. Haemoperfusion is effective in severe poisoning.

Glutethimide

This may produce sudden apnoea secondary to raised intracranial pressure. The presence of raised intracranial pressure may be revealed by papilloedema, which should be sought in poisoning with this drug. This sign may lag 48 h or more behind the development of raised pressure.

Urgent treatment is required with dexamethasone, 8 mg i.v. and 4 mg four times daily, supplemented with the osmotic diuretic mannitol; 200 ml of the 20% mannitol solution is infused over 30 min. Although effective, mannitol must be administered with care in the elderly, with monitoring of the central venous pressure to avoid the development of heart failure.

Antidepressant drugs

Monoamine oxidase inhibitors

These drugs prevent the breakdown of endogenous monoamines (Chapter 19, Section 19.3), and this is the basis of the hypertension which is their most important toxic effect. Severe hypertension may result if a patient on a monoamine oxidase inhibitor takes food with a high content of sympathomimetic amines like tyramine. Overdose may present a complex picture, including either hypertension or hypotension. The basis of the latter is not clear. Hyperreflexia and convulsions are also relatively common. Treatment is directed at the particular toxic effects which are prominent in individual patients.

Tricyclic antidepressants

These drugs inhibit noradrenaline reuptake in peripheral or central neurones, block parasympathetic muscarinic receptors and have a quinidine-like effect on the heart (Chapter 19, Section 19.3). Tachyarrhythmias may result. Alternatively, heart block and negative inotropic effects on the heart are also seen. Hypotension, especially orthostatic, is common. Ventricular fibrillation or other arrhythmias are not uncommon causes of death in tricyclic antidepressant poisoning. Electrocardiographic monitoring, if possible in an intensive care unit, is indicated after more severe tricyclic overdoses. Agitation and convulsions also occur frequently. Several of these effects are due to parasympathetic blockade and this can be countered with the cholinesterase inhibitor physostigmine (2 mg slow i.v. injection). Tachyarrhythmias may be controlled and the coma reversed quickly. The effect lasts for only about 20 min, when the dose of physostigmine can be repeated. This is a relatively specific antidote but unless administered with great care it is easy to induce severe cholinergic effects.

Analgesics

Salicylates

Only in severe overdose does aspirin cause central nervous system depression. A severely poisoned patient may be alert, garrulous and even aggressive. It is easy to underestimate the severity of salicylate poisoning on clinical grounds. A metabolic acidosis caused by the drug itself may be complicated by a respiratory alkalosis induced by hyperventilation. Aspirin may still be recovered from the stomach 12 h after ingestion because of the gastric stasis induced by the drug.

The efficacy of forced alkaline diuresis is such that the rate of aspirin excretion may be increased by a factor of 20. It should be considered when plasma salicylate concentration is greater than 3.5 mmol/l and the patient is clinically toxic. Some centres now favour haemodialysis for its beneficial effect on electrolyte and acid–base status.

Opiates

Overdose is sometimes seen in drug addicts who, because of the variable potency of the preparations to which they have access, may accidentally take an overdose. The most powerful opiates, such as morphine and diamorphine, are seldom used in deliberate self poisoning since they are usually administered parenterally. Pentazocine is available in tablet form, as is dextropropoxyphene. The latter has been widely prescribed in combination with paracetamol. In overdose this preparation may lead to profound respiratory depression caused by dextropropoxyphene and hepatotoxicity caused by paracetamol.

Opiates are unusual in having a specific and selective antagonist, naloxone (Chapter 18, Section 18.2). This is a competitive antagonist, reversing their respiratory depressant effects and itself lacking any depressant effect on the respiratory centre. Naloxone is given as a 0.4 mg dose i.v., repeated at 2–3 min intervals as required. High doses are sometimes required if large doses of synthetic opiates have been taken. The half-life of naloxone is shorter than that of most opiates and monitoring is required even after apparent complete reversal of the overdose.

Paracetamol (acetaminophen)

The main problem is hepatotoxicity. Paracetamol is metabolized by the liver. At therapeutic concentrations the major products are glucuronide and sulphate conjugates. A much smaller proportion is metabolized by the microsomal mixed function oxidases, with the product of this pathway being detoxified by combination with glutathione. However, in overdose, greatly increased amounts of paracetamol are metabolized by this secondary pathway, which exhausts glutathione stores and leaves an excess of a toxic metabolite. This then combines covalently with protein macromolecules in the liver to produce hepatic necrosis with a centrilobular pattern. If the patient survives, normal liver function is usually restored in a few months.

The best guide to the likelihood of the development of hepatic necrosis is the plasma level of paracetamol and the rate of decline, i.e. the half-life of the drug. A half-life of more than 4 h indicates saturation of the major routes of conjugation and potential toxicity. To wait for this information, however, requires a delay of more than 4 h from the patient's presentation before therapy is commenced. In practice, as a level of more than 1 mmol/l 4 h or more after ingestion suggests that hepatic necrosis is likely, treatment should be given. Figure 22.1 gives a guide to the management of paracetamol poisoning determined by plasma level and time after ingestion. To be effective, treatment must be begun as early as possible. It consists of either methionine given orally or *N*-acetyl cysteine given intravenously. Methionine enhances glutathione synthesis by the donation of thiol groups, while *N*-acetyl cysteine is hydrolysed *in vivo* to cysteine, a glutathionine precursor. Thus, additional glutathione is made available to combine with the toxic metabolite and thus prevents binding to liver. In general, oral methionine is the treatment of choice, mainly because it is less than 5% of the price of *N*-acetyl cysteine. However, the latter is useful in unconscious patients, such as those who take paracetamol in combination with dextropropoxyphene, or if vomiting is a problem.

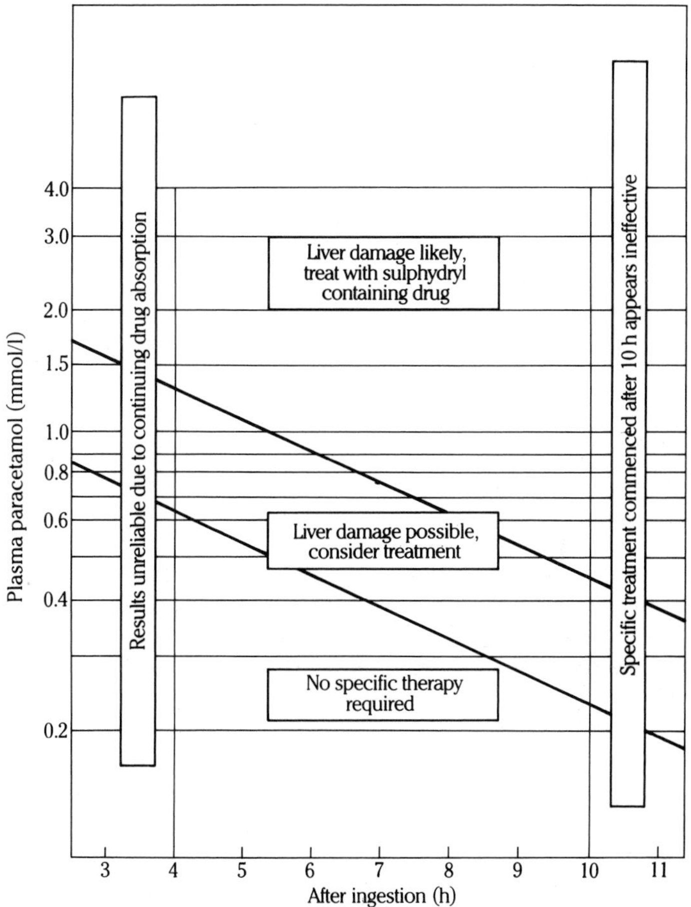

Fig. 22.1. Management of paracetamol poisoning.

Metal poisoning

Iron

The clinical presentation of iron poisoning may progress through three distinct phases:

1 Iron is astringent and initially produces a gastritis, which may be erosive and haemorrhagic. It is seldom a serious problem and the amount of blood loss is usually trivial. However, if vomiting and diarrhoea are severe they may lead to circulatory collapse.

2 Even in severe untreated poisoning, the initial gastritis usually resolves and the person's condition then appears satisfactory for 12–24 h or even longer. This quiescent phase represents the interval between initial local astringent effects on the gastric mucosa and the toxic effects of absorbed iron. If the patient first presents during this phase it is vital not to be misled into assuming that no further problems will arise simply because gastritis and diarrhoea have resolved.

3 If the natural course of the illness is not interrupted by treatment, the third stage is entered about 24–48 h post-ingestion. It is caused by widespread tissue poisoning by free iron, since the quantities absorbed following serious overdose may overwhelm the body's transfer and storage capacity. The prognosis is poor. Coexisting hepatic necrosis, cardiac and renal failure are further complicated by hypovolaemic shock resulting from a haemorrhagic enterocolitis. Central nervous system involvement follows, with the onset of convulsions and then coma.

Desferrioxamine is a specific antidote for iron poisoning. It acts as a chelating agent for iron combining with it to form the octahedral complex ferrioxamine. It not only binds free iron but also removes it from transferrin and ferritin. The complex formed is excreted in the urine, so adequate renal function is necessary. Otherwise, haemodialysis to remove ferrioxamine is indicated.

At presentation, the patient is given 2 g desferrioxamine i.m. and gastric lavage is carried out, using 1 g for each lavage; 5 g is then left in the stomach to prevent absorption of any residual iron. Further desferrioxamine is then administered by slow intravenous infusion, not more than 15 mg/kg/h to a maximum of 80 mg/kg/h. A more rapid infusion may cause anaphylaxis and a larger total quantity itself produces renal damage. Treatment is continued until satisfactory serum iron concentrations (200 mmol/l) are reached or until transferrin is no longer 100% saturated. Desferrioxamine may be given by repeated intramuscular injection but this may cause pain at the injection site.

Other metals

Other chelating agents (D-penicillamine, dimercaprol and sodium calcium edetate) are useful in acute or chronic metal poisoning, particularly lead, copper or arsenic.

Comment

In 10% of cases, self poisoning requires intensive treatment; the remainder recover with simple nursing measures. Treatment in most cases is supportive. Gastric lavage or induced emesis are unnecessary when only a small amount of relatively safe drug has been taken. There are only a few specific antidotes.

Methods of increasing elimination carry their own risks and are not universally effective. They should be reserved for cases of serious toxicity. Not every case requires psychiatric evaluation but sympathetic management and appropriate social advice and help may avoid a recurrence.

Appropriate treatment of poisoning is important to ensure that the effects of the toxin are minimized and that the treatment itself does not cause further morbidity. A number of centres maintain comprehensive databases and offer 24 h information and advice by telephone or computer link. One of these should be contacted in any case of doubt. Some contact numbers are listed below.

Birmingham:	West Midlands Poisons Unit 021-554 3801 Ext. 4109
London:	National Poisons Information Service 071-635 9191
Newcastle:	Regional Drug Information Unit 091-232 5131
Scotland:	Scottish Poisons Information Bureau 031-229 2477 031-228 2441 (viewdata)
Wales:	Welsh National Poisons Information Service 0222-709901

Chapter 23
Drug Prescription: Legal and Practical Aspects

Although a medicine and its active drug constituents can have a powerful effect in the treatment of disease and the alleviation of symptoms, the inappropriate choice of drug or the incorrect dose of an appropriate drug could lead to serious morbidity or even mortality. The choice of therapeutic agent must be based on information gained from clinical history, examination and any necessary further investigations. Other factors that influence the choice are the age of the patient and associated pathology (renal or hepatic disease).

Once the decision has been made, the patient must be supplied with the medicine or treatment. The importance of this stage has often been ignored both in practice and in the training of doctors. Poor communication by the medical practitioner is a major factor in poor compliance of the patient with instructions. Clear, unambiguous instructions to the patient are essential not only to indicate the dose and frequency with which the medicine is to be taken but also to reinforce any additional advice about diet, smoking and the level of social and physical activity.

In most countries there are restrictions on the availability of drugs. In the UK medicines are classified into three categories:

1 General sales list preparations are medicines that can be supplied by most retailers in supermarkets, etc. Some simple analgesics, e.g. aspirin and antacids, are widely available for sale. These preparations may be used excessively or inappropriately and can contribute to drug related morbidity either by direct toxicity or through drug interactions.

2 Pharmacy medicines, which may only be supplied by a registered pharmacist, may be supplied to a patient without a prescription from a registered medical practitioner. These 'over-the-counter' preparations may cause adverse effects and interact with other prescribed drugs.

3 Prescription-only medicines can only be supplied by a pharmacist on the prescription of a registered medical (or dental) practitioner.

Comment

Details of legal requirements vary in different countries. The ethical and practical responsibilities are universal.

23.1 LEGAL ASPECTS OF PRESCRIBING IN THE UK

Prescribing of drugs in the UK is regulated by the Medicines Act of 1968, the Misuse of Drugs Act of 1971 and the Misuse of Drugs Regulations of 1973, amended in 1985.

Controlled drugs

Under the Misuse of Drugs Regulations of 1985, drugs with a high abuse potential, drugs of addiction and other drugs with non-therapeutic psychotropic activity are categorized as controlled drugs. These drugs, which include narcotic analgesics, cocaine, barbiturates, amphetamines and related agents, can only be prescribed by registered medical practitioners. Controlled drugs are divided into five schedules which replace the previous schedules of the 1971 regulations.

Schedule 1 includes cannabis, hallucinogens and other non-medicinal drugs with an abuse potential and is not of therapeutic relevance.

Schedule 2 includes over 100 'controlled' drugs with greater or lesser medicinal uses, such as opiates (heroin, morphine, pethidine, etc.), cocaine, amphetamine and quinalbarbitone. There are limitations and conditions on the prescription of these drugs. The prescription must be in the required form (see below).

Schedule 3 includes a small number of minor stimulant drugs, such as diethylpropion, most barbiturates and the analgesics buprenorphine and pentazocine. Prescribing controls which apply to Schedule 2 also apply to drugs in this schedule. There are other differences relating to manufacture, possession and destruction but these are of no therapeutic relevance.

Schedule 4 is a new category which includes 35 benzodiazepines with an increasingly recognized abuse potential. At present there are no special limitations on the prescription of these drugs.

Schedule 5 includes weak narcotic analgesics and dilute preparations of morphine, such as a mixture of kaolin and morphine BP used for symptomatic treatment of diarrhoea. No special prescription or labelling restrictions apply.

Prescriptions for Schedule 2 controlled drugs must follow specific legal guidelines:

1 The prescription must be written in the physician's own handwriting.

2 The prescription must include the name and address of the patient.

3 The medicine or drug, the dosage form, e.g. 'tablets', the strength of the preparation, the dose and the quantity to be supplied or the total number of doses should be stated in figures and words, e.g. 10 (ten) mg.

4 The prescription must be signed and dated by the practitioner and include his address.

The requirements for controlled drug prescription are the basis of good prescription writing and should be used as a model for all prescriptions.

There are legal obligations on medical practitioners to report to the Home Office for registration of any patient who is believed to be dependent or addicted to controlled drugs. The legal aspects of drug regulation and the control of drug abuse are further reviewed in the *British National Formulary*.

23.2 PRACTICAL ASPECTS OF PRESCRIBING

It is obvious that while appropriate drug therapy can be of great benefit, inappropriate therapy is not harmless. On all occasions, there should be a positive reason for prescribing a drug. Drug treatment should never become a routine. In hospital it is still not uncommon to find 'routine' prescriptions for hypnotics, analgesics and purgatives without any consideration of individual need. Many patients and doctors expect a consultation to result automatically in the prescription of a medicine. Both of these procedures are undesirable and bad prescribing practice.

When drug treatment is indicated, it is mandatory that the most appropriate agent is given in the correct dose and in a regimen which results in optimum treatment with minimum adverse effects.

When the treatment has been selected, the doctor communicates his wishes to the pharmacist and the patient by his prescription. Accurate communication with the pharmacist is essential if the patient is to receive the desired treatment.

Prescriptions for medicine should be either typewritten or written legibly in ink (mandatory for controlled drugs) and in clear English. There is no justification for writing illegible or unintelligible prescriptions. The use of Latin or Greek terms or obscure abbreviations is anachronistic and liable to be misunderstood by nursing staff and/or patients.

When writing prescriptions, practitioners should:

1 Specify the patient's full name, address and age, although the legal requirements is 'age if under 12'.

2 Indicate clearly the drug or medicine. As discussed below, it is preferable to use the approved or generic name rather than the proprietary or brand name.

3 Specify precisely the strength of tablets, capsules or mixtures. It is good prescribing practice to indicate these in words and figures and mandatory for prescriptions of controlled drugs.

4 Indicate the dose frequency and total quantity to be supplied or the duration of treatment. Once again it is good practice to include these in words and figures as this is a legal requirement for controlled drugs.

5 Do not leave large blank spaces on the prescription, which may be filled in by forgery to obtain unauthorized supplies of abused drugs.

6 Sign the prescription, date it and indicate your name and address. Addition of a telephone number assists the pharmacist in contacting the prescriber in the case of a prescription for an unusual drug or dose regimen.

Approved (generic) or proprietary (brand) name prescribing?

Drugs available on prescription have approved or generic names. Individual manufacturers give their own preparations proprietary (brand or trade) names. A drug that is not covered by patent rights may be available in several proprietary formulations of the same generic preparation. There are obvious commercial pressures to encourage proprietary prescription. Proprietary names are usually short, snappy and memorable. They do not, however, necessarily give any indication of the active ingredients of the medicine. All marketed preparations have passed basic standards of purity and safety. They may differ in their formulation and this may affect absorption and distribution. Although there have been a few examples where formulation differences have led to marked changes in effect and toxicity, on the vast majority of occasions the minor pharmaceutical differences between formulations are irrelevant in clinical practice. It is good prescribing practice to use the generic name of drugs unless there is a very compelling reason for using brand names, e.g. when a combination tablet is being used or when a slow-release preparation of a drug with a narrow therapeutic range (e.g. theophylline) is being prescribed. In Britain proprietary prescription in general practice legally compels the pharmacist to provide that particular brand, with attendant inconvenience to the pharmacist and often delay to the patient. As proprietary preparations vary greatly in price, generic prescribing may result in a prescription of a less expensive preparation with attendant savings in the overall cost of drug treatment. Comparative costs of equivalent preparations can be readily assessed from the *British National Formulary*.

The *British National Formulary* is published by the British Medical Association and the Pharmaceutical Society of Great Britain twice a year and is provided free to practising doctors and medical students in the UK. All marketed medicines are listed systematically together with brief notes on adverse effects, contra-indications and details of dosage. It is a practical pocket reference manual. It should be used in conjunction with textbooks and monographs which provide background information on the rational basis of treatment and guidance on the choice of drug from a list of preparations. It should also be used in conjunction with formularies compiled and published at a local hospital or general practice level. These formularies are now very common and essentially serve to indicate which drugs will be readily available to prescribers in a particular locality or hospital.

Good prescribing practice

1 Familiarize yourself with a limited number of well-established drugs with known effects and side effects. Do not chop and change amongst equivalent preparations on whim or fancy. Avoid trying out new preparations simply because of novelty or extensive commercial promotion. Always prescribe by generic or approved names.

2 Try to devise a treatment regimen which allows drugs to be given once or twice daily. Try to reduce the total number of drugs being given to a minimum and encourage patients to take medicines at a convenient time or place in their daily routine. Avoid vague terms like 'with food' or 'after meals' as the frequency of drug taking may depend on the number of meals taken each day. However, if it is intended that a medicine, such as a non-steroidal anti-inflammatory drug, is taken with food, then state this and the frequency. Always avoid the use of 'as before' or 'as directed' and specify the dose and frequency. Do not prescribe 'as required' without stating the maximum dose and dose interval.

3 Check the dose carefully each time you prescribe. Do not trust to memory and be particularly careful when doses are in the microgram range or when prescribing for children and the elderly.

4 It is now routine practice in Britain to indicate to the patient on his prescription the name of the medicine. Avoid labels like 'the tablets' or 'the mixture'.

5 Use compound preparations and combination tablets only when there is an established therapeutic need for all the constituents, and where the combination of two or more drugs aids compliance.

6 Finally, always review drug prescriptions regularly: every day in hospital patients or weekly or monthly as appropriate in outpatients or general practice. When reviewing prescriptions ask the questions:

(a) Is the drug treatment still necessary?

(b) Is the optimum dose regimen being followed?

(c) Is the desired effect being achieved?

(d) Are there any symptoms or adverse effects which could be secondary to drug treatment?

Do not continue treatment by repeating prescriptions over long periods of time without assessing the response in the patient or, worse still, without seeing the patient.

Comment

The basis of good prescribing is a sound training in clinical methods and pathophysiology, which, together with an understanding of pharmacodynamic and pharmacokinetic properties of the drugs being used, permits maximum benefit to be achieved with the minimum risk of adverse effects. Prescriptions are legal documents. They should consist of clear, legible instructions to the pharmacist. Illegible, incomplete or ambiguous prescriptions are not only bad medicine, they are illegal.

23.3 EVOLUTION OF A NEW DRUG

Drug development aims to produce a novel therapeutic agent which is superior in efficacy to existing remedies and which causes less frequent or less severe adverse effects.

The development of a new therapeutic agent involves a multidisciplinary group in many years of works. Formerly, drugs were extracted from natural plant and animal sources. Therapeutic use was empirical and based on traditional experience. Over the last 80 years an impressive number of drugs have been synthesized chemically. With the development of genetic engineering and the production of monoclonal antibodies it is likely that even more agents will be produced artificially.

Synthetic techniques have produced pure substances. This has led to increased specificity of action and, in some cases, greater efficacy and reduced toxicity. Unfortunately new drug development is expensive, and only a few substances ($< 1\%$) of those developed are actually marketed and used in practice.

The range of novel chemical entities developed has occasionally led to unexpected toxicity. As a consequence most governments have established bodies to regulate drug marketing, e.g. the Committee on Safety of Medicines in Britain, and the Food and Drug Administration in the USA. These agencies supervise clinical research on new drugs and license new products. Although they serve to protect the public and are seen to do so, the statutory procedures that must be followed in applying for a licence for a new drug add greatly to the costs and time of development.

There is some evidence that the rate of introduction of entirely novel agents is slowing down. Whether this reflects economic pressure or diminished novel synthetic capacity or ability is not clear.

23.4 CLINICAL EVALUATION OF A NEW DRUG

Only after animal studies have proved efficacy and the toxicological studies have provided a measure of the possible risk can new drugs be given to humans. At this stage a further requirement is analytical evidence of chemical purity and pharmaceutical stability.

Evaluation in man can be considered in four phases. The relevance and extent of studies at these stages depends on the drug and its indications. Drugs for use in rare diseases, or in life-threatening and as yet untreatable states, may be evaluated in patient groups at an earlier stage than those with readily measurable effects on common diseases.

Phase 1

Phase 1 involves small scale studies in normal volunteers. These studies should determine whether the drug can be given to man without serious symptoms or toxicity and whether it has the desired pharmacological effects. These studies often begin with a dose ranging study, using 1/50 to 1/100 as the effective dose in animals and increasing until the desired effect, or adverse effects, are seen. These studies should only be performed on volunteers who are informed about the implications of the tests and who give their consent freely. Studies should include careful assessment of clinical, haematological and biochemical evidence before and after drug administration to identify pharmacological actions and adverse effects. Phase 1 studies should only be performed by experienced staff, under medical supervision, and in premises with appropriate resuscitative facilities and support.

Phase 2

Phase 2 studies determine whether the new drug has the desired effect on patients with the appropriate disease. In Britain these investigations can be performed only after submission of preclinical and Phase 1 study results to the Committee on Safety of Medicines. This body either issues a clinical trial certificate (CTC) or authorizes limited clinical trials under an exemption procedure (CTE). Phase 2 studies initially may be open, uncontrolled, dose ranging experiments but should include controlled studies under single or double-blind conditions. They may involve comparisons with inactive placebo or known active agents.

Phase 3

If the results of therapeutic efficacy and safety justify it, the next step is progression to large scale clinical trials to determine how the new drug compares in clinical practice with existing remedies, and to establish its profile of action and frequency of adverse effects.

After Phase 3 studies the evidence from all stages of development is assembled and, if the conclusions indicate a useful action, the drug may be submitted to the regulatory authorities with a request for a product licence.

Phase 4

A new drug is usually marketed after only a few hundred, or at the most a few thousand, patients have been exposed to it for a relatively short period (weeks or months). As discussed in Chapter 24, post-marketing surveillance is increasingly undertaken to assess efficacy and toxicity of new drugs on a larger scale. No uniform scheme for Phase 4 supervision has yet been established, but few doubt the necessity of collecting this information on low frequency adverse effects.

23.5 MARKETING AND PROMOTION

The rationale for the development of new drugs should be to provide better drugs; better in the sense of being more effective, safer or cheaper. Unfortunately, only a small proportion of 'new' drugs actually represent a truly novel development or application. More often, 'new' drugs at best incorporate modest molecular variations based on existing drugs, or pharmaceutical formulation changes which have a marginal effect on absorption, toxicity or efficacy. At worst they are copies of existing drugs or minor reformulations to extend patent rights and royalties.

Drug development is expensive. This is borne by the pharmaceutical industry, which justifiably expects to recoup the cost of development when the product is finally marketed. In some therapeutic areas where drugs are widely used, e.g. antibiotics, non-steroidal anti-inflammatory drugs, analgesics and antihypertensives, heavy investment in marketing and promotion has led to the use of undistinguished new drugs in place of equally effective, cheaper and established alternatives whose side effect profile is well known. Therapeutic fads and fashions should be avoided and prescribing practices changed only when good evidence of improved efficacy or reduced toxicity is available.

The physician needs guidance on critical assessment of what represents an important advance. Unfortunately, his most accessible source of information is the representative of the pharmaceutical manufacturer who has been specially trained and briefed to promote his particular new product; indeed, his livelihood depends on the ability to do so.

Practitioners must seek out alternative sources of information from district or regional information pharmacists, specialist clinical colleagues, postgraduate meetings and publications in the scientific literature. Publications, in themselves, can be misleading. Evidence from a few controlled studies published in well established journals subject to peer review are more reliable than bulky obscure proceedings of sponsored meetings to promote a particular drug.

Physicians should make an active attempt to determine in what way a new drug represents an improvement over existing therapy, and what is the price in terms of adverse effects and actual cost of the drug.

As new drugs may be marketed after studies in only a few hundred or thousand patients, special vigilance is required in the first few years of use to determine low frequency but potentially serious adverse effects.

Comments
New drug developments should be examined critically; objective evidence from several sources should be sought to highlight improved therapeutic efficacy and reduced toxicity in controlled comparison with established remedies.

23.6 COMPLIANCE WITH DRUG THERAPY

Approximately one-third of out-patients take their treatment as directed, one-third partly comply and one-third never comply. Poor 'compliance' is found in all socioeconomic and racial groups and there is no satisfactory method of predicting who will fail to comply with treatment. However, compliance is likely to be decreased in certain circumstances:

1 The very young and the very old.

2 Patients requiring long-term treatment.

3 Failure to understand that treatment is beneficial or that the disease is potentially dangerous.

4 Complexity of treatment. Prescription of too many drugs in different doses.

5 Difficulty of access to the drugs, for example, when a patient with rheumatoid arthritis is faced with a childproof container.

6 Adverse effects: although if these are genuinely unavoidable they might be tolerated if the treatment is seen to be beneficial.

7 Expense: this is likely to be a factor in those countries where medicines are purchased at their full value.

Detection of poor compliance

This is not easy. Doctors in general believe that poor compliance happens to other doctors' patients. There are, however, certain simple procedures which can help in detecting poor compliance:

1 Ask the patient how he or she is getting on with the medication and whether they are finding it easy to take the treatment as prescribed. A friendly enquiry of this nature might reveal poor compliance and the reasons for it.

2 Assessment of pharmacological effect. This is clearly easier for some drugs than for others. A patient receiving a beta-blocker, for example, should have a relative bradycardia. In general terms, failure to achieve a therapeutic goal should always raise the question of poor compliance.

3 Assessment of the rate of drug consumption. This has its limitations, as medication can be disposed of easily, but two approaches can be tried. In general practice the actual and expected rate at which repeat prescriptions are requested might show a gross disparity, suggesting that the medication is not being taken at the expected rate. The other approach is to count the number of tablets in the drug container and to calculate the number used.

4 Drug level monitoring is becoming increasingly available (Chapter 2). Its most definitive role in determining compliance is the finding of unexpectedly low levels or no drug at all in the plasma. Levels that are merely subtherapeutic might be the result of poor compliance but could also reflect abnormally low bioavailability or high clearance. Quantitative assessment can be made of many drugs in saliva. As a simple screening manoeuvre it may be useful to perform qualitative tests for the presence or absence of drugs in urine.

Improving compliance

There is no absolutely reliable method of ensuring compliance with drug therapy. However, the following may be helpful:

1 Patient counselling. Explain clearly to the patient, or relative where appropriate, why treatment is necessary and what is likely to be achieved by the treatment.

2 Keep the treatment regimen simple. Wherever possible use once or twice daily doses and try to avoid the need for a midday dose. Review drug treatment regularly to assess whether all treatment is still necessary.

3 Treatment schedule. Explain when the drugs should be taken and in what dose. In addition to explaining verbally write it down, as the patient may forget your instructions.

4 Outline possible adverse effects and encourage the patient to contact you before the next appointment if symptoms get worse rather than better.

5 Enquire at each follow-up about adverse effects and ask how your patient is getting on with the treatment in general. If adverse effects develop change the dose or the drug.

6 In elderly patients, or those disabled by arthritis, ensure that the drug is accessible and not in a childproof container.

7 If it is imperative that a drug be taken but there is a serious doubt about patient compliance, then slow-release intramuscular depot preparations are available. Examples include phenothiazines, progestogens and iron preparations.

Comment

There is little point in putting a lot of effort and money into reaching a diagnosis if the patient is not going to comply with the therapy. The natural history of the underlying disease is then the same as if you have never begun the diagnostic evaluation. Poor compliance should always be borne in mind and efforts made to ensure that treatment is taken as prescribed. Among the various methods for improving compliance, the one which is more important than all the others is patient counselling. Explain the reasons for drug therapy clearly to your patient and on subsequent review continue to ask sympathetically about the progress of treatment.

Chapter 24
Adverse Drug Reactions

24.1 DEFINITION AND MAGNITUDE OF THE PROBLEM

An adverse drug reaction can be defined as 'any undesired or unintended effect of drug treatment'. This definition is intentionally very broad and includes such effects as an acute allergic reaction to penicillin, severe hypoglycaemia after excessive insulin administration, osteoporosis after long-term corticosteroid therapy and rebound hypertension after discontinuing clonidine and phocomelia in the children of mothers exposed to thalidomide during early pregnancy.

It has been estimated that an average hospital medical patient receives between five and ten different drugs during a 10 day stay in hospital. During this time about 25% of patients experience one or more adverse drug effects, and 1% experience a life-threatening event due to drugs. Of these, the majority are patients who have tumours and develop pancytopenia as a result of cancer chemotherapy. Only one in a thousand medical patients suffers a life-threatening adverse drug effect in which the risks of therapy seemed in retrospect to outweigh the potential benefits. The potential for adverse reaction is even greater in general practice. Some 25% of acute medical admissions to hospital can be attributed in whole or in part to the adverse effects of drug therapy.

Older age groups receive a disproportionately high number of prescriptions for drugs and adverse drug reactions are particularly common in this group for pharmacokinetic, pharmacodynamic and social reasons.

Adverse drug effects can be classified in many ways. A useful approach to the problem is given in Table 24.1. In this scheme adverse effects are grouped into those that are predictable on the basis of the drug's known actions and those that are not. The former type usually occurs early in the course of treatment, is a common event which is dose related and is either recognized as a possibility before clinical trials begin or very shortly thereafter. By contrast, the latter type is usually infrequent, rarely recognized until widespread use of the medicine has occurred and need not necessarily be dose dependent.

Table 24.1. Adverse drug effects

Predictable reactions	*Unpredictable reactions*
Excess pharmacological activity	Allergic effects
Rebound response upon discontinuation	Genetically determined effects
	Idiosyncratic effects

24.2 PREDICTABLE ADVERSE REACTIONS

Excessive pharmacological effects

Predictable adverse drug effects are due to excessive pharmacological activity of the drug in question. This arises particularly with CNS depressants and with cardioactive, hypotensive and hypoglycaemic agents. Specific examples of this type of reaction are:

1 Respiratory depression in severe bronchitic patients given morphine or benzodiazepine hypnotics.

2 Hypotension resulting in stroke, myocardial infarction or renal failure in patients receiving excessive doses of antihypertensive drugs.

3 Bradycardia in patients receiving excessive digoxin.

Less obvious but equally important are predictable adverse effects when the particular pharmacological effect involved is not the one for which the drug was initially administered. For example, a patient receiving an antihistamine for the prevention of motion sickness may become drowsy.

All patients are at risk of developing this type of reaction if high doses are given. However, certain subgroups are particularly susceptible (Chapters 3 and 4) and include those with renal disease, liver disease, the very young and the elderly.

Withdrawal symptoms or rebound responses after discontinuation of treatment

This type of reaction is unusual in that it occurs in the absence of the causative agent. The abrupt interruption of therapy is followed by a characteristic withdrawal syndrome:

1 Extreme agitation, tachycardia, confusion, delirium and convulsions may occur following the discontinuation of long-term central nervous system depressants, such a barbiturates, benzodiazepines and alcohol.

2 Acute Addisonian crisis may be precipitated by the abrupt cessation of corticosteroid therapy.

3 Severe hypertension and symptoms of sympathetic overactivity may arise shortly after discontinuing clonidine therapy.

4 Withdrawal symptoms after narcotic analgesics.

In all these instances adaptation has occurred to the drug at the receptor level. This adaptation is usually associated with some tolerance to the effects of the drug, and a gradually increasing dose of drug may be necessary to sustain the initial effect. Withdrawal effects may be minimized by gradual withdrawal of the drugs involved or by substitution with longer-acting or less potent agents and gradual withdrawal.

24.3 UNPREDICTABLE ADVERSE EFFECTS

Allergic drug responses

Drug allergy or hypersensitivity are common adverse drug effects. Indeed, some clinicians regard this type of response as being the single most frequent adverse drug effect. Such reactions are unpredictable and are often not dose related. They occur only in a small proportion of the population exposed to the drug, and it is usually impossible to predict the individuals who will experience this response in advance. These reactions vary from mild erythematous skin reactions to major anaphylactic shock. An allergic adverse effect of a drug is characterized by the fact that:

1 The reaction does not resemble the expected pharmacological drug effect.

2 There is delay between first exposure to the drug and the development of a reaction.

3 The reaction recurs upon repeated exposure even to traces of the drug.

The drugs most frequently associated with allergic skin reactions are the penicillins, the sulphonamides and blood products.

Genetically determined effects

The major toxicity of some drugs is restricted to individuals with a particular genotype or genetic make-up. Thus patients with hereditary pseudocholinesterase deficiency are unable to metabolize the muscle relaxant succinylcholine and may develop prolonged paralysis and apnoea following its use (Chapter 18, Section 18.5). Similarly, individuals with glucose-6-phosphate dehydrogenase deficiency are at substantial risk of developing acute haemolytic anaemia after exposure to the antimalarial drug primaquine and to sulphonamides and quinidine. Some of the most common types of genetic abnormalities that may lead to drug toxicity are shown in Table 24.2.

Genetically determined acetylator polymorphism affects responses and adverse effects to isoniazid, hydralazine and procainamide. Such drugs are metabolized in the liver by the enzyme *N*-acetyl transferase. There is a bimodal distribution of acetylator capacity in the population, with some individuals being slow and others fast acetylators (Chapter 1). Slow acetylators of isoniazid given standard doses are much more likely to suffer from peripheral neuropathy than fast acetylators. The drug induced lupus syndrome is much more common in slow acetylators receiving hydralazine or procainamide. Adverse effects of hydralazine and also gold salts and D-penicillamine are linked to the specific histocompatibility antigens. In the future, tissue typing may help to predict susceptibility to drug toxicity.

Table 24.2. Some genetically determined types of drug toxicity

Defect	Toxic drug	Symptoms
Pseudocholinesterase deficiency	Succinylcholine	Paralysis, apnoea
Glucose-6-phosphate dehydrogenase deficiency	Sulphonamides, quinidine, primaquine	Haemolysis
Acetylator polymorphism	Procainamide, hydralazine	Systemic lupus (in slow acetylators)
	Isoniazid	Neuropathy (in slow acetylators)
Hepatic prophyria	Barbiturates	Symptomatic porphyria

Idiosyncratic drug reactions

The term idiosyncrasy is used primarily to cover unusual, unexpected or bizarre drug effects that cannot readily be explained or predicted in individual recipients. Also included in this type of reaction are drug induced fetal abnormalities such as phocomelia (limb deformity), which developed in the offspring of mothers receiving thalidomide in early pregnancy.

Drug induced malignant disease is fortunately rare and may be considered an idiosyncratic drug effect:

1 Analgesic abuse may rarely cause cancer of the renal pelvis.

2 Long-term oestrogens without coincidental progestogens may induce uterine cancer.

3 Immunosuppressive drugs may induce lymphoid tumours.

4 Intramuscular iron preparations may cause sarcomata at the site of injection.

5 Thyroid cancer may develop in patients who have received ^{131}I-therapy in the past.

24.4 DISCOVERY OF DRUG INDUCED DISEASE

Before a new drug is released for widespread use the manufacturer must obtain a licence from the appropriate government authority (Committee on Safety of Medicines in the UK, Food and Drug Administration in the USA, Department of Drugs in Sweden, etc.). It is likely that over 3000 healthy volunteers and patients will have received the drug in supervised trials before permission for general marketing is given, unless the drug is for a rare disease when experience may be much smaller. By this stage most of the pharmacological effects are known. Adverse effects resulting from excess pharmacological activity may be well documented. That is, however, not the case for unpredictable toxicity. Such adverse effects are often not identified until it has been subjected to much more widespread use. Only after several years was it recognized that the β-receptor blocking drug practolol could cause an oculomucocutaneous syndrome when taken regularly over a long period. Likewise, thalidomide had been marketed for several years before its potential for causing severe limb deformities (phocomelia) in the offspring of mothers taking it in early pregnancy was appreciated.

In order to identify unexpected adverse drug effects, several different approaches have been adopted:

1 Cohort study. This is used when groups of drug recipients are followed to evaluate outcomes after drug exposure.

2 Spontaneous report of suspected adverse drug reactions. This occurs when prescribers report suspected reactions to a central agency which investigates, collates and reviews the resulting information.

3 Review of vital statistics. This occurs when epidemiologists review national or regional statistics to note any unusual epidemics of diseases or uncommon disorders.

4 Case control study. This is used when patients with suspected drug induced disease are compared with a reference population.

Each approach has its strengths and weaknesses but the different types of study are complementary.

Cohort studies

These generally allow the detection of events occurring with a frequency of greater than 1 per 500 exposed. Various types of cohort study have been conducted to detect and quantify drug toxicity. The duration of follow-up varies from weeks to decades.

Short-term clinical trials

These are expensive to conduct and time consuming. They are usually done early in the lifetime of a drug and are confined to patients who have no disorders other than those relevant to the drug in question. Thus the approach is useful only in detecting and quantitating common acute adverse drug effects in otherwise healthy subjects.

Long-term clinical trials

These are formidable undertakings and are rarely conducted. They are expensive to organize and maintain. They are confined to medications which are used on a long-term basis, e.g. oral contraceptives, antidiabetic drugs and antihypertensive drugs. When successful they give useful information both on acute and delayed effects of drug treatment. However, there are often problems in maintaining the integrity of the study cohort and in demonstrating that satisfactory randomization of the treated and control groups has been carried out.

Post-marketing surveillance of established drugs

Studies in which a group of recipients is identified and observed for possible adverse effects are now being conducted more frequently. The periods of observation are usually brief (days or weeks) and the size of the cohorts small (rarely more than 2000). Such studies are useful for quantifying known acute effects after short-term exposure to drugs and for identifying subgroups of the population who are at greatest risk of toxicity, e.g. elderly, those with renal impairment, liver disease, etc.

Post-marketing surveillance of new drugs

This approach is relatively new. It aims to review a large cohort of 10 000 or more recipients of a drug newly released onto the market and to follow such individuals for a substantial period: at least one and preferably several years. When successful, such studies have the potential for detecting both acute and delayed toxicity following short- or long-term exposure. Once again a major problem is to maintain the integrity of the study cohort. Although less expensive to conduct than a long-term clinical trial, such studies are nevertheless likely to be confined to those new drugs used for prolonged periods in large numbers of patients.

These studies give not only an indication of what reactions may occur but also some idea of the frequency with which they may be expected.

Spontaneous reports of suspected adverse drug reactions

In the USA, the UK, Scandinavia and most Western European countries there are agencies that collect information about suspected adverse drug effects. For example, in the UK, the Committee on Safety of Medicines has an adverse reaction subcommittee which encourages physicians to report suspected adverse drug reactions on a standard form. The resulting information is analysed regularly to determine whether or not any unusual patterns of reports are emerging. Unfortunately it has a relatively low response rate, particularly from hospital based physicians.

Spontaneous reporting has been useful in confirming whether or not a newly suspected reaction is widespread in the community. This approach, however, only assesses the number of suspected reactions. There is no estimate of the frequency of reactions because it gives no details of the numbers exposed to the drug in the population from which the reports were received.

Vital statistics

A review of national or regional healthcare statistics should be, in theory, a useful way of detecting an unsuspected epidemic of an unusual condition or a marked increase in prevalence of a common condition. This might prove to be so if the collection of such statistics were sufficiently accurate and if the data processing and review undertaken were sufficiently rapid. At present this approach is not practical. In the west of the USA an epidemic of uterine cancer occurred during the 1970s. This was well documented in the regional statistics but no-one appreciated its significance until isolated reports linking long-term oestrogen use to uterine cancer were published. By then the major epidemic was already under way. An efficient and informed review of the vital statistics could well have led to the discovery of this problem 2 or 3 years earlier. Regular perusal of accurate regional vital statistics could indicate conditions which showed an unexpected increase and therefore which might be drug induced.

Case control studies

The drug consuming habits of patients with a suspected drug induced disease are compared with those of a reference population who do not have the suspect disease. This approach is increasingly being used to detect and quantify drug related disease. It is particularly useful in showing associations between drug use and rare diseases where the risks of developing the disease are less than 1 in 500 persons exposed. Under those circumstances, it would be prohibitively expensive and complex to attempt to follow a cohort of recipients, and it is easier to start at the suspected disease and work back to the drug exposure.

In case control studies the results are expressed as relative risks: for example, the risk of being a cigarette smoker in a series of patients with lung cancer compared to the risk in reference patients without lung cancer. This information is insufficient to assess the actual risk of getting lung cancer if one is a smoker. Calculating such a risk requires additional information not usually available to those conducting the case control study.

There are major limitations to case control studies:

1 While they may show associations between diseases and drug use, they do not prove that these associations are causal.

2 They are difficult to conduct in practice since they can be subject to bias either as a result of the type of reference population studied or of foreknowledge of the hypothesis under review by the interviewer.

3 It is important to confine interest to newly diagnosed cases in order to avoid distortion of drug consuming habits as a consequence of awareness of the presence of a significant disease. For example, when assessing the association between chronic renal failure and analgesic abuse, it would not be advisable to look at previously diagnosed cases of renal failure since such patients are likely to have been advised to avoid drugs in general and analgesics in particular. A case control study which included previously diagnosed cases of renal failure amongst the cases could therefore produce a result which did not show any drug association with analgesic abuse even if, in reality, analgesic abuse was indeed associated with significant risk of chronic renal failure.

Using these techniques it is likely that the ability to detect serious drug related toxicity will greatly improve in the 1990s. Provided that these limitations are appreciated and the resulting information is handled efficiently, this approach has much to offer, particularly when we are dealing with rare or delayed drug effects.

24.5 REDUCTION OF THE RISK OF ADVERSE EFFECTS

Many powerful drugs are now available. It is hardly surprising that occasionally untoward effects are produced. With a better knowledge of the pharmacological mechanisms whereby drugs exert their effects, and their toxicity, and the pathophysiology of diseases, it is likely that in the future drug therapy may become safer. The risks of developing adverse drug effects can be reduced by observing simple rules:

1 Always include a detailed drug history as part of the clinical history or consultation.

2 Only use drug treatment when there is a clear indication for it and there is no non-pharmacological alternative.

3 Avoid multiple drug regimens and combination tablets whenever possible.

4 Pay particular attention to drug dose and response in the young, the old and those with coexisting renal, hepatic or cardiac disease.

5 Review the need for continuing treatment regularly and stop drugs which are no longer necessary.

Index